Director's Forum

1st Edition

Editors

Robert J. Weber, RPh, PharmD, MS, BCPS, FASHP
The Ohio State University Medical Center and College of Pharmacy

Michael D. Sanborn, MS, RPh, FASHP
Baylor Health Care System

Scott Mark, PharmD, MS, MPH, MBA, FASHP
University of Pittsburgh Medical Center and School of Pharmacy

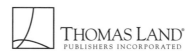

THOMAS LAND®
PUBLISHERS INCORPORATED

Thomas Land Publishers, Inc.
St. Louis, Missouri

Published by Thomas Land Publishers, Inc.
255 Jefferson Road
St. Louis, MO 63119-3627

www.thomasland.com
www.hospitalpharmacyjournal.com

ISBN: 978-0-615-41464-5

To order this book: www.tlpstore.com

Note to Reader

The authors and publisher have made every effort to ensure the accuracy and completeness of the information presented in this book. However the authors and publisher cannot be held responsible for the continued currency of the information, any inadvertent errors or omissions, or the application of this information. Therefore, the authors and publisher shall have no liability to any person or entity with regard to claims, loss, or damage caused or alleged to be caused, directly or indirectly, by the use of the information contained herein.

Foreword

Effective pharmacy leadership has never been more critical than today, not just by the director, but at all levels—assistants, coordinators, operation managers, and supervisor.

Pharmacy leaders are facing the "perfect storm" of challenges:

- Continuing pressure to reduce or contain costs while providing additional revenue for the organization's bottom line, and promoting accurate medication billing that can survive external audit;
- Increasing demand of services related to additional people in health care insurance plans and the aging of baby boomers, which is leading organizations to build or enlarge facilities, and hence, new pharmacy space;
- Ensuring a fail-safe patient medication system while implementing new technology (eg, patient care area automated dispensing cabinets, robotic dispensing devices, computerized physician order entry, electronic medical record, and bar code medication administration);
- Enhancing the pharmacy practice model to ensure all patients receive the appropriate level of patient-centered clinical services, 24/7;
- Maintaining an engaged workforce, developing leaders for the future, and being the local employer of choice.

Needless to say, these challenges raise many questions and lots of "need to knows." As time is of the essence, where can leaders go for pharmacy-specific information? Over the course of pharmacy service development, pharmacy leaders have assisted each other by sharing experiences, ranging from intravenous admixture programs and unit dose systems to clinical services.

For answers to your questions and a starting point for your "need to knows," I highly recommend this comprehensive compilation of *Director's Forum* columns from the *Hospital Pharmacy* journal. This column, initiated in January 2006 and continuing today, has brought thoughtful discourse to the issues of pharmacy leadership via the collaboration of Robert Weber, Michael Sanborn, and Scott Mark. As stated in the first published column, its purpose stands as *"A series of articles designed to guide pharmacy leaders in establishing patient-centered services in hospitals. We hope to answer key questions that pharmacy directors face and provide others with information to foster growth in pharmacy leadership. The articles in this column will build on one another and, when put together, will serve as a 'tool kit' to develop patient-centered pharmacy services in hospitals of all sizes."*

I applaud these authors as contemporary leaders, not only for conceptualizing and implementing this column but also for continuing to provide relevant topics and discussions.

I would like to highlight a few topics from these columns to stimulate your exploration of this compilation.

- Core competencies in drug distribution, medication order review, essential departmental data, financial management, and regulatory compliance
- Technology: developing pharmacy information system infrastructure, planning for central pharmacy automation, making the most of unit dose dispensing automation, effective use of smart pumps, and implementing a bar-code medication administration system
- Advanced programs: pharmacy-based immunizations, investigational services, anticoagulation management, residency training, medication management therapy services, and REMS
- Personnel management: succession planning and progressive discipline, innovative roles for pharmacy technicians, and reduction of staff turnover

This publication is useful for current pharmacy leaders and for all pharmacists as they evaluate and improve their practices. In addition, selected columns are a must for incorporation into all PGY-1 and PGY-2 residencies per leadership. Likewise, pharmacy students in appropriate courses and during their IPPE (Introductory Pharmacy Practice Experience) and APPE (Advanced Pharmacy Practice Experience) will benefit from selected columns.

It is a genuine pleasure to present these columns in one spot as the "tool kit" originally intended by the authors.

—Sara J. White, MS, FASHP
(Ret.) Director of Pharmacy
Stanford Hospital and Clinics
Pharmacy Leadership Coach

Contents

Automation/Technology

Core Competencies in Hospital Pharmacy Practice

Drug Policy

Human Resources Management

Management and Leadership

Medication Safety

Patient Services and Related Issues

Automation/Technology

Establishing a Plan for Central Pharmacy Automation

Thomas W. Glowa, PharmD, BCPS, * and Robert J. Weber, MS, FASHP[†]*

The *Director's Forum* series is written and edited by Michael Sanborn and Robert Weber and is designed for guiding pharmacy leaders in establishing patient-centered services in hospitals and health systems. Another specific goal of this column is addressing many of the key challenges that pharmacy directors currently face, while also providing information that will foster growth in pharmacy leadership and patient safety. Previous *Director's Forum* articles have discussed various aspects of pharmacy technology implementation and utilization. This feature reviews the steps and strategies for implementing and evaluating automation in a central pharmacy area supporting a decentralized pharmaceutical model.

INTRODUCTION

The current state of the economy has escalated pressure on health care organizations to determine methods of cost reduction while maintaining safety and quality. As stated previously in the *Director's Forum* column, hospital pharmacy costs represent approximately 7% to 10% of a hospital's operating budget and pharmacy personnel account for nearly 20% of the pharmacy budget.[1] Medication errors significantly affect patient safety, particularly those that occur in the pharmacy dispensing process. The traditional system—pharmacy dispensing in which a pharmacy technician fills a medication order and a pharmacist verifies its accuracy—is prone to error. For example, a study of the pharmacist's interception of dispensing errors by pharmacy technicians determined that the rate of interception was 79%. Of the 140,755 medication doses filled at an academic medical center in a 7-month period, 5,075 medication errors occurred, with 1,055 doses (21%) missed by the pharmacist and dispensed to patients.[2]

Costs of medication are a continual and substantial challenge to hospital pharmacy directors. In its yearly published analysis, the American Society of Health-System Pharmacists (ASHP) provides a projection of drug costs for the upcoming year to assist directors in preparing the pharmacy budget.[3] For 2009 the authors predicted an increase of drug expenditures of 1% to 3% in hospitals, 0% to 2% in outpatient settings, and 1% to 3% in clinic-administered drugs. The authors listed the new drugs released by the US Food and Drug Administration (expected approval of 14 drugs in 2009) and discussed the various factors that likely would influence drug expenditures, such as drug safety concerns, generic drugs, Medicare Part D, and changes in the drug supply chain. The projected expenditure data provide compelling evidence that pharmacy directors must not only implement an effective formulary system but also provide for effective control of inventory and purchasing practices of new and high-cost medications.

Regulatory requirements pose added challenges to the pharmacy director. The United States Pharmacopeia standards for compounding intrave-

*Clinical Pharmacist, Pittsburgh Center for AIDS Treatment, University of Pittsburgh Medical Center; [†]Executive Director of Pharmacy, University of Pittsburgh Medical Center; Associate Professor and Chair, Department of Pharmacy & Therapeutics, University of Pittsburgh School of Pharmacy, Pittsburgh, Pennsylvania.

nously administered drug products incorporate facility changes and an expanded and detailed quality assurance mechanism. In addition, diligent controls of narcotic dispensing in the pharmacy are a fundamental step in effectively managing narcotic control in the organization.

Finally, there is a continuing shortage of pharmacists. According to the 2007 ASHP national survey of pharmacy practice in hospital settings, it is estimated that 6.4% of full-time equivalent hospital pharmacist positions remain vacant, with an overall turnover rate for pharmacists of 7.7%.[4] Relatively few programs are available that train highly qualified pharmacy technicians, and there are no consistent national requirements for the education, training, and certification of technicians.[5]

In response to workplace issues of cost, quality, and workforce, pharmacy directors must establish a strategy and implement programs that control medication inventory and efficiently use personnel. Most often this strategy involves analyzing a hospital's central pharmacy operations and determining how technology can help solve these workforce issues. The objective of this article is to provide the pharmacy director with a guide for designing and implementing pharmacy automation that supports a patient-centered pharmacy service. The specific aims of this article focus on designing a patient-centered pharmacy by (1) determining the central pharmacy needs for automation, (2) describing the varied automation employed in a central pharmacy, (3) listing indicators for evaluating the effectiveness of central pharmacy automation, and (4) describing elements used to demonstrate a positive return on investment (ROI) for central pharmacy automation.

DETERMINING CENTRAL PHARMACY AUTOMATION NEEDS

Determining the breadth and scope of automation in the central pharmacy area depends on the service, quality, and efficiency goals set for the pharmacy operation. Committing to a patient-centered pharmacy practice model is the single most critical variable that determines types of central pharmacy automation. For example, at the University of Pittsburgh Medical Center a decentralized pharmacist and technician team provides a comprehensive pharmaceutical care approach.[6] As a result, the goal of the central pharmacy automation is to prepare and dispense doses "in batch." Furthermore, establishing an efficient system with a goal for zero tolerance of medication dispensing errors is necessary. For the purposes of this article, central pharmacy automation design that accommodates a decentralized pharmacy service model is described.

According to a 2007 national survey on pharmacy informatics, many automated dispensing solutions are implemented in hospital pharmacies.[7] In a survey of 4,112 hospital pharmacy directors, 10.1% of hospitals are using robots to dispense medication and 12.7% are using automated pharmacy carousel systems (APCS or carousels); most hospitals are planning for acquisition of such technology in the future.

Central pharmacy dispensing traditionally involves a procedure in which a pharmacy technician retrieves a medication from a shelf and places the medication in a patient-labeled cassette or bag. A pharmacist verifies the medication before its delivery to the nursing unit. Hospital pharmacies also may employ a decentralized dispensing process involving storage of medications in an automated dispensing cabinet (ADC) on the nursing unit. In this scenario a pharmacy technician picks a medication from a shelf. Then a pharmacist checks the medication before the technician delivers the medication to the nursing unit and restocks the medication in the cabinet. When it is time for administration of a patient's medication, the nurse accesses the medication from the unit-based cabinet and administers the drug.

Both processes are fraught with the potential for human error, primarily because they rely on visual inspection as the sole mechanism for detecting mistakes. Neither process provides adequate inventory management and time for performance of clinical functions by a pharmacist. Maintaining a manual, perpetual inventory system is nearly impossible for most hospital pharmacies because of the number and types of medication dispensed.

Transitioning from manual and decentralized systems to more centralized or hybrid pharmacy automation systems appears a promising avenue toward improving the accuracy of the dispensing process, tightening inventory control, and increasing the time available for performance of clinical activity by pharmacists. Centralized pharmacy automation options for dispensing include bar-code scanning, robotic dispensing, carousels, narcotic management, and automated decision-support systems. In many instances an integrated combination of these solutions may be used.

AUTOMATION THAT SUPPORTS A DECENTRALIZED PHARMACY MODEL
Central Pharmacy Bar Coding

Bar-code technology involves the placement of a unique identifier on a medication in the form of a bar-code that is readable by an optical scanner. The bar-code on the medication typically contains the National Drug Code number, which is a 10-digit, 3-segment number that incorporates the drug manufacturer or distributor; the specific strength, dosage form, and formulation; and the package size and type. The bar-code also may be customized so that it contains additional information, such as the expiration date of the medication. In many cases the manufacturer applies the bar-code to the unit-dose packaging. However, many medications require repackaging of each individual dose if the manufacturer has not applied a bar-code or if it is not readable by the optical scanning system used by the scanner. When interfaced with the pharmacy information system, scanning of the bar-code can detect a mismatch between the medication scanned and the medication ordered; a mismatch triggers an audible or visual alarm that alerts the user of the scanner, ensuring that the correct medication, dose, and dosage form are dispensed. However there are several limitations and "workarounds" with regard to this technology, as shown in **Table 1**.

It has been shown that pharmacy-based bar-code technology can reduce dispensing errors and adverse drug events (ADEs).[8] A 36% reduction in dispensing errors and a 63% reduction in potential adverse events was observed in a 735-bed tertiary care academic medical center after implementation of bar-code technology.

Table 1. Limitations of a Bar-Code System in a Central Pharmacy

Limitations	Work-arounds
Mislabeling: Incorrect bar-code placed on packaging	Bypass scanning step
Lack of a bar-code	Performing steps out of sequence: Filling and dispensing medication and scanning afterwards
Unreadable bar-code: Crinkled, torn, smudged, or covered up by another label	Disabling alarms
Technology failure: Scanner malfunction, power failure, wireless connectivity problems	Time-saving efforts: Affixing commonly used bar-codes to a sheet of paper for rapid scanning
Mix-up of medication after scanning	No policy for failure to scan

The study followed 3 configurations of bar-code technology. The first involved a 2-day fill process in which medication doses were manually stocked, retrieved, and scanned during the filling process. The second involved a bar-code–assisted stocking and retrieval system using a carousel in which medication doses were scanned before stocking the carousel and retrieved as directed by the carousel and 1 dose per batch was scanned during filling. The third process involved manual stocking and retrieval of medication doses and scanning of only 1 dose per batch. Of the 3 configurations, those with the best rate of decrease in ADEs were the processes in which all medication doses were scanned at filling (93% to 97% relative reduction) or using a carousel dispensing system (86% to 97% relative reduction). The configuration in which only 1 dose per batch was scanned led to a lower reduction in dispensing errors (60% relative reduction) and a 2.4-fold increase in potential ADEs. Limitations of the study included its open nature, the necessary exclusion of controlled substances, and, for ethical reasons, the inability to observe actual ADEs as a result of dispensing errors. The study demonstrated the benefit of implementing bar-code technology

and recommended that every dose be scanned in the dispensing process.

Ideally, bar-code technology should be used whenever and wherever a medication is handled in the pharmacy. The bar-code should be scanned or the medication should be bar-coded whenever it is received from the wholesaler. Medications also should be scanned when they are stocked on the shelf, retrieved from the shelf for filling, and verified by the pharmacist for dispensing. Furthermore, following all of these steps will improve overall bar-code reliability if point-of-care medication administration scanning is employed.

Robotics Technology

Devices used in implementing centralized pharmacy automation include robotic dispensing systems and APCS. Bar-code scanning drives robotic dispensing systems. The most common configuration uses a robot for filling patient-specific medications. A robot also can be used for picking medications for restocking in an ADC. Robots interface with the pharmacy information system to provide accurate filling of individual patient-specific cassettes, storage rings, or envelopes based on a medication profile. The accuracy of a robotic dispensing system exceeds that of the visual picking of a drug from the shelf by a pharmacy technician and verification by a pharmacist. A robot can operate 24 hours a day—filling medications, crediting returned medications, or restocking medications—to reduce both pharmacy technician and pharmacist labor and time.

Reducing the time for required pharmacist check of doses enables pharmacists to spend more time on clinical activity, such as medication therapy management. Many regulations by state boards of pharmacy allow for reduced pharmacist checking of medications dispensed by a robot. Typically, intermittent quality control checks are performed. The use of robotic dispensing also can lead to more effective inventory management. A perpetual inventory of a medication can be maintained, and the robot can interface with the pharmacy wholesaler to automatically order a medication when the level falls below the minimum quantity. Expired medication costs can be reduced because many robots use stock rotation algorithms to prevent medications from expiring. In addition, a robot can check the expiration date of a medication and set aside medications that are expired or about to expire. Because of its superior accuracy, missing medications also can be reduced.

Limitations of the accuracy of a robotic dispensing system parallel that of bar-code technology. The correct bar-code must be applied to a medication. The bar-code must be readable by the optical system of the robot; the robot will reject the medication dose if the bar-code is not readable. In such a case, a dose will not be dispensed to the patient and additional repackaging will be required. Medications

used by the robot must be adequately stocked to avoid missing medication. Although a robot may have the capacity to store and fill many tens of thousands of medications, storage of some medications on the robot will not be possible and such medications will require an alternative filling process.

Medication Carousels

APCS have many of the benefits of robotic dispensing systems and are also based on bar-code technology. Medication carousels are ergonomically efficient, high-capacity medication storage and retrieval systems. Carousels typically provide bar-code–based and "pick to light" medication stocking and retrieval. The carousel ideally interfaces with the pharmacy information system. When a medication order is processed, a bar-code label is printed and scanned by the pharmacy technician. Like the robot, the carousel shelving rotates and the bin with the appropriate medication is lit. When the technician removes and scans the medication, the quantity is deducted from inventory. The carousel can maintain a perpetual inventory and automatically send a purchase order to the wholesaler when a medication's inventory falls below par. Furthermore, carousels can interface with ADCs, filling medications when levels in the cabinets fall below par. Scanning also is required when restocking the medication; expiration dates of medications can be tracked, helping avoid dispensing of expired medications and reducing inventory costs. Carousels offer more efficient storage than traditional shelving because they have a high storage capacity in a smaller footprint. Because of this benefit, floor space and storage capacity in the pharmacy can be maximized, and carousel implementation typically results in reclaiming department square footage.

Medication errors can be further reduced by placing "look-alike sound-alike" medications in different positions on the carousel to ensure the impossibility of picking up one medication instead of another. Different doses of the same medication should not be placed next to one another; they can be placed in different positions on different shelves if desired. The carousel will automatically rotate shelves and highlight the correct medication. Scanning of the bar-code ensures that the correct medication is removed. Oswald and Caldwell investigated whether dispensing error rates decreased after implementing an APCS at a 613-bed acute tertiary care university hospital.[9] The rate of dispensing errors was observed in 3 areas of pharmacy operation: first-dose or missing medication fill, ADC fill, and interdepartmental request fill. The rate of dispensing errors to ADCs was modestly reduced by APCS, but the carousel had no effect on error rates when dispensing first doses or missing medications. This study had many limitations. The first was that the carousel was not interfaced with the pharmacy information system for the filling of first doses and missing doses. It was required that technicians manually enter first doses and missing medications into the carousel system. Secondly, the checking of the carousel medications was limited to specific pharmacists in the study period compared with the previous practice of multiple pharmacists checking medications. Also, the study was an observational study only and no statistical tests were performed. The

authors concluded that the best role of the carousel was the restocking of medications to ADCs; however, many departments would likely choose to include additional dispensing activities to improve department efficiency and patient safety.

Narcotic Control Systems

Because of security concerns, controlled substances are not dispensed through a robotic or carousel system. However, centralized options for tracking of controlled-substance usage are available. Perpetual controlled-substance inventory records can be maintained using a computer system interfaced with ADCs on the nursing units. The system may be combined with ADCs dedicated for controlled-substance use or other commercially available hardware (eg, *NarcStation-RX*, McKesson Automation, Pittsburgh, PA) in the pharmacy for additional security. The interface with ADCs allows automated restocking of medications in the cabinets when levels decrease be low par. Access to controlled substances can be limited in the pharmacy and compliance with US Drug Enforcement Administration and state rules and regulations can be increased. The software possesses the ability to record and track waste, recalled medications, and expired medications. Inventory management functions can be performed: the software can generate purchase orders or record the transfer of a controlled substance to another institution. The system can assist with compounding medications with controlled substances, and it can be used to record waste associated with compounding. A final benefit is that most software includes controlled-substance disposition tracking to ensure that medications that are issued from the department are ultimately stocked in their assigned location.

Bar-code technology also can be combined with narcotic management systems. Scanning of a medication barcode can be required at the point of restocking a cabinet. When a bar-code is scanned, the appropriate storage location (drawer and pocket) within the cabinet opens to ensure correct filling and restricted access solely to the pocket being filled. Ideally, narcotic management systems are combined with ADCs, but they also may be used with nursing or specialty units with traditional locked medicine cabinets.

Narcotic management systems possess the ability to track controlled-substance usage. Trends can be identified and cabinet inventory amounts can be adjusted accordingly. Because all transactions are electronically recorded, the administration activity of nurses and the dispensing activity of pharmacists can be tracked. Reports of activity by drug, unit, and nurse or pharmacist can be automatically prepared and analyzed to detect diversion. Controlled-substance inventory records and transaction reports can be maintained in a single database. The creation and maintenance of users' identities within the system can be restricted to avoid the creation of fake user names for fraudulent access to the system.

Automated Decision-Support Systems

Automated decision-support tools are available for reducing medication errors and ADEs, managing inventory, and increasing pharmacist's clinical interventions. Traditionally, hospital pharmacies have relied on basic decision-support tools at the point of order entry into the pharmacy information system, such as drug-allergy checking, duplicate therapy checking, and drug-drug interaction checking. Advanced decision-support tools such as renal dosing support, drug-disease interaction support, and support for compliance with clinical guidelines and hospital clinical initiatives have been built into computerized prescriber order-entry systems.

Automated decision-support tools are also available to evaluate the effectiveness of the dispensing process. Automated decision-support systems are rule-based systems that can recommend solutions to repetitive management problems and can significantly improve the overall efficiency of the automated technology.[10] The value of automated decision-support systems derives from their ability to analyze data coming from different sources. Information can be imported from automated dispensing devices, such as ADCs, robots, or carousels, and processed by automated decision-support software. The software can provide graphical or statistical reports in relationship to predetermined bench marks selected by the institution. Furthermore, automated decision-support software can provide information for improvement of inventory management. Data on the current supply of a medication can be derived by the software from all automated devices and evaluated. Inventory trends can be identified and monitored. Decision-support software also can be helpful for identifying trends in narcotic usage—with both dispensing and administration. The data can be analyzed to detect specific user deviations compared with average usage, and large deviations from the norm can be helpful in identifying potential diversion situations. This can be done in real time. Use of a certain drug by nurses can be plotted; and if a nurse deviates from the norm, the nurse can be followed more closely. Data can be collected, processed, and used later for prosecution.

Compliance with clinical guidelines and hospital initiatives can be monitored using automated dispensing equipment data. For example, dispensing of a preferred drug from all automated devices can be compared with that of a nonpreferred drug. Because activity can be narrowed down to a specific nursing unit and/or cabinet, patients who receive the nonpreferred drug can be identified, as well as the prescribing physician. Depending on the capabilities of the equipment, the indication for the drug also can be identified. A cost analysis may then be performed on the information gathered to develop a plan for either curtailing the use of the nonpreferred drug or converting the nonpreferred to a preferred drug.

The space available in any automated device is limited, therefore performance must be regularly optimized with decision-support software. Data derived from automated sources can be used to add or remove a medication from a robotic dispensing system. If medication utilization in an ADC, robot, or carousel has changed significantly, consideration should be given to available storage quantities and whether the medication is better suited for a different type of available automation (eg, moving a high-volume medication from an automated cabinet to the robot).

Oftentimes, medication-use trending functions must be performed manually using information that is not necessarily current. Automated decision-support software can be useful because it provides a real-time snapshot of the current inventory of medications throughout the hospital. Current pricing information from the wholesaler can be incorporated to provide a complete up-to-date cost analysis quickly and accurately. These data can then be compared with historical data to identify trends.

EVALUATING EFFECTIVENESS OF CENTRAL PHARMACY AUTOMATION

ASHP has developed an approach for improving the medication-use process in health systems.[11] The effectiveness of automation can be assessed using the following elements: feasibility, financial return, and quality and safety return. Feasibility is defined by the convenience of implementing the automation project. Elements of feasibility that must be considered include the addition of staff and the financial investment required. Quality and safety are evaluated based on the reduction of dispensing errors. The financial impact of the automation is determined by its ROI.

Consideration of the value of centralized pharmacy automation related to both pharmacy staff efficiency and improvement to the accuracy of the medication-use process is important. Pharmacist and technician time saved through central pharmacy automation can often be redeployed to patient-centered professional activities. Other cost-benefit examples include the use of bar coding to prevent the costs of medication errors or using a robotic dispensing system to free additional pharmacist time for conducting medication reconciliation on a patient care unit.

RETURN ON INVESTMENT FOR CENTRAL PHARMACY AUTOMATION

Central pharmacy automation is a long-term investment, with the hospital pharmacy manager and financial administrators determining whether the investment results in a positive ROI. Calculating the ROI represents a way of measuring the financial value of a project. As resources become scarcer in hospitals, using the ROI analysis can help justify important central pharmacy automation. In developing the ROI, the director also must provide information on the specific financial return, as well as other indirect benefits to the organization. These other benefits could involve improving patient safety, raising patient satisfaction scores, or improving compliance to a regulatory standard. The key indicators, with explanations, used in calculating a typical ROI are shown in **Table 2**.[12]

To further explain some of these terms, the cost of central pharmacy automation should be "fully loaded" and include the costs for hardware, installation, software licenses, and infrastructure changes (computer networking, training, etc). The useful life of the automation is estimated by focusing on the primary operating purpose of the investment. For example, as a result of continual technological advances, computer hardware usually has a useful life of 3 years, even though the actual device may continue to work for several more years. The net present value (NPV) of the automation expense is used for appraisal of the value of long-term projects; it is a way of comparing the value of money now with the value of money in the future. A positive NPV indicates a positive ROI because the value of money saved on a project in the future exceeds the present value of that money.

A positive incremental cash flow means that an organization's cash flow will increase with the acceptance of the project. Profitability index and modified internal rate of return are used to determine the attractiveness of a project. The profitability index gives insight to the value derived from each dollar invested. The lowest acceptable profitability index is 1.0, and a higher ratio increases the desirability of a project. The modified internal rate of return assumes that the positive cash

Table 2. Definitions of Elements in a Return-on-Investment Analysis

Useful life of investment	Length of time the investment is used for its primary operating purpose
Cost of investment	Amount necessary for purchasing a product
Incremental cash flow	Additional operating cash flow that an organization receives from taking on a new project
Reinvestment rate	Rate at which cash flows may be reinvested
Net present value (NPV)	Comparing the value of money now with the value of money in the future
Profitability index	The relationship between the benefits and costs of a project; also known as the benefit-cost ratio
Modified internal rate of return	Interest rate received for an investment consisting of payments and income that occur at regular periods
Payback period	Time necessary for the return on investment of a project to repay the sum of the initial investment

Memorial Hospital

Return on Investment Analysis - Medication Carousel and Decision Support Software

This template calculates the key financial indicators of a capital investment.

Directions
1. Enter the data requested in the yellow highlighted cells only.
2. Enter all numbers as positive values (i.e. expenses should be entered as positive amounts).
3. Utilize a 3% inflation rate each year for all revenues and expenses (except depreciation expense).
4. Fringe benefits are calculated at 22% of salaries.

Key Financial Indicators (1)

Useful Life of Investment - 10 year maximum*	5	Net Present Value of 5 Year Cash Flow	$47,622
Cost of Investment	$275,000	Profitability Index (2)	1.17
5 Year Incremental Cash Flow	$435,000	Modified Internal Rate of Return (3)	10.9%
Reinvestment Rate	8.0%	Payback Period	3.6

* Should represent best estimate of useful life for the primary operational purpose of the investment. Maximum useful life to use is 10 years

	Cost	Year 1	Year 2	Year 3	Year 4	Year 5	Total	Residual Value (4)
Financial Savings								
Technician Labor Efficiency-2.5 FTE's		80,000	82,000	84,000	86,000	88,000	420,000	
Pharmacist Labor Efficiency-0.5 FTE		46,000	48,000	50,000	52,000	54,000	250,000	
Inventory Reduction		150,000	10,000	10,000	10,000	10,000	190,000	
Total Savings		276,000	140,000	144,000	148,000	152,000	860,000	
MEDICATION CAROUSEL								
Hardware & Software		275,000					275,000	
Maintenance Services Fee		0	20,000	20,000	20,000	20,000	80,000	
Installation, Implementation, & Training		40,000					40,000	
DECISION SUPPORT								
Software		20,000					20,000	
Maintenance			2,000	2,000	2,000	2,000	6,000	
Installation, Implementation, & Training		2,000					2,000	
Sub-total Expenses		337,000	22,000	22,000	22,000	22,000	423,000	
Incremental Cash Flow		-61,000	118,000	122,000	126,000	130,000	437,000	$0
Incremental Cash Flow including Residual Value							437,000	$437,000
Depreciation Expense								
Equipment - 5 yr life	273,000	39,000	39,000	39,000	39,000	39,000	195,000	
Computer Hardware - 3 yr life	2,000	667	667	667	0	0	2,000	
Total Depreciation Expense	275,000	39,667	39,667	39,667	39,000	39,000	197,000	
Incremental Operating Margin		-$100,667	$78,333	$82,333	$87,000	$91,000	$340,000	
Cumulative Incremental Net Cash Flow	($275,000)	($336,000)	($218,000)	($96,000)	$30,000	$160,000	$162,000	
Cumulative Incremental Net Cash Flow including Residual Value								$162,000
Present Value of Cash Flows		-$56,481	$101,166	$96,848	$92,614	$88,476	$322,622	$0
Present Value of Cash Flows including Residual Value								$322,622

(1) Financial Indicators within this box are based on a 5 year useful life.
(2) Profitability index is the ratio of the present value of future cash flows divided by the initial investment.
(3) Modified Internal rate of return assumes that cash flows from the project are reinvested at the reinvestment rate.
(4) Residual value represents the estimated amount of cash received for the project assets if sold after 5 years (factored into the key financial indicators above).

Figure 1. Sample return on investment for central pharmacy automation. FTE = full-time equivalent.

flows are immediately reinvested until the end of the project. Of course, the shortest possible payback period is the most desirable for any project. **Figure 1** shows an ROI for a medication carousel. When developing an ROI, linking the numbers in the ROI to specific data sets is important so that the contents of the ROI can be validated. For example, the costs of construction may link to a spreadsheet that lists, in detail, all of the items included in estimating the construction costs.

CONCLUSION

Automating the dispensing functions of the central pharmacy provides the opportunity for improving quality and focusing the efforts of the pharmacist on patient-centered activities. The pharmacy director must use central pharmacy automation in a way that meets the mission and vision of the pharmacy service. The pharmacy director must establish a good business and clinical case for the expense of the automation. If central pharmacy automation is implemented and effectively justified in hospitals, achieving patient-centered pharmacy services will be a reality.

REFERENCES

1. Weber RJ. Core competencies in hospital pharmacy practice: department financial management. *Hosp Pharm.* 2006;41(7):689-694.

2. Cina JL, Gandhi TK, Churchill W, et al. How many hospital pharmacy medication dispensing errors go undetected? *Jt Comm J Qual Patient Saf.* 2006; 32(2):73-80.

3. Hoffman JM, Shah ND, Vermeulen LC, et al. Projecting future drug expenditures—2009. *Am J Health Syst Pharm.* 2009;66(3):237-257.

4. Pedersen CA, Schneider PJ, Scheckelhoff DJ. ASHP national survey of pharmacy practice in hospital settings: prescribing and transcribing—2007. *Am J Health Syst Pharm.* 2008;65(9):827-843.

5. Manasse HR Jr. Ensuring the competence of pharmacy technicians. *Am J Health Syst Pharm.* 2007;64(8):816.

6. Weber RJ, Skledar SJ, Sirianni CR, Frank S, Yourich B, Martinelli B. The impact of hospital pharmacist and technician teams on medication-process quality and nurse satisfaction. *Hosp Pharm.* 2004;39(12):1169-1176.

7. Pedersen CA, Gumpper KF. ASHP national survey on informatics: assessment of the adoption and use of pharmacy informatics in U.S. hospitals—2007. *Am J Health Syst Pharm.* 2008;65(23):2244-2264.

8. Poon EG, Cina JL, Churchill W, et al. Medication dispensing errors and potential adverse drug events before and after implementing bar code technology in the pharmacy. *Ann Intern Med.* 2006; 145(6):426-434.

9. Oswald S, Caldwell R. Dispensing error rate after implementation of an automated pharmacy carousel system. *Am J Health Syst Pharm.* 2007;64 (13):1427-1431.

10. Sanborn M. Making the most of unit dose dispensing automation. *Hosp Pharm.* 2007;42(6):572-577.

11. Vermeulen LC, Rough SS, Thielke TS, et al. Strategic approach for improving the medication-use process in health systems: the high-performance pharmacy practice framework. *Am J Health Syst Pharm.* 2007;64(16):1699-1710.

12. Shim JK, Siegel JG. *Schaum's Outline of Financial Management.* New York, NY: McGraw-Hill; 2007. ∎

Making the Most of Unit Dose Dispensing Automation

Michael Sanborn, MS, FASHP *

Pharmacy directors are faced with a myriad of options when it comes to unit dose automation. The goal of this *Director' Forum* article is to outline the most common types of automation available, summarize the advantages and disadvantages of each, and review considerations surrounding optimization, maintenance, and patient safety.

BACKGROUND

Today there are many choices associated with unit dose dispensing automation and a common question is, "What type of automation is best for my facility?". The answer to this question is as varied and complex as each of the sites in which we practice. The solution depends on a variety of factors, including hospital logistics, staffing, financial resources, the existing technology platform, and most importantly, the desired goals associated with the automation need. An important foundation for the decision-making process is the development of an automation strategic plan that addresses each of these areas combined with a careful analysis of the available technology solutions.

Across the country, automated dispensing technologies continue to gain significant market share in hospitals and health systems. For example, the number of hospitals reporting the use of centralized pharmacy automation has more than tripled in 6 years, from 4.5% in 1999 to 15% in 2005.[1] Likewise, facilities reporting the availability of decentralized automated dispensing machines (ADM) continues

to grow (49.2% to 71.8%) during the same period. Larger hospitals tend to be more automated than smaller hospitals, with more than 90% of hospitals over 300 beds reporting some type of centralized or decentralized automation. Uniquely, however, pharmacy directors were evenly split when asked if they envisioned a centralized versus a decentralized drug distribution system in the future.[1]

Which half of the directors are correct in their predictions? Time will tell, but the reasons for the perceived disagreement are multi-fold. For example, hospital logistics play a key role in the types of automation that are best suited for a particular facility. The availability of pneumatic tube systems and other means of medication delivery must be considered when evaluating potential automation solutions. Distance considerations and ease of access from the dispensing point to the patient care unit will also influence automation decisions.

Another market force driving the uptake of dispensing equipment is changing and emerging technology. Options associated with centralized automation have significantly increased over the last 10 years with the advent of carousel applications in pharmacies and the increase in patient-specific automated packaging systems. Much of this growth has been fueled by the increasing need for bar-coded medications. Decentralized

*Corporate Director Director of Pharmacy, Baylor Health Care System, Dallas, Tex.

automation, on the other hand, has experienced many enhancements over the years, including patient profiling, improved security measures, and an increased variety of storage configurations, but the base technology has remained fairly constant.

The standardized HL7 (Health Level 7) data format has dramatically simplified interface development between pharmacy information systems and automated technologies, and this is seldom still a significant consideration regarding vendor selection. However, many vendors that market a variety of automation options are creating enhanced interfaces that allow their technologies to work more seamlessly with one another by selecting the most appropriate device for specific dispensing or replenishment task.

In 1998, the American Society of Health-System Pharmacists published comprehensive guidelines on the safe use of automated medication storage and distribution devices.[2] These guidelines apply to virtually all types of automated devices and are worth careful review as part of the decision-making process. It is important to note that any type of automation is merely a tool used in an effort to improve the efficiency of the medication-use process, and there are essentially three models associated with unit dose medication distribution technology. They include decentralized dispensing, centralized automation, or a hybrid of these two types. Each of these will be discussed in detail, but other important elements that require deliberation include optimization and maintenance, patient safety considerations, and return on investment.

DECENTRALIZED AUTOMATION

Decentralized pharmacy automation, as we know it, was first introduced in 1989 and has since rapidly expanded. These devices are commonly referred to as ADMs, and can be placed in virtually any patient care area to assist with the dispensing of medications. Initially, they were designed to assist pharmacists with controlled substance tracking and floor-stock medication control. ADM use has since been expanded to serve as a dispensing mechanism for 90% or more of medications used in a particular patient location. These cabinets have also been adapted for use in more unique environments where medications are used, such as in operating rooms, controlled substance vaults, ambulatory clinics, and as "night cabinets" for use when a pharmacy is closed.

There are a number of vendors of decentralized automation, and each offers a varying array of device configurations and options. It is beyond the scope of this article to compare and contrast each vendor, but evaluating and selecting an appropriate automation partner is a critical step in any automation plan. Important considerations include equipment functionality, reliability, service response (which may be different from region to region), and of course, economics.

There are many advantages to decentralized ADMs, which have given rise to their market dominance as a pharmacy automation solution. Some of these advantages include improved turn-around time due to the near immediate availability of medications, reduced opportunities for pilferage over an open floor-stock system, and improved charge capture. Nursing time associated with controlled substance counts is dramatically reduced since it is typically unnecessary to count every medication after every shift. Additionally, ADMs have the potential to reduce the restocking time that is often associated with returned medications from a unit dose cart-fill system; however, this time savings must be counterbalanced with the new functions associated with cabinet restocking. The tracking and reporting capabilities that ADMs provide can also be quite useful, and they have shown to improve the detection of narcotic diversion.[3] Finally, ADMs have been used to effectively improve patient safety and provide pharmacy services after a hospital pharmacy is closed, and this function can be further enhanced through remote site review of medication orders prior to vending a medication from the cabinet.

An important point regarding the ADM that is often overlooked is that, pragmatically speaking, it is a nursing tool more so than a pharmacy tool. True, it automates medication dispensing, which falls under the purview of the pharmacist, but in most hospitals, more than 90% of the transactions related to an ADM are performed by nursing personnel. Therefore, it is wise to solicit nursing input when evaluating ADM solutions or when making modifications to existing functions. Additionally, nursing time associated with cabinet use should also be considered when determining machine configurations for each area with an effort to prevent unnecessary "queuing" at the station during common administration times.

Patient safety considerations with ADMs are multifold, but vendors continue to incorporate new safeguards to reduce the potential for errors. Evidence showing both increases and decreases in the rate of medication errors after ADM implementation is available and further underscores the importance of effective planning and risk mitigation with any technology.[4-7] Pharmacy-mediated opportunities for errors associated with these systems include filling units with incorrect medications, mixing products or strengths in the same location during restocking, not removing expired medications, and not assigning appropriate par levels to reduce situations where a drug is needed but not available. Fortunately, most ADM manufacturers have now incorporated bar-code scanning technology to significantly improve cabinet restocking accuracy.

There are also nursing-related error opportunities, including not double-checking a medication upon removal or when returning unused medications, paying inadequate attention to product labels, entering the wrong patient data when gaining access to an ADM, or bypassing the profile system. Additionally, many nurses will try to minimize the amount of time spent using the cabinet by removing multiple medications—sometimes enough for use during an entire shift—for multiple patients during a single cabinet session. This is a dangerous practice and bypasses important patient safety features that are part of an effective medication-use system.

An important safety requirement related to ADMs is eliminating override medications; a situation where access to a medication is permitted prior to a pharmacist's review of the prescriber's order. The Joint Commission mandated this requirement several years ago in response to the high-error potential associated with this practice. Errors associated with overrides are significant, and have been reported to be as high as 11.7%.[5] Despite this fact, as much a 13.3% of medications in US hospitals are withdrawn on an override basis, which is an improvement over previous years, but still provides a significant opportunity for further progress.[1] Nevertheless, ADMs can improve overall compliance with Joint Commission standards.[8,9]

CENTRALIZED AUTOMATION

Centralized unit dose automation has also been available to pharmacies for many years and has continued to evolve. Initially, these systems consisted of strip packaging machines that could be integrated with the pharmacy information system to produce patient-specific unit dose medications for distribution via medication cassettes. These types of advanced packaging devices have seen an increased surge in popularity as pharmacists look for solutions that can provide bar-coded unit-of-use packaging.

Another type of centralized automation utilizes advanced robotic technology and bar-code symbology to identify packaged medications and select them for an individual patient. These medications can then be stored in a medication cassette or an envelope labeled with the patient's name. When it was developed in the late 1980s, this type of technology was unique, since it not only automated the traditional cart-fill process but could also manage both the first-dose dispensing function and the return process. The system can also be configured to handle most types of drug packages, including tab-

lets, capsules, syringes, prepackaged liquids, vials, ampules, and patches.

A third type of centralized automation uses carousel technology, which was adapted from conveyor-shelf storage units traditionally used in the manufacturing industry.[10] These devices offer excellent capacity and inventory control capabilities and can often store 2,000 to 3,000 various-sized items in a vertical or horizontal rotating shelf format. In these types of systems, the carousel is interfaced with the pharmacy information system and when a medication order is received, the shelving system within the carousel rotates to the ordered drug one item at a time. Lighted prompts guide the user to the proper medication, and the appropriate number of dosage units are removed and placed into a bag labeled with a bar-coded, patient-specific sticker that is generated by the carousel software. This type of system can be used to store a large percentage of the total pharmacy inventory.

Like ADMs, there are advantages and disadvantages to centralized automation. A significant advantage is that medication selection associated with these systems is automated and bar-code driven, reducing the potential for human error.[11] Because they inherently use bar codes to dispense medications, they also offer unique compatibility for bedside bar-code scanning systems. Some of them can automatically screen for outdated medications, dramatically reducing the likelihood of dispensing an outdated drug. The systems are also "inventory friendly" because they can be configured to contain a relatively small amount of inventory on hand (vs ADMs, which typically increase inventory values by adding multiple storage locations), use stock rotation algorithms, and can be configured to automatically reorder medications based on current use. In many states, it is also possible to use centralized robotic technology to reduce the amount of time pharmacists spend checking medications by implementing quality assurance protocols that check only a small percentage of robot-dispensed doses.

Disadvantages of centralized technologies can differ from facility to facility. Oftentimes, the logistical challenges of a traditional cart-fill system remain, such as delivering medications, transferring medications when a patient is moved to a different location, and assuring the return of medications to the pharmacy when a patient is discharged. A centralized system does not address unit-based storage requirements, and medication pilferage and "borrowing" for other patients are potential problems. From a safety perspective, centralized technologies have proven to be very effective; however, it is possible for a human operator to introduce an error into the system[12] by assigning an incorrect bar code or packaging a medication incorrectly, and because this type of error is unrecognizable to the automation, it can be replicated several times. Finally, since these systems are pharmacy-based, there are often space considerations that must be addressed.

THE HYBRID MODEL

Many hospital pharmacies and health systems have decided to use a hybrid automation system that employs both centralized and decentralized dispensing technologies. The goal behind this hybrid model is to maximize the benefits of both types of systems while minimizing the potential disadvantages. This type of distribution system also allows for automation of the largest percentage of drug distribution tasks, and it is especially beneficial for larger hospitals (more than 200 beds).

For example, a hospital may choose to operate a centralized robotic system so that patient-specific, bar-coded medications can be dispensed to each patient care area. The same facility may also deploy ADMs to manage controlled substances, floor stock items, and prescribed "as needed" medications. This symbiotic automation platform has other benefits, since interfaces exist that will allow the centralized robot (or a carousel) to pick medications for an ADM, dramatically reducing the time required to restock and further minimizing opportunities for filling errors.

A hybrid model provides enhanced flexibility to modify the dispensing model based on a particular drug product; however, it can create additional distribution system challenges. Interface development and machine coordination for multiple systems can be difficult. Additionally, because there is more extensive use of different types of automation, integrating all of the technologies to create a seamless dispensing process can be time-consuming during implementation.

OPTIMIZATION IS KEY

Regardless of the type of automation in place, the most important aspect of effectively applying the technology is optimization. Virtually all automation projects that have failed have done so due to lack of optimization and process improvements. As previously stated, the technology is merely a tool, and how it is "designed, understood, and implemented determines the use and the benefits realized."[13] Without appropriate planning, process redesign, and a focus on enhanced effectiveness, automation can essentially make bad processes happen automatically. Likewise, the efficiency of automation functioning at peak performance can deteriorate over time as changes occur in prescribing habits or the hospital's patient population. Additionally, automation does not always lead to improvements in patient safety, and according to the United States Pharmacopeial Convention (USP), nearly 20% of medication errors reported are due to problems with computerization or automation. In fact, there were over 8,000 errors reported with ADMs in 2003, and nearly 70% involved an incorrect drug or dosage.[14]

Effective optimization can have a dramatic impact on user satisfaction, operational costs, human resource requirements, and patient safety. For all automation, it is important to balance the need for just-in-time inventory with patient utilization to prevent shortages. Data from the automated device(s) should be analyzed at least quarterly. In addition to inventory par values, low-use items, and medications used but not stocked should be reviewed. Medication locations should also be assessed periodically to separate look-alike, sound-alike medications and to enhance device functionality.

Reviewing large amounts of dispensing data and other transactions can be tedious and time-consuming; however, the time savings generally pays off multifold for all end users and provides additional patient safety improvements. Optimization is typically much easier for centralized automation versus decentralized ADMs

due to the sheer number of inventory line items that must be evaluated and modified. With a centralized robot, for example, there may be 700 to 800 line items used for daily dispensing, whereas a series of 40 ADM cabinets each containing 250 line items requires 10,000 total line items to be reviewed.

At our 1,000-bed university teaching hospital, for instance, we use a hybrid dispensing model and have 84 ADM locations, carousel technology, and a dispensing robot. Prior to 2003, only minimal efforts had been undertaken to optimize the decentralized cabinets. A small workgroup was created that evaluated data available from the ADM transaction activity (eg, withdrawals, returns, refill activity, stockouts, low-use items) with a primary focus of improving user satisfaction and reducing the workload associated with the technology. The team met biweekly and reviewed these data and made changes to cabinet inventories, medication configurations, and restock/delivery schedules. Over a 6-month period, the results were significant.

As an illustration, the initial average stockout rate for all cabinets was 10.4 stockouts/cabinet/week with some areas experiencing as many as 23 stockouts per week. This was a major point of dissatisfaction for both nursing and pharmacy and created a significant amount of rework to address the daily drug shortages. Over the course of 6 months, the ADM team was able to decrease the stockout rate by 91.6% (see **Figure 1**). Another improvement identified was related to cabinet restocking activity, which had a significant impact on pharmacy workload and the manpower needed to maintain the ADMs. Initially, our

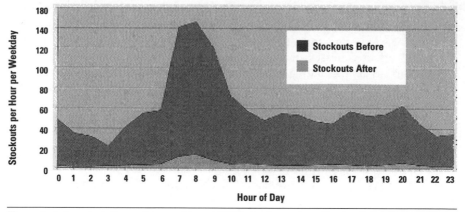

Figure 1. Automated dispensing machines (ADM) stockout rate at Baylor University Medical Center before and after optimization (ADM stockouts by time of day).

average number of cabinet restocks per week was 15.4 since most of our high-use cabinets were programmed to be refilled two to three times per day. By adjusting inventory levels and par values, it was possible to reduce refill frequencies to once daily for high-use cabinets and to every other day in some areas, which lowered our overall ADM restocks/cabinet/week to 6.8 (see **Figure 2**).

FINANCIAL CONSIDERATIONS

An important consideration for any pharmacy technology project is overall cost and return on investment (ROI). Most automation vendors will perform a facility-specific ROI calculation for their equipment that often includes inventory cost improvements, waste reduction, labor savings, and other potential cost reduction or avoidance opportunities. It is impor-

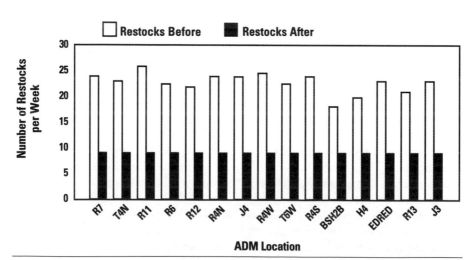

Figure 2. Automated dispensing machines (ADM) refill activity at Baylor University Medical Center before and after optimization (restock activity for the top 15 units).

tant to review this information carefully to assess both its accuracy and feasibility. It is often helpful to enlist a representative from the hospital's finance department to assist with the ROI. This step can ensure compatibility with the hospital's requirements for a business plan and financial model, and may also generate additional proponents for the project.

Many ROI projections are not fully realized due to less than ideal implementations or as a result of inappropriate expectations. With ADMs for example, there is no question that they will save a significant amount of nursing time versus a traditional manual floor stock system; however, there may not be a requisite reduction in nursing staff in favor of reallocating their time to patient care responsibilities. This is still a positive gain for the hospital, but does not result in hard-dollar savings that can offset the cost of the equipment. It is also possible to have a net increase in FTE requirements associated with an automation project if the system is implemented inefficiently. The literature offers some examples of these mixed results,[7,8,15-19] and if possible, it is important to validate projected ROI calculations with other similar facilities.

Negotiating aggressive technology pricing is another important aspect of the purchase. Typically, the hospital's group purchasing organization will have prenegotiated prices with preferred vendors; however, it is sometimes possible to negotiate even lower costs. It is also important to consider the entire cost of the project as part of a larger automation plan. For instance, the initial capital outlay for a centralized dispensing robot can be significant, but in a large hospital it is often less than the combined annual costs of a decentralized dispensing system. Another benefit of a hybrid model is that it can actually be less costly than a fully decentralized system, since it reduces the total number of ADM and auxiliary units needed, which can offset the cost of the centralized automation.

SUMMARY

Dispensing automation has become a mainstay in almost every hospital pharmacy in the country. There is a wide variety of choices available today, and each type of technology continues to expand and evolve. It is important to evaluate automation choices carefully, because decisions in this area often have a lasting impact on the department and can significantly affect hospital staff and patients. Regardless of the type of system chosen, ongoing optimization is critical to maximizing return on investment.

REFERENCES

1. Pedersen CA, Schneider PJ, Scheckelhoff DJ. ASHP national survey of pharmacy practice in hospital settings: dispensing and administration—2005. *Am J Health Syst Pharm.* 2006;63:327-345.

2. American Society of Health-System Pharmacists. ASHP guidelines on the safe use of automated medication storage and distribution devices. *Am J Health Syst Pharm.* 1998;55:1403–1407.

3. Crowson K, Monk-Tutor M. Use of automated controlled substance cabinets for detection of diversion in US hospitals: a national study. *Hosp Pharm.* 2005;40:977-983.

4. Skibinski K, White B, Lin L, Dong Y, Wu W. Effects of technological interventions on the safety of a medication-use system. *Am J Health Syst Pharm.* 2007;64:90-96.

5. Kester K, Baxter J, Freudenthal K. Errors associated with medication removed from automated dispensing machines using override function. *Hosp Pharm.* 2006;41:535-537.

6. Oren E, Shaffer ER, Guglielmo BJ. Impact of technologies on medication errors and ad-

verse drug events. *Am J Health Syst Pharm.* 2003;60:1447-1458.

7. Klibanov OM, Eckel SF. Effects of automated dispensing on inventory control, billing, workload, and potential medication errors. *Am J Health Syst Pharm.* 2003;60:569-572.

8. Garrelts JC, Koehn L, Snyder V, Snyder R, Rich DS. Automated medication distribution systems and compliance with Joint Commission standards. *Am J Health Syst Pharm.* 2001;58:2267-2272.

9. Rich DS. Automated dispensing devices. *Hosp Pharm.* 2000;35:666-670.

10. Kolar GR. Outsourcing: route to a new pharmacy practice model. *Am J Health Syst Pharm.* 1997;54:48-52.

11. Ragan R, Bond J, Major K, Kingsford T, Eidem L, Garrets JC. Improved control of medication use with an integrated bar-code-packaging and distribution system. *Am J Health Syst Pharm.* 2005;62:1075-1079.

12. Cohen MR. Error despite robotics? *Hosp Pharm.* 2004;39:1021-1022.

13. Lee P. Ideal principles and characteristics of a fail-safe medication-use system. *Am J Health Syst Pharm.* 2002;59:369-371.

14. Thompson CA. Technology hasn't eliminated medication errors yet, USP reports. *Am J Health Syst Pharm.* 2005;62:243-245.

15. Schwarz H, Brodowy B. Implementation and evaluation of an automated dispensing system. *Am J Health Syst Pharm.* 1995;52:823-828.

16. Shirley KL. Effect of an automated dispensing system on medication administration time. *Am J Health Syst Pharm.* 1999;56:1542-1545.

17. Lee LW, Wellman GS, Birdwell SJ, Sherrin TP. Use of an automated medication storage and distribution system. *Am J Hosp Pharm.* 1992;49:851-855.

18. Guerrero RM, Nickman NA, Jorgenson JA. Work activities before and after implementation of an automated dispensing system. *Am J Health Syst Pharm.* 1996;53:548-554.

19. Klein EG, Santora JA, Pascale PM, Kitrenos JG. Medication cart-filling time, accuracy, and cost with an automated dispensing system. *Am J Hosp Pharm.* 1994;51:1193-1196. ∎

Implementing a Bar-Code Medication Administration System

Robert J. Weber, MS, FASHP*

The *Director's Forum* series is written and edited by Michael Sanborn and Robert Weber and is designed for guiding pharmacy leaders in establishing patient-centered services in hospitals and health systems. Another specific goal of this column is addressing many of the key challenges that pharmacy directors currently face while providing information that will foster growth in pharmacy leadership and patient safety. Bar-code medication administration (BCMA) is an important medication safety program for hospitals, and the involvement of the pharmacy director in its implementation and evaluation is critical. This installment of the *Director's Forum* describes the necessary steps for implementing and evaluating a BCMA program.

INTRODUCTION

Growing evidence of the number of medical errors that occur throughout the US health care system has prompted an increased interest in using technology to improve safety. Medication errors, which occur at a rate ranging from 19% to 36% in hospitals and over half of which occur during medication administration, are a significant concern for patients, health care organizations, and clinicians.[1] Bar-code medication administration (BCMA) systems are an example of technology being employed to reduce medication administration errors. These systems electronically compare a patient's identity and medical information (eg, in an electronic medication order) against a bar-coded medication, alerting the nurse of the potential for a medication administration error. It is hypothesized that these alerts, if properly interpreted and acted on by nurses, will help prevent medication administration errors. Furthermore, the Institute of Medicine recommends using BCMA systems to ensure the timeliness and accuracy of medication administration.[2] Several studies have shown that bar-coding systems reduce medication dispensing errors and adverse drug events in a hospital pharmacy (by 63%), in addition to reducing medication administration errors (by 50% to 60%) (University of Pittsburgh Medical Center, unpublished data, 2004).[3]

Despite these predictions, a recent survey by the American Society of Health-System Pharmacists shows that a small percentage of hospitals have implemented BCMA technology.[4] The reasons for this limited implementation may include the expense of bar-code systems and, more importantly, the significant efforts required for evaluating and changing the medication-use process to maximize the use of bar-code technology.

There is a paucity of literature that describes the steps necessary for implementation and evaluation of a BCMA system by an organization. A report describing the practical aspects of bar-coding medication provides some guidance to the mechanics and suggests that reliable processes must be in place for patient and caregiver identification, as well as for medication bar coding.[5] In addition, a recent report highlights work-arounds

Chief Pharmacy Officer, University of Pittsburgh Medical Center; Associate Professor and Department Chair, University of Pittsburgh, School of Pharmacy, Pittsburgh, Pennsylvania.

Director's Forum **21**

in BCMA systems that threaten their effectiveness.[2] Because of the barriers to implementation of BCMA systems, such as the cost of the aforementioned processes and the exposed workarounds, communication by organizations of the impact that these systems have on preventing medication errors is vital.

This article presents the University of Pittsburgh Medical Center's (UPMC's) experience in implementing a system for BCMA. The specific aims of this article include (1) establishing the conceptual framework for using bar-code systems as part of an organization's safety plan, (2) designing a multidisciplinary process for selecting a bar-code system, (3) installing the computing infrastructure for support of bar coding, (4) establishing an inventory control system that ensures nearly 100% bar coding of medications, (5) revising pharmacy and nursing medication processes to enhance functionality, and (6) developing quality indicators for bar-code systems. Information is provided on a real-world experience that informs pharmacy directors who are seeking to make their medication systems safer using BCMA.

BACKGROUND

The UPMC Presbyterian hospital is a 647-bed academic medical center affiliated with the University of Pittsburgh Schools of the Health Sciences, with nationally recognized patient care programs in critical care medicine, organ transplantation, orthopedics, geriatrics, cardiology, and internal medicine. Prior to implementation of BCMA, the system for medication dispensation at UPMC Presbyterian was a fully automated bar-code process employing robotics (McKesson Automated Health-care, Inc., Pittsburgh, Pennsylvania), medication carousels, and an integrated electronic health record (Cerner *PharmNet* and Cerner *HNA Millenium*, Kansas City, Missouri) that provided pharmacists with ready access to patient medical record data, including progress notes, laboratory results, and allergy information. The system for nursing medication administration comprised a paper medication administration record (MAR) that relied on manual implementation by the nurse of the best practices for medication, including allergy and duplicate medication screening, along with timely and accurate medication administration. Currently, UPMC Presbyterian implements a comprehensive interdisciplinary medication safety program that uses an evidence-based model and supportive data from the United States Pharmacopoeial Convention's *MEDMARX*, recognized as one of the most credible medication error reporting systems.[6]

CONCEPTUAL FRAMEWORK

The goal of UPMC Presbyterian with regard to medication-patient safety is elimination of medication errors through the systematic reporting, analysis, and sharing of medication error information and problem-solving strategies across the organization. The institution's framework for medication-patient safety focuses on using reporting systems and other data sources to identify problems, as well as implementing evidence-based interventions to improve safety in medication prescribing, administering, and dispensing. The framework is endorsed by the institution's executive management and trustees, with

Table 1. Drugs Associated With Serious Administration Errors at University of Pittsburgh Medical Center Presbyterian

Morphine, oxycodone, hydromorphone
Phenytoin
Tacrolimus
Warfarin
Metoprolol
Calcitonin-salmon
Lactulose glyburide, glimepiride
Insulin

all planning for medication safety focused on designing programs that are consistent with this framework.

BCMA was compatible with the organization's medication safety conceptual framework. Because a bar-coded medication dispensing system (*Robot-Rx*, McKesson) and an integrated electronic health record with emerging decision-support capabilities were already in place, UPMC Presbyterian was well positioned for establishing the BCMA program. Moreover, the program was regarded as an enhancement of the current medication safety system through the continued use of new technology.

Data from the organization's medication error reporting system was used to examine BCMA's potential impact on safety. Serious medication errors—as defined by the National Coordinating Council on Medication Error Reporting and Prevention index—were reviewed for an 8-month period prior to implementing BCMA.[7] Using this index greatly enhanced the ability to identify the breadth and scope of system problems, as indicated by *near misses* (categories A and B) and *sentinel serious events* (categories D through I). Analysis revealed

a potentially significant impact from BCMA's prevention of serious medication administration errors associated with high-risk medications (opiates, antibiotics, medications for diabetes and cardiovascular conditions, etc). Table 1 lists the drug products associated with serious medication administration errors that were determined potentially preventable through use of BCMA.

IMPLEMENTATION STEPS
Bar-Code Medication Administration System Selection

Selecting a BCMA system requires a multidisciplinary approach, including hospital leadership, physicians, nurses, pharmacists, and information system specialists. At UPMC Presbyterian, a steering committee with representatives from each of these areas was developed that conducted site visits, reviewed BCMA system demonstrations from vendors, and developed specific criteria for selection. Table 2 describes some of the criteria that were developed for selection of a BCMA system.

Establishing Computing Infrastructure

The Steering Committee evaluated the current information system infrastructure and purchased equipment that promoted portability (eg, wireless connections, computer carts) and integration with the institution's electronic health record. This required a systematic "swap out" of computer devices, as well as facility upgrades, to accommodate wireless connections and handheld BCMA scanners. These processes take time but are a necessary part of the work plan for implementing BCMA systems. Another consideration in using wireless devices is the

Table 2. Selected Criteria for Choosing a Bar-Code Medication Administration System

Nursing satisfaction with usability
Pharmacy satisfaction with usability
Availability and usability of portable, wireless BCMA equipment (eg, handheld scanners)
Ability to integrate with the existing hospital computing infrastructure
Usefulness of the alert system in BCMA (eg, reduced "nuisance" alerts, ability of nursing/pharmacy to easily deal with alerts)
Connectivity and integration with current pharmacy automation (eg, unit-based cabinets, robotics)
Amount of implementation support (in hours, days, or weeks) by the vendor
Integration and compatibility with hospital's existing bar-code scanning systems
Compatibility with the hospital pharmacy's medication packaging system
Types of and accessibility to system reports (eg, scanning compliance by nurse/nursing unit, avoided errors)
Ability to extract data for reviewing quality indicators for the BCMA system
Ongoing support of the system (eg, routine maintenance, emergency calls)
Amount of process redesign necessary to implement BCMA

BCMA = bar-code medication administration.

impact on the security of the information system data. Developing a "single sign-on," or one sign-on password, for access to multiple applications (including BCMA) was critical in encouraging user compliance at UPMC Presbyterian. Handheld BCMA devices (from Cerner) that were easy to read and operate were selected for the project. Finally, patients' bar-code–readable wristbands were evaluated for durability and scanning capability.

Medication and Patient-Specific Bar-Code Processes

The unit-dose medication system is widely accepted as the standard for medication use within health systems. This system employs an individually packaged dosage, which is available as a commercial product or as an extemporaneously packaged item, for administration to patients. Although these systems promote safety by reducing confusion over the proper drug and dosage for administration, they do not necessarily prevent all potential medication administration errors. For example, if a medication is available as a given dosage strength and an alternative strength is ordered, the nurse may use the commercially available dosage form and modify it to give the ordered dose (eg, furosemide 10 mg order administered as one-half of a furosemide 20 mg tablet). To eliminate this potential for error, UPMC Presbyterian has developed a system that provides the immediate medication container for nearly 100% of the hospital's drug formulary.

Most hospital pharmacy computer systems use the national drug code (NDC) as a unique identifier for drug products. The NDC identifies the drug, formulation, strength, package size and type, and the drug's manufacturer. Manufacturers that place bar codes on their products embed the NDC information in the bar codes; however, there is currently no published database that lists the readability of a manufacturer's bar codes by specific software systems, making the initial preparation for bar-code medication packaging a labor-intensive process. UPMC Presbyterian accomplished this process by using the BCMA software for validation of the drug products requiring bar coding through scanning the pharmacy inventory to determine whether each product could be read by the BCMA system and revising the inventory shelf labels to indicate which products contained bar codes that were recognized by the BCMA software. Because the bar-code readability of drug products varies, the process of properly labeling the inventory storage bins in a pharmacy prevents the ordering of products that are not recognized by the BCMA system.

The assessment of the drug formulary at UPMC Presbyterian showed that approximately 49% of the available drug products were recognized by the BCMA system. Extemporaneous packaging by the pharmacy was required for the drug products without a commercially available bar code or those not recognized by the BCMA system. There are a variety of methods for packaging that allow medication administration as unit-of-use at the patient's bedside. **Figure 1** represents the packaging process implemented by UPMC Presbyterian to ensure 95% to 100% availability of bar-code medications.

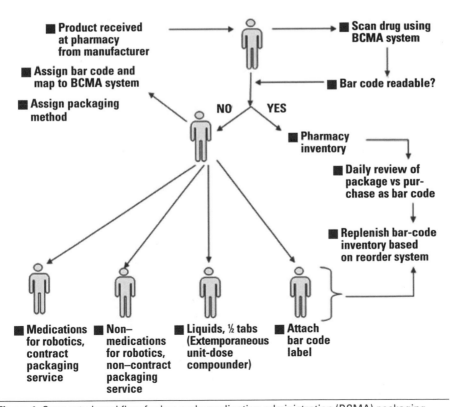

Figure 1. Suggested workflow for bar-code medication administration (BCMA) packaging.

Medication Processes Redesign

Implementing a BCMA system requires an evaluation and revision of the current medication process workflow. Developing a process for which patient identification occurs as the first step is vital to the accuracy of the BCMA system. This is done by scanning patients' wristbands to verify their identities. Specific procedures must be developed based on the following medication processes:

1. Physician review of medications on the BCMA electronic record
2. Medication scanning practices
3. Medication administration practices
4. Availability of unit-dose medications ready for BCMA administration
5. Order verification and review procedures

An example of clarifying medication scanning practices is illustrated in an observational study conducted by Koppel et al.[5] The study identified work-arounds for medication scanning, including scanning without visual check of the MAR, not scanning patients first to verify their identities, administering medication without using the BCMA scanner, placing bar codes for medications on paper or other documents, and scanning the medication bar code after the medication was removed from its package. Organizations should use this reference to develop effective medication administration rules in a BCMA system.

Developing Quality Indicators for Bar-Code Medication Administration

BCMA systems are designed for prevention of medication errors by alerting nurses to the potential for a medication administration error. There is a scarcity of literature on the impact of bar-code medication systems on compliance to safety processes and on their ability to prevent medication errors. A study by Poon et al. demonstrated a reduction in medication errors in the pharmacy as the result of implementing a BCMA system.[3] At UPMC Presbyterian, the goal in developing quality indicators was evaluation of the compliance to key safety processes, as well as better understanding of how the alert system could be revised and refined. Quality indicators focused on the following areas:

1. Bar code scanning compliance to ensure accurate patient identification
2. Percentage of medication administration warnings that actually prevent an error
3. Observation of medication administration practices
4. Staff satisfaction with the BCMA system.

Table 3 lists potential quality indicators that can be used when evaluating a BCMA system.

LESSONS LEARNED

As discussed earlier, data have been published on work-arounds associated with the BCMA systems. (See Koppel et al. for further information.) This section briefly reviews some of the lessons learned at UPMC Presbyterian during implementation of a BCMA system.

First, with respect to planning and implementing BCMA, significant variations in the medication ordering and administration processes were observed within the hospital, including how the MAR was used and how medication order information was entered into the pharmacy computer

Table 3. Quality Indicators for a Bar-Code Medication Administration System

Outcome	Indicator	Data Source	Metric (Numerator/ Denominator)	Frequency
Process outcome to ensure compliance with patient identification procedures and reliability of BCMA software	Bar-code scanning compliance	BCMA software	Number of medications scanned/Medications mapped to BCMA software	Weekly
Process outcome to assess the ability of the BCMA system to identify medication errors	Prevented error warning effectiveness	BCMA software	Number of error warnings/Number of prevented medication errors	Daily
Clinical outcome indicator to measure the effectiveness of the BCMA system in reducing medication errors	Observed medication error rate	Blinded observation of medication administration and comparing of medication administration to physician's written order	Number of medication errors, with no more than 1 error per dose/Number of observed medication administrations × 100%	Quarterly
Clinical outcome indicator to measure the effectiveness of the BCMA system in reducing serious medication administration errors	Incidence of serious medication administration errors	*MEDMARX* medication error reporting system	Number of medication administration errors in NCC MERP categories D through I/Number of doses dispensed	Monthly
Process outcome to determine nurse satisfaction with the safeguards of the BCMA system	Nurse satisfaction	Survey nurses to rate their perceived safety of the medication administration system according to a Likert scale (1 = strongly disagree; 5 = strongly agree)	Average Likert score from the nurse survey[a]	Quarterly

[a]There is no denominator for this metric; BCMA = bar-code medication administration; NCC MERP = National Coordinating Council on Medication Error Reporting and Prevention.

system. For example, if human insulin was ordered by a physician, it usually was done so as a detailed order with dosage based on the patient's blood glucose level. Nursing staff then documented the detailed human insulin order on the previously used handwritten MAR, and the pharmacy entered the human insulin order into the pharmacy ordering system with the simple designation "as directed"—because the pharmacy used the computer system as a product-dispensing system. Because the BCMA system used information from the pharmacy computer system to populate the electronic MAR (e-MAR), this practice provided the nurse with inadequate information for safe administration of the insulin. Consequently, medication order entry practices had to become more patient focused and had to consider the medication administration practices of the nursing staff. During the initial implementation of BCMA in UPMC Presbyterian's pilot units, there were many instances in which the medication order entry into the pharmacy computer system and the resultant order on the e-MAR did not contain all of the parameters necessary for administration of the medication by the nurse. The pharmacy medication order entry discrepancies were a continual problem as the institution expanded its implementation; this may have been the result of not making the pharmacy more aware of the nursing medication administration process. A key lesson learned from the implementation experience was the importance of establishing a focus group of pharmacists and nurses who could review the current medication administration process, as well as identifying the information required by the nurse to ensure effective pharmacy medication order entry.

Another example of medication order discrepancies was associated with the assignment of medication administration times. Because pharmacists were entering medication orders outside of a given nursing unit, they were often unaware of the most appropriate medication schedule for a patient, so they used a standard medication administration time. This practice created errors in medication administration times and delayed therapy where it was clinically warranted. Thus, a focus group of pharmacy and nursing personnel should be established to determine whether the use of standard medication administration times is beneficial.

As UPMC Presbyterian evaluated the effectiveness of BCMA, the institution quickly learned that the warning system for potential errors triggered by scanning a patient's wristband or a medication bar code affected the users' perceptions of the BCMA system. As a result, it was suggested that the warnings and alerts be examined and simplified to eliminate nuisance alerts.

Developing a steering committee to address the planning, implementation, and operational issues for BCMA is an effective strategy. In terms of information sharing, the Steering Committee at UPMC Presbyterian generated support for BCMA as a part of the safety culture and increased general awareness of errors as systems problems as opposed to individual fault. The Steering Committee designed a plan that included pharmacy, nursing, and information system personnel who provided direct support to users during the first 10 to 14 days of each unit's BCMA implementation. This support was integral in building the confidence of the nursing and pharmacy staff in using the BCMA system.

BCMA serves as an important catalyst for preventing medication administration errors. UPMC Presbyterian has asked users questions about the value of the BCMA system in the care of their patients to gauge organizational acceptance of this program, and it is clear that the degree to which individual clinicians adopt and implement the BCMA system depends on their belief in the system's ability to support a safe medication administration system and to increase the efficiency of their work. The BCMA system functions in as close to real-time as possible so that errors are prevented before they reach the patient. To continue promoting acceptance and understanding of the BCMA system, organizations must develop methods of sharing information about the errors it has prevented.

CONCLUSION

The success of BCMA implementation at UPMC Presbyterian depended on the organizational commitment of resources and a viable plan for reducing barriers to safer practices. BCMA use underscores the need for a continued emphasis on developing the functionality of and enhancing practitioners' use of the system. This can be accomplished by focusing on (1) adding system functionality to effectively screen for related events in medication administration, (2) continually eliminating nuisance alerts, (3) revising order-entry practices to make them consistent with the approved standard administration times and methods of nurse medication administration, (4) revising order-writing practices for inclusion of proper route of administration and dosage forms to meet specific patient needs, and (5) addressing process issues related to bar-code packaging and scanner functionality service. Implementing an effective BCMA system will help further promote the hospital pharmacy's role in developing a patient-centered pharmacy.

ACKNOWLEDGMENTS

This article is dedicated to the memory of Mark T. Hopkins, former Chief Information Officer for UPMC Presbyterian Shadyside, who died of cancer in November 2007. Mark's vision for computing infrastructure and information system integration, as well as his tireless efforts in implementing UPMC's BCMA system, was an inspiration to us all.

REFERENCES

1. Barker KN, Flynn ED, Pepper G, et al. Medication errors observed in 36 health care facilities. *Arch Intern Med.* 2002;162(16):1897-1903.

2. Institute of Medicine. *Preventing Medication Errors.* Washington DC: The National Academies Press; 2007.

3. Poon EG, Cina JL, Churchill W, et al. Medication errors and potential adverse drug events before and after implementing bar code technology in the pharmacy. *Ann Intern Med.* 2006;145(6):426-434.

4. Pedersen CA, Schneider PJ, Schecklhoff DJ. ASHP national survey of pharmacy practice in hospital settings—dispensing and administration—2002. *Am J Health Syst Pharm.* 2003;60(1):52-68.

5. Koppel R, Wetterneck T, Telles JL, Karsh B-T. Work-arounds to bar-code medication systems: their occurrences, causes and threats to patient safety. *J Am Med Inform Assoc.* 2008;15(4):408-423.

6. Leape, LL. Reporting of adverse events. *N Engl J Med.* 2002;347(20): 1633-1638.

7. National Coordinating Council for Medication Error Reporting and Prevention (NCC MERP) taxonomy of medication errors. NCC MERP Web site. http://www.nccmerp.org/pdf/taxo2001-07-31.pdf. Accessed October 8, 2008. ∎

Electronic Prescribing

Robert J. Weber, MS, FASHP, * and Scott M. Mark, PharmD, MS, MEd,*
FASHP, FACHE, FABC†

The *Director's Forum* series is written and edited by Michael Sanborn and Robert Weber and is designed for guiding pharmacy leaders in establishing patient-centered services in hospitals and health systems. Another specific goal of this column is addressing many of the key challenges that pharmacy directors currently face, while also providing information that will foster growth in pharmacy leadership and patient safety. As the use of electronic prescribing grows in health systems, pharmacy directors must be positioned to assist their organizations in a variety of ways when implementing and evaluating these systems. This installment of the *Director's Forum* provides a brief primer to electronic prescribing and its implications for improving the patient-centered provision of hospital pharmacy services.

INTRODUCTION

Improving patient safety has become a key objective of health care in the last several years. In particular, medication safety has the specific goals of integrating error-reduction programs as part of an organization's workflow (eg, culture changes), reducing the number and severity of adverse events from medication errors, and implementing technology to automate safe practices. Several automated approaches have been employed to ensure that no harm comes to patients. Examples of effective medication safety technology include robotic medication preparation and dispensing, barcode medication administration, and use of medication carousels and automated dispensing cabinets.[1]

Electronic prescribing, or e-prescribing, is the most recent technological advancement in medication safety. E-prescribing involves the use of computers for ordering, modifying, reviewing, and transmitting drug orders or prescriptions. An advantage of e-prescribing systems is the availability of decision support, which is an information database that reviews an electronic prescription entry and alerts the prescriber if the entry will result in a medication error. E-prescribing systems have been increasing in use in hospitals since the early 1990s. A recent review of hospital-based e-prescribing notes that this technology has been useful in reducing medication adverse events.[2]

E-prescribing has grown in the outpatient setting as well. The Veterans Administration reports that the use of dangerous drugs to treat illness in older veterans (eg, benzodiazepines, narcotics, anticoagulants) was improved significantly with e-prescribing.[3]

The success of e-prescribing has prompted consumer groups and federal officials to mandate implementation of e-prescribing systems in hospitals, clinics, and physician practices. One ardent supporter of e-prescribing is the Leapfrog Group, which is composed of influential US industries that pay for health care services for their employees.[4] Companies participating in Leapfrog, such as AT&T, General Electric, Boeing, and IBM, are spending billions of dollars for employee health care to support a system that is, in their view, dysfunctional, un-

*Executive Director of Pharmacy, University of Pittsburgh Medical Center; Associate Professor and Chair, Department of Pharmacy and Therapeutics, University of Pittsburgh School of Pharmacy; †Director of Pharmacy, University of Pittsburgh Medical Center; Assistant Professor and Vice Chair, University of Pittsburgh School of Pharmacy, Pittsburgh, Pennsylvania.

structured, and unsafe. As a result, they require that their paid health care organizations implement technology to improve patient safety. The Center for Medicare and Medicaid Services (CMS) will require e-prescribing as a condition of participation at some point in 2009. Furthermore, in community pharmacies, using e-prescribing systems for handling CMS prescription claims has significantly benefited pharmacy benefits managers and retailers.[5]

Pharmacy directors must think strategically about the role of technology in their medication safety plans. Specifically, the pharmacy's involvement in e-prescribing is vital to its success. A practical guide to e-prescribing, as well as a helpful resource for pharmacy directors with regard to implementation of this technology, is a handbook by Jack E. Fincham, *e-Prescribing: The Electronic Transformation of Medicine.*[6] The aims of this article are to define e-prescribing and describe its components, to illustrate how e-prescribing improves patient safety, and to outline the steps in implementing an e-prescribing system. This article presents pharmacy directors with a frame work for developing and implementing an e-prescribing system to promote a patient-centered pharmacy service.

E-PRESCRIBING DEFINED

As stated earlier, e-prescribing involves using a computer device for ordering, modifying, reviewing, and transmitting prescription orders. The processing of prescriptions using the traditional method (eg, written orders) differs from e-prescribing in both the community and hospital settings. The computer setup for e-prescribing can involve a laptop, a desktop PC, a handheld device with prescribing software, or another device such as customized ordering and bar-code scanning hardware. The required computer equipment for implementing hospital-based e-prescribing is listed in **Table 1**.

E-prescribing in Hospitals

In the hospital setting, traditional methods of order processing involve a physician or another caregiver handwriting an order, after which the order is placed in a "pickup" bin for the pharmacy or placed in a pneumatic tube system for delivery to a pharmacy area. Once the order has reached the pharmacy area, a technician or pharmacist enters the order into a pharmacy computer system. The medication order is entered in a way that requires that the pharmacist use

Table 1. Computer Equipment Needed for E-Prescribing

Windows-compatible PC
64 to 128 MB of RAM (computer memory); hard disk space of at least 20 MB
Internet connection or connection to the institution's network
Computer processing speed of at least 200 mHz
Wireless network or Internet connection
Printer and computer monitor
E-prescribing software (eg, Cerner, TDS Eclipsys)
Capability of downloading software to a personal digital assistant (eg, *Blackberry*, *Palm Pilot*)
Palm OS or *Windows Pocket PC 2003* operating systems for handheld computers
USB ports for downloading information to the handheld computer

Adapted from Fincham JE, *e-Prescribing: The Electronic Transformation of Medicine*. Boston, MA: Jones and Bartlett Publishers; 2009.

pull-down menus for patient location, drug, dose, frequency, time scheduling, and label generation. Entering the medication order into the pharmacy computer system triggers various alerts, such as dose limits, drug allergy warnings, drug interactions, and drug preparation considerations. The pharmacy computer system can then populate other hospital systems to share medication data. Examples of other systems that might share this data include nursing medication administration records, physician task lists, physician-specific e-mail accounts, and financial billing software. This sharing of data often requires employing software that interfaces 2 computer systems; this interface must be routinely monitored and maintained for information security and integrity.

E-prescribing in hospitals involves physicians using hospital software (vendor or "homegrown" applications) to enter medications, which differs from the pharmacy order-entry process. Physician order entry entails selecting a patient name and accessing a pull-down menu of appropriate medication order sentences. An *order sentence* is a prebuilt medication order that includes the drug name, dose, and frequency. Following are examples of order sentences:

- Furosemide 80 mg PO daily
- Metoprolol XL 100 mg PO twice daily
- Cefazolin 1 g in 50 mL of dextrose 5% and water 1 hour preoperatively and 48 hours after surgery
- Phenytoin extended-release capsules 300 mg PO at bedtime

As physicians enter medications into the computer software, various alerts, or "decision-support" informa-tion, appear to guide safe prescribing. Examples of decision support include drug availability with formulary alternatives, dose checking, dose adjustments for renal and hepatic disease, allergy warnings, drug interactions, and significant safety warnings (eg, black box warnings).

E-prescribing in Community Practice

With the traditional method of prescribing in community pharmacies, prescriptions are delivered by a patient and a pharmacist enters the prescription order into a system containing software that checks for all of the appropriate prescribing warnings and that also submits the prescription for authorized payment to a prescription insurance provider. Certain agencies, referred to as *pharmacy benefits managers*, are hired by insurance companies to monitor compliance to formularies, prescribing limits, payments to pharmacies, and co-payments by patients. The pharmacist receives verification or denial of payment, and on verification, a prescription label prints or selected pharmacy automation is signaled to fill the prescription.

E-prescribing in the community setting involves physicians using computer software to electronically transmit, through an interface, prescriptions to a pharmacy for filling and delivery to patients. Prescriptions are checked by the software for medication safety and formulary compliance and are then received by the pharmacy's computer for filling. This process eliminates direct handling of the prescription by the patient, and in a mail-order pharmacy environment, this process removes the patient from the pick-up process as well. Pharmacies receiving e-prescriptions from physicians must undergo certification of their computer software for compliance with privacy and data integrity standards. In addition, outpatient prescription data can be housed in data warehouses that allow access by physicians. SureScripts-RxHub, which provides access of prescription data between pharmacies and physicians, is an example of a data warehouse.[7] An application of Surescripts-RxHub, called RxHub *MEDS*, allows viewing of outpatient prescriptions by physicians while patients are admitted to a hospital setting.[8]

E-prescribing systems in hospitals may be separate, stand-alone products or part of an electronic medical record. In addition, other applications of information technology (IT) may be in separate systems, such as radiology, laboratory, or pathology software. Regardless of the configuration of e-prescribing systems, interoperability is required, which ensures that information from differing systems can be incorporated into the prescribing process. To make interoperability successful, standardization of terminology and information is necessary so that disparate systems can effectively "talk" with one another.

BENEFITS OF E-PRESCRIBING

Since IT became a mainstay of the medication-use process, it has been demonstrated that e-prescribing systems are beneficial to patient safety. Understanding the traditional risk points in the medication-use process illuminates the ways in which e-prescribing can improve safety. These risk points include hand writing legibility, drug name confusion, dosing errors, and physician lack of knowledge on current prescribing guidelines.

Handwriting Legibility

Mistakes and mishaps related to handwriting have resulted in serious medication errors. Several case examples illustrate these types of errors, as in the following:

- An issue with physician handwriting resulted in the interpretation of a *Reminyl* order as *Amaryl*.
- Unclear writing of "QD" sometimes results in QID drug administration.
- Unclear writing of directions causes administration of prophylactic antibiotics without a stop date.
- Multiple abbreviations may represent the same concept, which leads to confusion of meaning.
- Dose concentration and strength prescribing are, at times, unclear.

E-prescribing eliminates handwriting errors by providing clear directions for prescription orders. In addition, properly constructed medication order sentences can prevent confusion on duration of therapy or other criteria for administering medications (eg, "Hold metoprolol if BP < 100 systolic").

Drug Name Confusion

Errors related to drug name confusion involve brand and generic names that look or sound alike, as well as confusing word derivatives and symbols. As with handwriting errors, e-prescribing prevents these errors by providing a clear, computer-generated order that can be easily interpreted by staff.

Dosing Errors

Critical errors that lead to serious adverse events are related to overdosing and underdosing of medications. Examples of this include failing to reduce doses for patients with renal dysfunction and failing to indicate appropriate stop dates for medications. Two case examples are intravenous colchicine prescribed indefinitely, resulting in refractory neutropenia, and dosing of gentamicin at 80 mg every 8 hours in a 93-year-old patient, resulting in acute tubular necrosis. The patient safety movement in US health care was instigated by a series of serious dosing errors with chemotherapy. E-prescribing prevents dosing errors by using interoperability of systems to link clinical information (eg, serum creatinine, age, body surface area) to the medication order and to alert the prescriber of the potential for error.

Physician Lack of Knowledge on Current Prescribing Guidelines

The practice of medicine is constantly changing, with new drugs and new uses of current drugs affecting the way disease is treated. Examples of changing guidelines include the treatment of hypertension (The Seventh Report of the Joint National Committee on Prevention, Detection, Evaluation, and Treatment of High Blood Pressure guidelines), anticoagulation (American College of Chest Physicians guidelines), and antiinfectives (Infectious Disease Society of America [IDSA] guidelines). Prescribing errors of this nature are prevented with e-prescribing by physicians having access to the most current practices for specific, often costly, and adverse reaction–prone medications.

IMPLEMENTATION STEPS
E-prescribing System Selection

Selecting an e-prescribing system requires a multidisciplinary approach that includes hospital leadership, physicians, nurses, pharmacists, and information system specialists. Developing a planning committee, which includes representatives from each of these areas, that conducts site visits, reviews system demonstrations from vendors, and develops specific criteria for selection is important. The pharmacy director should take an active role in this committee to ensure that safe medication practices are integrated into the e-prescribing system. Table 2 describes some of the criteria for selection of an e-prescribing system.

Establishing a position in the pharmacy department that specializes in IT may be beneficial for successful implementation and maintenance of an e-prescribing system. There are a growing number of postgraduate didactic and residency training programs in

Table 2. Criteria for Selecting an E-prescribing System in a Hospital

Nursing satisfaction with usability
Pharmacy satisfaction with usability
Physician satisfaction with usability (eg, medication selection menus)
Availability and usability of portable, wireless handheld devices
Ability to integrate with the existing hospital computing infrastructure
Usefulness of the alert system within the e-prescribing system (eg, reduced "nuisance alerts," ability of physician to deal easily with alerts)
Amount of implementation support (in hours, days, or weeks) by the vendor
Degree of interoperability with existing hospital information systems
Types and accessibility to system reports (eg, e-prescribing compliance)
Ability to extract data for reviewing quality indicators for the e-prescribing system
Ongoing support of the system (eg, routine maintenance, emergency calls)
Amount of process redesign necessary to implement e-prescribing
Integration with outpatient prescribing systems

pharmacy IT that can be contacted to recruit qualified pharmacists.

Establishing Computing Infrastructure

An institution's current information system infrastructure must promote portability as much as possible when purchasing equipment for e-prescribing (eg, wireless connections, handheld devices, computer carts). This may require a systematic "swap out" of computer devices, as well as facility upgrades to accommodate wireless connections, and so on. These processes take time and must be included in the work plan for implementing e-prescribing. One particular consideration for use of wireless devices is the security of the e-prescribing data. The organization must have a security plan that protects patient health information and facilitates an efficient prescribing process for physicians.

Medication Processes Redesign

Implementing an e-prescribing system requires evaluation and revision of the current medication process workflow because order entry will no longer be conducted by the pharmacy. The medical staff must have adequate input and authority in developing the processes for order entry. Specific procedures should be developed for the following medication processes: medication order sentences and e-prescribing order sets, graphic user interface for physicians, e-prescribing alert system, and pharmacy order verification and review procedures.

Medication order sentences and order sets direct the appropriate prescribing of medications in the e-prescribing system. Examples of this include duration of therapy for antibiotic drugs; guidelines for anticoagulation; guidelines proposed by the IDSA; use of aspirin, beta-blockers, and angiotensin-converting enzyme inhibitors in heart disease; and sedation practices in the intensive care unit. The pharmacy director can solicit the department's clinical pharmacists and drug information specialists to work closely with the Pharmacy and Therapeutics Committee to gain appropriate approval for prescribing guidelines that serve as the basis for medication order sentences.

The screen displays and the number of "mouse clicks" necessary for entering an order are important considerations. Developing complex screens and cumbersome order methods will frustrate physicians and potentially slow adoption of e-prescribing.

If not properly designed, the alert system for e-prescribing can lead to physician dissatisfaction. The most common alerts involve allergies, therapeutic duplication, and drug interactions, all of which may involve distracting alerts (eg, aspirin and warfarin drug interaction in a patient with a normal international normalized ratio who takes aspirin on a regular basis). As a patient is discharged, ordering medications for fulfillment in an outpatient pharmacy promotes proper medication reconciliation. The alerts for this practice should focus on health plan formulary adherence. The physician approval required for nonformulary medications may unnecessarily delay delivery of important medication to patients.

A frequent and important question regarding implementation of this technology concerns the change in the role of the pharmacist as a result of e-prescribing. Many organizations see e-prescribing as a method for reduction of pharmacy full-time staff; the pharmacy director must be proactive in developing a practice model that fully engages the pharmacist in patient-centered care.

The pharmacists' role in computerized prescriber order entry is verification of the physician-entered medication according to institution standards. E-prescribing is different from pharmacy dispensing in that it does not activate the pharmacy dispensing process (eg, generate a label for preparation, bill for the medication). As a result, the pharmacist must review the entered order for appropriateness and assign a drug product to the order. For instance, after receiving a prescription with an order sentence that states "furosemide 80 mg PO daily," the pharmacist verifies the order based on review of the patient's medical record, chooses "furosemide 80 mg tablet" from a drop-down formulary menu, and prints a label to dispense the medication or sends a message that initiates dispensing of the medication from robotics or a unit-based automated medication station. From a productivity standpoint, verification and dispensing in an e-prescribing system does require pharmacist time, and this should be considered when revising pharmacy workflow after implementing e-prescribing.

Enhancing the patient-centered aspect of pharmacy service is an important opportunity that is presented to pharmacy directors with the implementation of e-prescribing. For example, physicians most likely will rely on the pharmacy for help in answering questions related to e-prescribing; this provides an opportunity for discussion of patients' drug-related problems with physicians. Furthermore, the pharmacist time saved during the e-prescribing process can be used to pro vide other patient-centered phar-macy services, such as patient medication education, pharmacokinetic dosing services, medication reconciliation, immunizations, and anticoagulation management.

Developing Quality Indicators for E-prescribing

E-prescribing systems are designed to prevent medication errors by alerting the physician of the potential for a prescribing error. As hospitals implement e-prescribing systems, administrators and others will want to know the return on their sizable investment. Quality indicators should be focused on physician compliance in using the e-prescribing system, medication errors associated with e-prescribing, and physician and staff satisfaction with the e-prescribing system.

LIMITATIONS OF E-PRESCRIBING SYSTEMS

E-prescribing systems have limitations, and they allow for differing types and severities of medication errors and adverse events. A fundamental example is that of a physician entering medications for the wrong patient. Preventing this type of error requires system alerts (eg, age, dosing considerations, drug duplication) that are not directly related to patient identification and that require an intuitive review and analysis by the ordering physician. Physicians must be diligent in using the e-prescribing system in a safe and systematic fashion to prevent serious errors.

With respect to planning for and implementing e-prescribing technology, significant variations in the medication ordering and administration process may exist in the hospital, especially with regard to the methods used for ordering medications. For instance, a nursing unit or a certain procedure may rely on verbal orders from physicians. Although discouraged in hospitals, development of a process for handling verbal orders may be necessary. Ultimately, medication order-entry practices must change to promote e-prescribing by physicians. A physician champion in this effort is vital to physician buy-in for the system. As a result, a key lesson for implementation is establishment of a focus group of physicians, pharmacists, and nurses who can review the current medication ordering and administration process and amass the required information for safe medication order entry.

Another example of a medication order discrepancy is associated with assigning medication administration times. Because pharmacists are verifying medication orders outside of a given nursing unit, they are often unaware of the most appropriate medication schedule for a patient and, therefore, use a standard medication administration time. This practice causes errors in medication administration times and may delay therapy where clinically warranted. Again, a focus group of physician, pharmacy, and nursing personnel is beneficial to reach a consensus on the use and implementation of standard medication administration times.

Developing a steering committee that addresses these planning, implementation, and operational issues for e-prescribing is essential for success. In terms of information sharing, the steering committee employed in e-prescribing implementation can foster support of e-prescribing as a part of the safety culture of an institution and can increase general awareness of errors as systems problems versus individual fault. The steering committee can charge an implementation plan that consists of pharmacy, nursing, and information system personnel who provide direct support to users during the first 10 to 14 days of each unit's e-prescribing implementation. Building the confidence of the physician, nursing, and pharmacy staff in using the e-prescribing system is vital.

E-prescribing serves as an important catalyst for preventing medication prescribing errors; the degree to which individual clinicians adopt and implement the e-prescribing system depends on their view of the system in promoting safe medication use and increasing the efficiency of their work. Organizations should survey physicians about the utility of the e-prescribing system in the care of their patients to gauge organizational acceptance of the program. Clearly, the e-prescribing system functions in as close to real time as possible because errors are prevented before they reach the patient. To promote acceptance and understanding of use of the e-prescribing system in a more effective way, organizations must develop methods for sharing information about errors prevented and for further analyzing the system causes of these errors.

CONCLUSION

The success of e-prescribing systems depends on organizational commitment of resources and an organized plan for reducing barriers to unsafe practices. E-prescribing systems underscore the need for a continued emphasis on developing the functionality of and enhancing practitioners' use of new technology. This can be accomplished by focusing on the addition of system functionality to effectively screen for prescribing errors, continuation of eliminating of "nuisance" alerts, revision of order-entry practices for consistency with the approved standard administration times and methods of nurse medication administration, and re vision of order-writing practices to improve the safety and efficiency of e-prescribing. The pharmacy director has an important role in adopting e-prescribing by emphasizing the part this technology plays in patient safety, providing expertise to help develop and implement e-prescribing, and assisting in evaluating its effectiveness.

REFERENCES

1. Kelly WN, Rucker TD. Compelling features of a safe medication-use system. *Am J Health Syst Pharm*. 2006;63(15): 1461-1468.

2. Eslami S, de Keizer NF, Abu-Hanna A. The impact of computerized physician medication order entry in hospitalized patients—a systematic review. *Int J Med Inform*. 2008;77(6):365-376.

3. Pugh MJ, Fincke BG, Bierman A, et al. Potentially inappropriate prescribing in elderly veterans: are we using the wrong drug, wrong dosage, wrong duration? *J Am Geriatr Soc*. 2005;53(8): 1282-1289.

4. Computerized physician order entry. The Leapfrog Group Web site. www.leapfroggroup. org/for_hospitals/leapfrog_hospital_survey_ copy/leapfrog_safety_practices/cpoe. Accessed January 11, 2009.

5. E-prescribing. Centers for Medicare and Medicaid Services Web site. http://www.cms. hhs.gov/EPrescribing/. Accessed January 11, 2009.

6. Fincham JE. *e-Prescribing: The Electronic Transformation of Medicine*. Boston, MA: Jones and Bartlett Publishers; 2009.

7. SureScripts-RxHub: National Patient Health Information Network. http://www.rxhub.net/. Accessed January 11, 2009.

8. RxHub *MEDS*. SureScripts-RxHub Web site. http://www.rxhub.net/index. php?option=com_content&task=view&id=33 &Itemid=44. Accessed January 13, 2009. ∎

Developing a Pharmacy Information System Infrastructure

Michael Sanborn, MS, FASHP*

This *Director' Forum* article will focus on the development of a pharmacy information system infrastructure, including the importance of system design and operation, strategic planning for technology improvement, and the emerging role of the pharmacy informaticist. Today these systems are an integral part of virtually every pharmacy operation and essential to effective patient care.

The pharmacy information system (IS) as we know it was first described in the literature in the 1970s and has evolved dramatically since that time from simple patient profile systems to advanced, integrated medication and patient information databases. Most pharmacists cannot imagine practicing in an environment without a pharmacy IS, yet some hospital pharmacies still lack basic pharmacy IS. In a 2003 survey of Florida acute care hospitals, Warner et al. (2005) found that 14.7% of responding facilities did not have a pharmacy IS and approximately half of these facilities were planning to implement a system within 2 years.[1] The survey also found varying availability of other health technologies such as computerized patient records, medical information retrieval systems, and automated pharmacy dispensing systems.

Historically, investment and innovation in health care information systems has lagged behind technology advancements in other industries. Fortunately, this gap is narrowing. The increased prominence of patient safety has propelled newer health care technology applications, such as computerized provider order entry (CPOE) and bedside bar-code medication administration (BBMA) scanning, to the forefront, and hospitals across the United States are investing millions of dollars into these areas. For example, in 1999 approximately 46% of hospitals still utilized handwritten medication administration records (MAR), but their use has steadily decreased to only 24% in 2005.[2] The implementation of fully-electronic MARs has replaced both handwritten and printed MARs in more than 20% of hospitals. These numbers demonstrate, however, that there is still much to accomplish.

Pharmacy directors must have a proficient knowledge of health care technology and IS. This starts with an understanding of the hospital's IS in general, followed by an understanding of medication-use information interrelates with the hospital system. Felkey (1997) described a four-layer IS hierarchy within a health system that included a foundation layer of transaction processing, information management, decision support, and advanced applications.[3] This hierarchy is applicable to both the hospital IS and to the department of pharmacy IS. In many hospitals, the pharmacy IS operates as a "stand-alone" application that is interfaced to other hospital systems to share patient data and transaction information. Some health care systems have employed

*Health System Pharmacy Director, Baylor Health Care System, Dallas, Texas

software solutions in which clinical applications (eg, laboratory, pharmacy, radiology) are fully integrated into a single product and traditional interfaces are not necessary for these systems to communicate. A common clinical data repository provides the necessary patient information to each of the clinical applications.

Whether stand-alone or integrated, either of these pharmacy IS scenarios must be continually optimized to provide improved patient care. Of equal importance is that as technology continues to advance, so does its complexity. Pharmacists today are faced with an increasing number of technology options, including a range of automated dispensing systems, compounding devices, order-scanning software, "smart" infusion pumps, intervention-documentation programs, CPOE, BBMA, and advanced clinical decision support tools. Effectively leveraging these technologies can result in a host of essential data elements, trending capabilities, and research, all of which have been described in a previous *Director's Forum* article.[4]

Successful pharmacy leadership requires an active knowledge of each of these advancing health care technologies, as well as an evolving plan to integrate these systems into daily practice with a focus on continuously improving the medication-use process and patient care. The first step in this process is developing a strategic pharmacy IS plan.

DEVELOPING AN IS STRATEGIC PLAN

The most critical step in creating a pharmacy IS infrastructure is developing and maintaining a strategic plan. It is often said that if you do not know where you are going, you are never going to get there, and this ax-iom is absolutely true for IS progress around medication use. An important precursor to generating the pharmacy plan is to better understand the health system's plans related to information technology. Hospital IS departments often have detailed strategic plans with short- and long-term goals, and the pharmacy director must be familiar with these plans as well as be able to tactically align and integrate pharmacy's plans with those of the health system. Additionally, the plan should be clearly aligned with the overall mission and initiatives of the hospital and account for the availability of resources, such as operational and capital funding and the personnel necessary to execute the initiatives. The hospital's IS support structure and its effectiveness surrounding pharmacy applications is another important consideration.

In many instances, the important elements of a strategic plan are already known prior to the former planning process, but formal planning helps to clarify and prioritize pharmacy technology initiatives and allows for effective dissemination of departmental IS goals. Such operational strategic plans often start with an analysis of the strengths, weaknesses, opportunities, and threats (SWOT). A candid evaluation of these areas serves as a useful framework for reviewing strategy, position, and direction for the department. The planning process forces department leadership to look beyond day-to-day activities and assess what needs to be accomplished over the course of the next 3 to 5 years.

As an example, in 2003, Bay-lor University Medical Center and its three sister hospitals on the same campus embarked upon a SWOT analysis and strategic planning process surrounding the pharmacy IS infrastructure. At that time, key strengths included a diverse and accomplished clinical pharmacy staff, several internal department IS resources, and a desire by hospital and new pharmacy leadership to improve systems and patient safety; weaknesses included a core IS system that had been implemented suboptimally (one of the four hospitals was functioning without a pharmacy IS, the stand-alone system did not have a lab interface, and several purchased enhancements had not been installed), a labor-intensive dispensing technology platform, poor physician-order communication to the pharmacy via thousands of paper faxes daily, a cumbersome intervention documentation system, and limited capital planning associated with the pharmacy enterprise. Opportunities existed to leverage strong physician support and newly available and emerging technologies to improve the medication-use process. There were also several pharmacy IS components that had already been purchased but not implemented. The threats identified were minimal and mostly internal to the department, but also included the threat of doing nothing.

The resulting Baylor strategic plan prioritized the need to optimize the existing pharmacy IS by fully implementing core technologies and expanding the IS to include all of the Baylor hospitals on campus. A laboratory interface was also prioritized and financially justified. After this was accomplished, a goal was set to implement advanced decision support tools utilizing the new lab interface within the pharmacy IS to alert pharmacists to potential patient problems through electronic patient screening. A digital order-scanning system and a complete overhaul of the dispensing systems were also identified, justified, and scheduled for implementation. The initial timeline for execution of the full plan was estimated at 24 months, but was completed approximately 6 months ahead of schedule. Positive outcomes associated with plan completion included: improved patient monitoring and screening,[5] significant labor reduction, user satisfaction, patient safety benefits associated with automated dispensing equipment, and dramatically improved order processing and pharmacy workflow.[6] Enhancements to the pharmacy IS infrastructure also allowed for several important operational improvements, including decentralized pharmacist services.

The strategic plan should be a "living" document that is continually updated and modified based on progress. This ongoing evaluation and planning is just as important as the development of the initial plan. This will ensure the department is moving in the desired direction and will also reinforce the importance of careful planning and execution of goals and objectives. It also serves as an opportunity to continually look for ways of strengthening the pharmacy technology infrastructure.

SYSTEM SELECTION, DESIGN, AND OPERATION

Oftentimes, pharmacy leadership is able to evaluate, select, and design certain pharmacy technologies, although in some instances IS decisions are driven on behalf of the health system. In either case, it is important for pharmacy to be an integral part of the selection process and then to embrace the decision and move forward. Clark et al. (1999) discussed the importance of not only selecting the appropriate system features and functions, but then taking responsibility for achieving the full benefit of the system.[7] This is an important distinction and often serves as a common failure point for many IS projects. It is rare for any piece of health care technology to work at its optimum level on the first day of implementation. In most cases, as long as hardware and software are validated and purchased from a reputable vendor, it is not the technology that fails but rather the leadership surrounding its implementation.

Selection of a particular piece of technology should always involve a thorough, objective evaluation and comparison of available solutions as they relate to the needs of the department. This process is often formalized through an RFP (Request for Proposal) process, whereby specific hospital requirements are developed in advance and then forwarded to the potential vendors. Site visits by key personnel and other on-site demonstrations are extremely valuable in determining whether a particular piece of technology is a good fit for the organization. Once responses to the RFP are analyzed and the selection is made, the contracting process is another critical step towards project success. There should be clear delineation of the deliverables, expected timelines, vendor expectations, and service/support requirements.

Prior to implementation, careful planning and system design work must take place, and effective project management is vital to success. This planning must take into account the needs of clinicians, staff members, patients, and others that may be affected by the project. An analysis of current and future state is important, and performance benchmarks should be set in advance to measure the overall success of the implementation. Necessary implementation resources should be determined, and realistic but aggressive time-lines should be finalized. An educational plan and revised policies and procedures must also be developed and implemented.

Once the system has been implemented, ongoing maintenance and support can often be relinquished to the hospital's IS department and/or the vendor. System optimization, however, is one of the most critical, yet commonly overlooked areas of system operation and it must occur throughout the life cycle of the product. For example, pharmacist alerts decision support algorithms within an IS system can be extremely useful in preventing adverse drug events. However, in many instances, the total quantity of alerts generated during a given time period can cause a pharmacist (or physicians, in the case of CPOE) to bypass alerts that could indicate a significant potential for patient harm. Working with the IS vendor to reduce the number of nuisance alerts and providing unique identifiers for the most significant alerts are potential optimization steps that are critical to reducing the likelihood of this problem.

Other examples of optimization opportunities include stock-outs associated with automated dispensing cabinets, bar-code read failures with handheld medication scanners, and dose range adjustments within smart infusion-pump drug libraries. In each of these instances, careful study of the problem or opportunity followed by system changes and enhancements can greatly improve functionality and user satisfaction.

THE ROLE OF THE PHARMACY INFORMATICIST

As the technology surrounding computerized medical information has evolved, so has the role of the pharmacist in this area. Recently, the American Society of Health-System Pharmacists (ASHP) published a formal statement summarizing the role of the pharmacist in medical informatics.[8] This document provides a useful summary of important IS applications and initiatives, and then details the pharmacist's responsibility with respect to these technologies. To a great extent, hospital pharmacists have been actively using computerized health information longer than any other medical profession (initially as a means to provide detailed patient medication lists), and this level of familiarity and expertise creates a unique opportunity for the pharmacist as an informaticist.

Informatics has been defined as "the study, invention, and implementation of hardware, software, and algorithms used to improve communication, understanding, and management of information."[9] A pharmacist informaticist applies this definition to the practice of pharmacy and patient care. By definition then, this role goes beyond that of a system administrator or "super user" and involves the development, integration, and optimization of systems that utilize drug information, patient data, and information technology to enhance patient care and medication use.

Many facilities do not have the resources available to employ a full-time pharmacy informaticist. In this instance, it is critical to identify an individual within the department that can serve as the IS expert with the key responsibility of optimizing pharmacy systems. Oftentimes this responsibility falls to the pharmacy director or a supervisor, but just as frequently it can be a staff pharmacist with an aptitude for technology.

An important question surrounding the function of the informatics pharmacist is where to obtain necessary education to develop an expertise in pharmacy IS applications and technology. Unfortunately, very few pharmacy schools offer such advanced training, and most informaticists are "home grown." They have developed their expertise out of sheer necessity and a desire to influence information use, pharmacy practice, and patient care. As the health care community continues to elevate the role of these individuals, new opportunities for informatics education and training are evolving, including ASHP-accredited informatics residencies.

SUMMARY

Technology applications in health care continue to advance at a rapid pace. Pharmacist involvement in medical informatics and technology development, implementation, and optimization are essential to the ongoing improvement of medication-use systems and patient care. Strengthening the pharmacy IS infrastructure is a critical aspect of such improvements. The pharmacy director must take a leadership role within the organization to ensure effective and safe utilization of health information.

REFERENCES

1. Warner A, Menachemi N, Brooks RG. Information technologies relevant to pharmacy practice in hospitals: results of a statewide survey. *Hosp Pharm.* 2005;40:233-239.

2. Pedersen CA, Schneider PJ, Scheckelhoff DJ. ASHP national survey of pharmacy practice in hospital settings: dispensing and ad-

ministration—2005. *Am J Health Syst Pharm.* 2006;63:327-345.

3. Felkey BG. Health system informatics. *Am J Health Syst Pharm.* 1997;54:274-280.

4. Weber RJ. Core competencies in hospital pharmacy: essential department data. *Hosp Pharm.* 2006;41:582-587.

5. Sanborn MD, Sheehan V, Dillon T. Pharmacist Response to Advanced Decision Support Medication Alerts [abstract]. ASHP Midyear Clinical Meeting. Orlando, FL. December 7, 2004.

6. Sikri S, Sansgiry SS, Sanborn MD, Flinn M. Effect of a remote order scanning system on processing of medication orders. *Am J Health Syst Pharm.* 2006;63:1438-1441.

7. Clark T, McBride J, Zinn T. Achieving a computer system's benefits. *Hosp Pharm.* 1999;34:534-535.

8. American Society of Health-System Pharmacists. ASHP statement on the pharmacist's role in informatics. *Am J Health Syst Pharm.* 2007;64:200-203.

9. Pharmacy Informatics Group. Informatics. Available at: http://www.pharmacyinforma ics.com/informatics.html. Accessed March 23, 2007. ■

An Innovative Solution to Pharmacy Department Information Sharing

Matthew W. Eberts, PharmD, MBA*; Scott M. Mark, PharmD, MS, MEd, FASHP FACHE†; and Robert J. Weber, MS, FASHP‡

The *Director's Forum* series is written and edited by Michael Sanborn and Robert Weber and is designed for guiding pharmacy leaders in establishing patient-centered services in hospitals and health systems. Another specific goal of this column is addressing many of the key challenges that pharmacy directors currently face, while also providing information that will foster growth in pharmacy leadership and patient safety. Previous articles in this series have discussed the many different aspects of pharmacy management and leadership challenges. This feature addresses an innovative solution to pharmacy department information sharing.

INTRODUCTION

The physical cause of the February 1, 2003, Space Shuttle Columbia disaster was a breach in the thermal protection system caused by a piece of insulating foam that separated from the external tank seconds after launch.[1] The follow-up investigation revealed that organizational failures, including a poorly designed communication system, contributed to the accident. Several individuals within NASA felt that additional information needed to be gathered following the launch and wanted photos taken of the space shuttle. The message did not make it through the bureaucratic and convoluted NASA structure, and no pictures were taken. Without a "hardwired" system for sharing information, one can see why the system was ineffective.

Communication failures in the pharmacy negatively impact the department's ability to care for patients. Consider the following scenarios as examples. Why was the day staff unaware that a medication had stocked out overnight? Now they have a critical medication infusion running "dry" and no medication to prepare a new infusion bag. Why did the central pharmacist verify an order that the unit-based pharmacist was trying to clarify? Now a medication is verified at a suboptimal dose. Why did the pharmacy use the remainder of a limited supply antibiotic for a patient who didn't meet the criteria? Now a patient who truly needs the medication is unable to receive it. The examples continue, and they demonstrate that a system of communication that ensures information is being communicated in the right fashion and to the right people (eg, it is "hardwired") is fundamental to successful patient-centered pharmacy services.

Even the best designed process or initiative will fail if the message is not heard by the front-line staff. As George Bernard Shaw observed, "The single biggest problem with communication is the illusion that it has taken place."[2] A real-life example of a breakdown in communication occurred in the pharmacy at University of Pittsburgh Medical Center (UPMC)

*Pharmacy Manager, UPMC Presbyterian, University of Pittsburgh Medical Center; †Director of Pharmacy, University of Pittsburgh Medical Center; Assistant Professor and Vice Chair, Department of Pharmacy & Therapeutics, University of Pittsburgh School of Pharmacy; ‡Executive Director of Pharmacy, University of Pittsburgh Medical Center; Associate Professor and Chair, Department of Pharmacy & Therapeutics, University of Pittsburgh School of Pharmacy.

Presbyterian Shadyside, the 1,093-bed flagship hospital of the UPMC. In an effort to increase medication safety, the department streamlined sizes and strengths of various medications. This information was communicated in a variety of ways, including e-mails to the staff, discussions at staff meetings, and postings on 2 department bulletin boards. After the first few days of implementing this new initiative, some of the medication strengths and sizes that were eliminated began appearing back in stock and in the automated dispensing cabinets. During follow-up conversations with the staff determining why the initiative wasn't followed, staff remarked, "Nobody told us!"

The goal of this article is to provide the pharmacy director with strategies for using technology to improve communication in their departments. The aims of this article are to review the key elements of good communication system, to describe the experience at the UPMC in determining the best ways to communicate in the department, and to suggest strategies and identify challenges in implementing UPMC's communication solution. Effectively communicating departmental information will keep all members focused on the common goal of providing patient-centered hospital pharmacy services.

ELEMENTS OF A GOOD COMMUNICATION SYSTEM

Conventional communication systems in pharmacy departments range from simple meetings to Web sites. The most commonly used methods are listed in **Table 1**, along with the disadvantages or barriers they create. Though each method is important, each has limitations that prevent it from meeting all the department's

Table 1. Common Methods of Departmental Communication

Method	Barriers
E-mail	Not all staff actively read e-mail No central storage of information
Web site	Requires IT support to start and maintain "Pull" system vs "push" system
Shared drive	Unable to "push out" information Information can be difficult to find
Meetings	Not all staff can attend Scheduled vs just-in-time

information-sharing needs. Each of these methods should be used synergistically; the method of communication that dominates depends on the communication needs of a given situation.

Elements of a good communication system include the following: communicates messages directly to staff and archives messages in a searchable format; stores informational documents (ie, meeting minutes, educational program handouts, schedules); directly links to essential information (ie, drug information, formulary, intravenous [IV] guidelines, department Web site); hosts projects by allowing team members to share files, assign tasks, centralize feedback, and track progress; connects department members by hosting message boards and blogs; and houses historical information in retrievable format.

One of the strongest correlations to employee burnout is not having the resources necessary to perform an assigned task.[3] Often in hospital pharmacy the resources exist but the system breaks down when the employee is not able to locate the information in a timely manner. Successful information sharing requires that information be available to staff "just in time," regardless of job function or physical location.

CASE STUDY IN DEVELOPING EFFECTIVE DEPARTMENTAL COMMUNICATION
Background
UPMC Presbyterian is a tertiary-care, 801-bed academic medical center spread across 2 buildings. The pharmacy department employs a decentralized unit-based pharmacist model and dispenses medications from 2 centralized pharmacy facilities. The department consists of 155 full-time equivalents (FTEs) that cover a variety of shifts. The department is closely affiliated with the University of Pittsburgh School of Pharmacy, and faculty members from the school work in consort with pharmacists at the hospitals. Importantly, some of the department's management is located several floors away from the central pharmacy operations, making communication difficult at times. In addition, the operational programs, particularly those of the Pharmacy and Therapeutics Committee, create new practices and guidelines for the safe monitoring and dispensing of medication.

Description of the Problem
Because of the complex nature of the pharmacy department, there was a chasm at times in communication. The department needed to effectively facilitate information sharing throughout the department. Barriers to sharing information included 24/7 operation, decentralized staff, the high volume of information to share, and the number of different places information was stored. The department needed a communication and information-sharing tool that could ensure that important information was communicated to appropriate staff members, store information in a single searchable location, facilitate hands-off communication between front-line staff, and support department projects by allowing department members to contribute and review the information at times that worked for them.

Understanding Variation in Department Communication
The pharmacy department used different communication tools, including meetings, e-mails, a department Web site, and a shared data drive. Despite these tools, communication was often scattered and inconsistent. None of these options provided an optimal "hardwired" solution.

Focus Areas to Improve Communication
Table 2 lists the highest priority issues that needed improvement, along with the needs of each specific problem.

Solution: Implement Microsoft SharePoint
Microsoft SharePoint is a Web-based application that allows com-

Table 2. Priority Areas to Improve Departmental Communication

Area	Needs
Ancillary department ordering	Create electronic process
	Provide more efficient system for charge backup
	Decrease technician resources required
Charge pharmacist report	Communicate important issues between front-line staff
	Information archived and searchable
	Information pushed out to staff
Document storage	Searchable storage solution
	Archive information
	Keep documents in 1 place

prehensive content management and facilitates information sharing.[4] At UPMC, the *SharePoint* server is managed by the information services division, and they are able to create individual *SharePoint* sites as requested by end users. *SharePoint* sites are controlled at the department level. The department is able to determine the look and feel of the site, as well as the content. Managing a site requires only basic computer skills; it is not necessary to know computer programming or HTML to build and maintain a *SharePoint* site. Each site is customizable in regards to who has access to the site and what level of functionality they have when using the site.

SharePoint functions as a push and/or pull tool relative to information management. The site is able to store documents and links, and is able to host message boards and custom content. In addition to being a storage area to pull information from, *SharePoint* is able to push out information in the form of e-mail. The site can control what information will be e-mailed and to whom the e-mails will be sent. *SharePoint* contains an enterprise search tool that allows users to search the site's content for specific information. The pharmacy's *Share-Point* site provides the following functions.

Announcements

The announcements function is used to distribute information to the staff. The information is added to the department *SharePoint* site, with the option of e-mailing it to the department. The advantage of using *SharePoint* for this function versus sending out a traditional e-mail is that the announcement is stored on the site for future reference and can be searched when

necessary. When patient-controlled analgesia (PCA) barcoding went live, the *SharePoint* site was used to send information to the staff regarding the new process and the schedule for in-service events. In addition to sending that knowledge to the staff's e-mail accounts, it was also housed on the site for easy reference.

Document Storage

The *SharePoint* site serves as a repository for documents and stores them in an organized and searchable format. This function allows users to search the documents by name and/or content. Some of the documents stored on the site include meeting minutes, manager rotations, contact information, slides from educational programs, procedural information, internal references, and staff communications. Regarding the PCA barcode project, the slides used for the in-service events are stored on the site for reference and as a training resource for new staff.

Links to Important Information

Pharmacy staff has access to many different knowledge sources. The challenge staff members face is finding the information they need when they need it. Our *SharePoint* site has direct links that allow for point-and-click access to drug information, policies and procedures, department schedules, formulary information, medication error reporting, IV guidelines, material safety data sheet forms, and anticoagulation guidelines, among others. Because these resources are stored in different areas, they were not always at the fingertips of the staff. Now, from 1 location, the department *SharePoint* site, the staff is

1 click away from these tools. Compared with the department Web site, *SharePoint* is easier to add, update, and delete links.

Charge Pharmacist Report

The pharmacy department assigns a charge pharmacist each shift. This person is a staff pharmacist who, in addition to normal pharmacist functions, is charged with being the first step in the escalation chain for issues such as calloffs, information technology (IT) failures, drug shortages, etc. At the end of their shift, these issues are communicated to the department via the charge pharmacist report. The report is essentially a hand-off communication tool. The report captures specific information, such as computer issues, staffing issues, order issues, and what has been done to resolve the situation. The report is e-mailed to the staff each shift and it is stored on the *Share-Point* site for future reference. **Figure 1** displays an example of the department's online charge pharmacist report.

Host Department Projects

The site has been utilized as a forum for staff-driven pharmacy projects. For example, we have hosted a formulary cleanup project through the site. In an effort to hide from view items that were no longer relevant in the pharmacy information system, a forum was created for staff to enter the specific items they felt should be hidden. A group of staff members reviewed the list and, as appropriate, assigned the task to the IT team for removal from view. The process is completed entirely in *SharePoint*, and the staff can track the progress of each entry. *SharePoint* allows staff mem-

bers to participate despite the shift they work or their ability to attend meetings. In the first week, over 100 items were hidden from view.

Staff Message Boards

The department's *SharePoint* site has the functionality to host message boards. These can be used by the staff for idea sharing or resource gathering. Message boards have served as a forum for interesting clinical discussions, organizing department activities, and discussing UPMC-specific processes. For example, the message boards were utilized to facilitate a discussion on decreasing IV waste. Staff members were able to start discussion threads and provide follow-up ideas, such as reorganizing the storage of returned IVs and processes to get returned medications rotated into the stock more quickly.

Ancillary Department Ordering Site

The *SharePoint* site serves as the ordering system for ancillary departments that order medications from the pharmacy. The pharmacy department provides approximately $300,000/month in medications to ancillary units. Prior to utilization of the *Share-Point* site, we received orders via a system of faxes, e-mails, and phone calls. The paper orders were used to process and bill the accounts, and then served as the backup documentation for disputed charges. Managing the process required 1 FTE of technician time, and the process was plagued with missed collections. Now the departments place and track their orders via the *SharePoint* system. The ancillary sites receive e-mail updates as their orders are processed and are eventually ready for pickup. The site

*Confidential: Patient Informati... has been added

Modify my alert settings | View *Confidential: Patient Informati... | View Charge Pharmacist Report

Report Date/Time::	9/14/2009 7:00 AM
Shift Report for::	Night
::COMPUTER ISSUES:::	No
::INVENTORY ISSUES:::	No
WILL CALL -meds arriving via will-call::	No
::ORDER ENTRY ISSUES:::	No
::ROBOT ISSUE:::	No
::DELIVERY ISSUES:::	No
::STAFFING ISSUES:::	Yes
STAFFING - Issue #1::	On Coming Shift - LATE
STAFFING - Issue #1 Actions::	No adjustments were made - oncoming shift to address
STAFFING - Issue #1 Employee Name::	Joe Smith
STAFFING - Issue #1 Details::	delivery - estimating 7:30AM.
::OTHER ISSUES:::	Yes
OTHER - Issue #1 Description::	Lidocaine nerve block bags will expire tomorrow. Please try to use this supply first.

Figure 1. Example of charge pharmacist report.

provides easy reports for entering the billing into the pharmacy information system and provides a searchable system for backing up our charges as necessary. Since implementation, collections are at 100% and the process is run with 0.5 FTEs. The process for ordering has been simplified, as depicted in **Figure 2**.

Inventory Issues

Keeping up with product shortages, stock outs, and recalls was a source of frustration for the department. The *SharePoint* site is utilized to communicate a variety of inventory issues. For example, if a medication stocks out, a communication is created informing the staff of the stock out, estimated time it will be resolved, details regarding any will-calls, and the plan of action until the stock out is resolved. *SharePoint* is able to push this information to the staff but also store it centrally so if a staff member is curious about the status of a medication, the information can be easily located.

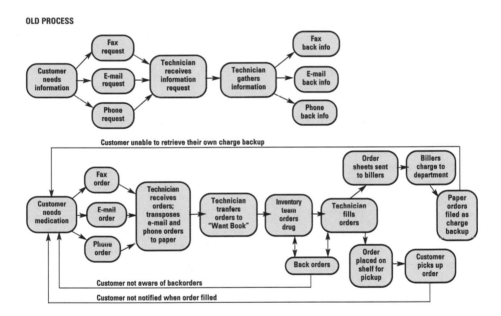

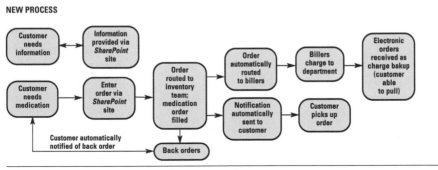

Figure 2. Revised departmental ordering using SharePoint.

Department Calendar

SharePoint is able to host a calendar. This calendar is used to post dates for upcoming pharmacy events such as staff meetings and educational programs.

Staff Feedback

The department's *SharePoint* site has been well received, as evidenced by the nearly 100% completion rate for the charge pharmacist report and the strong response to department projects such as removing items from view.

Lessons Learned

Prior to designing a *SharePoint* site, gain knowledge of the functionality the software. *SharePoint* is a powerful application with a lot of different tools. Unless one knows what all the different tools do, they may not be using the best tool for the job. Importantly, the site should be tested with your staff; during the designing process utilize a selected group of staff members to test the site and make improvement recommendations. Having the site vetted prior to implementation means the site will create a better first impression with the department. It is very important to ensure "buy-in" by the staff early in this process to guarantee success.

Strategies and Challenges in Implementing SharePoint

The first step to implementing a *SharePoint* site is access to the software. *SharePoint* can be purchased at the corporate, hospital or department level. If purchasing the product is not the best option departments can utilize *SharePoint* hosting sites. For a set fee, the host will establish a *SharePoint* site that end users can then customize for their needs. Alternative products to *SharePoint* such as *Basecamp* and *Central Desktop* are available. In order to successfully build a *Share-Point* site, one must identify the department's information-sharing problems. With this knowledge, determine the best *SharePoint* tool to address the issue. Once this outline is complete, the site building can begin.

The site is only useful if the department members incorporate it into their workflow. It is important to invest an adequate amount of time educating and demonstrating the site to the department. Once the staff begins using the site and sees the benefits it provides, they will become the biggest supporters and share the message with others.

CONCLUSION

Experienced leaders have learned that traditional information-sharing tools are not sufficient if the goal is to implement change, provide just-in-time knowledge, foster collaboration, or educate staff. The challenge of providing this information grows as pharmacy departments expand responsibilities and continue to decentralize. Important issues such as these require a more dynamic information-sharing platform for the message to stick. When the Institute of Medicine released *To Err Is Human* in 1999, people were outraged to learn that as many as 98,000 people die in hospitals each year because of medical errors.[5] Many medical errors can be avoided by the implementation of an effective communication tool. The UPMC Presbyterian Shadyside Pharmacy *Share-Point* site has provided a solution to the department's challenge of effectively sharing information between a large, decentralized staff. Keeping all of the staff members on the same page using a communication tool such as *SharePoint* will help to successfully achieve the goals of a patient-centered pharmacy department.

REFERENCES

1. Columbia Accident Investigation Board. *Columbia Accident Investigation Board Report, Volume 1*. Washington, DC: Government Printing Office; 2003.

2. George Bernard Shaw quotes. Thinkexist.com Web site. http://en.thinkexist.com/quotation/the_single_biggest_problem_in_communication_is/155222.html. Accessed September 15, 2009.

3. Demerouti E, Bakker AB, Nachreiner F, Schaufeli WB. The job demands-resources model of burnout. *J Appl Psychol*. 2001;86(3):499-512.

4. *Microsoft Office SharePoint* Server 2007: What is *SharePoint*? Microsoft Web site. http://sharepoint.microsoft.com/Pages/Default.aspx. Accessed September 14, 2009.

5. Kohn LT, Corrigan JM, Donaldson MS, eds. *To Err Is Human: Building a Safer Health System*. Washington, DC: National Academy of Sciences; 2000. ■

Get Smart: Effective Use of Smart Pump Technology

Michael Sanborn, MS, FASHP, * *and Tammy Cohen, BS, PharmD, MS†*

The *Director's Forum* series is written and edited by Michael Sanborn and Robert Weber and is designed for guiding pharmacy leaders in establishing patient-centered services in hospitals and health systems. Another specific goal of this column is addressing many of the key challenges that pharmacy directors currently face, while also providing information that will foster growth in pharmacy leadership and patient safety. Previous *Director's Forum* articles have discussed various aspects of pharmacy technology implementation and utilization. This feature focuses on the effective integration of smart pump technology to maximize patient safety benefits.

Smart or intelligent infusion pumps can integrate traditional infusion pump technology with decision-support functions based on predetermined clinical guidelines for intravenous (IV) drug administration. These clinical guidelines—often referred to as the *drug library*—provide upper-and lower-range limits for individual IV medications. To use the pump, a nurse selects the appropriate drug from the library, enters the infusion rate (and patient weight, if appropriate), and, if the information is within the preapproved limits, starts the infusion. If the data entered are outside of the acceptable range, either a hard-stop or soft-stop warning is generated by the pump. Hard stops require reentry of the dose information that conforms to the preapproved limits before starting the infusion. Soft stops allow the infusion to proceed without reentry after reviewing the alert.

As modifications are needed, the drug libraries can be updated by directly connecting the pump to a computer and downloading the information, or the database can be updated over a wireless network. Newer technology also is being developed that integrates bar-code technology on each IV bag, which will automatically program the pump based on the current physician's order. In most cases, smart infusion pumps also track and record usage data that can be retrieved and analyzed as part of an ongoing medication safety effort.

At a recent conference convened to discuss the prevention of patient harm and death from IV medication errors, striking information was presented on the seriousness of IV errors.[1] For example, according to United States Pharmacopeia *MEDMARX* data, harmful and fatal errors are nearly 3 times more prevalent with parenteral medications than with other routes of administration, and 58% of these errors occur during the process of IV administration. One of 3 high-priority IV medication safety practices recommended at the summit included the use of intelligent infusion devices with the dose-limiting feature enabled.

BACKGROUND

Recent surveys suggest that the purchase and utilization of smart pump technology continues to grow.[2,3] Use of intelligent infusion devices in hospitals rose from 32.2% in 2005 to

---

*Corporate Vice President, Baylor Health Care System; †Director of Clinical Pharmacy, Baylor Health Care System; Director of Pharmacy, Baylor Heart and Vascular Hospital, Dallas, Texas.

44% at the end of 2007. Hospitals reported increases in utilization regardless of size (see **Figure 1**). The most recent data suggest that the pharmacy is responsible for the ongoing maintenance of the drug library in nearly 70% of hospitals.[3]

Interestingly, just under 30% of hospitals with smart pumps use wireless technology to update their drug libraries, and less than half are using infusion pump event logs for quality improvement purposes.[3] It also has been found that nearly half of those facilities not currently using smart infusion pumps have plans to implement them in the future.

There are data suggesting that these facilities should reconsider their willingness to purchase such technology. A growing body of evidence shows that smart infusion pumps actually reduce errors.[4-13] However, as with most technology, there are significant variations in overall effectiveness depending on how the pumps are implemented. For example, Rothschild et al found no measurable improvement with smart pump technology in an intensive care unit (ICU) setting, whereas Larsen et al observed a statistically significant 73% reduction in IV infusion rate errors in a tertiary care pediatric hospital in conjunction with drug-concentration standardization.

The fundamental difference in these studies is the degree in which the user could bypass the drug library or ignore pump alerts and thereby circumvent the intended safety features of the infusion pumps. Poor compliance with the available safety features mitigates the benefits of this technology. Behavioral and technological factors must be addressed for smart pumps to achieve their potential for medication safety improvement.[14]

A retrospective, 16-month review of the impact of smart pumps on anticoagulant infusion errors was recently conducted at Brigham and Women's Hospital.[8] The authors identified significant error reductions using both hard and soft limits (501 and 362

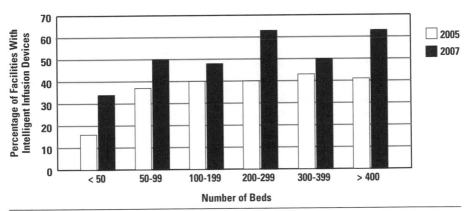

Figure 1. Smart pump adoption by hospital bed size. (Adapted from Pedersen CA, Schneider PJ, Scheckelhoff DJ. ASHP national survey of pharmacy practice in hospital settings: dispensing and administration—2005. *Am J Health Syst Pharm.* 2006;63[4]:327-345 and Pedersen CA, Gumper KF. ASHP national survey on informatics: assessment of the adoption and use of phar-macy informatics in U.S. hospitals—2007. *Am J Health Syst Pharm.* 2008;65[23]:2244-2264.)

alerts, respectively) in the drug library. Under-dose alerts were the most common error identified, followed by overdose alerts, with many 100-fold and greater dosing errors avoided. Duplicate therapy errors were also identified.

There are several key areas of focus that must be considered to maximize the patient benefits of this technology. These areas include vendor selection, technology implementation, and ongoing monitoring and maintenance of the technology. Each of these areas is discussed here, as well as a review of lessons learned during the ongoing use of smart infusion pumps.

VENDOR SELECTION

There are a number of vendors who market smart infusion pumps, and as with most capital purchases, selection is typically dependent on a variety of factors. If an organization is planning for the purchase of these devices, a multidisciplinary team of evaluators should be assembled. Representatives from pharmacy, nursing, the medical staff, biomedical engineering, materials management, anesthesia, and patient safety should be considered for inclusion on the team. Depending on the organization, there may be other groups whose participation should be invited. A financial analyst, for example, might be helpful when reviewing the impact of any bids that are received.

When considering the purchase of smart pumps, site visits and evaluations of other facilities that have already implemented the technology can be quite valuable. Most vendors and group purchasing organizations can provide a list of users for various products. Some important elements that should be considered before and during the site visit include the following:

- Overall functionality and ease of use
- Drug library development requirements
- Maximum and minimum fluid delivery rates
- Hard-and soft-stop functionality
- Alarms and alerts
- Override capabilities and limits
- Wireless versus nonwireless application
- Data capture and reporting capabilities
- Frequency of software and hardware update and enhancement
- Device reliability, service performance, and propensity for recalls
- User acceptance, satisfaction, and utility
- Adaptability to unique environments (eg, neonatal ICU [NICU], procedure areas)
- Integration of large-volume patient-controlled analgesia, and syringe pump systems
- Implementation and training assistance
- Contractual and cost issues

The vendor's plan for ongoing research and development is an other factor that should be considered. If integration with point-of-care barcode scanning is not currently available, understanding the time-line for that technology release is important. Likewise, future integration with the electronic medication administration record also should be investigated.

There are companies that provide detailed product overviews and cost information, such as MD Buyline (www.mdbuyline.com) and KLAS (www.klasresearch.com). These reports are typically fee-based, but most facilities subscribe to 1 or more of these databases and can access this information. Some group purchasing organizations also may provide these types of comparisons.

In late August 2008, KLAS reviewed 5 vendors of smart pump technology, including B. Braun, Baxter, Cardinal Health, Hospira, Sigma, and Smiths.[15] This review provided an update to an analysis that was conducted in 2007. KLAS interviewed over 200 health care professionals regarding their experiences with smart infusion pump vendors across 40 different indicators with a focus on large-volumetric pumps with dose-calculation software. The review found that wireless technology has been the greatest advancement in smart infusion pump technology, but wireless medication orders from the pharmacy to a smart pump are not yet taking place with any commercially available pump (however, some "homegrown" interfaces were identified).[16] Significant differences were found between various vendors.

Due diligence is essential in selecting a satisfactory infusion pump vendor. The pharmacy can often be a key contributor to vendor selection, and because pharmacists are typically responsible for ongoing drug library maintenance, data analysis, and overall monitoring, such input is essential.

IMPLEMENTATION

There are a handful of articles that describe the implementation of smart pump technology in hospitals.[11,17,18] The Baylor Health Care System implemented this technology across 13 hospitals in the Dallas–Fort Worth area starting in early 2005. The sys-tem found that the combined implementation factors described here are important for successful employment of smart pump technology.

Notably, development of the smart pump library and subsequent implementation of smart pump technology is significantly more straightforward if efforts already have been made to standardize drug concentrations across the hospital. With most vendors, there are typically few limitations on the number of drugs and concentrations that can be included in the library; however, failure to streamline the number of allowable concentrations for a particular IV medication in advance may lead to errors associated with improper concentration selection.[19]

A successful smart pump implementation must be a multidisciplinary initiative including, at least, nursing, pharmacy and biomedical engineering. Library development and maintenance typically can be managed by a pharmacist, and routine operations and nursing practice issues can be managed by nursing. Biomedical engineers can assist with the initial upload of the library, as well as participate in the technical aspects of library updates over time. When developing the library there are several factors that should be considered, such as library organization, medication concentrations, and dosing units.

The first concern should be the structure of the library. A library may be divided into several sections that can be thought of as "file folders." The sections can be organized by types of medication (emergent drips, antibiotics, fluids, etc), areas of the hospital (eg, medical-surgical unit, ICU, oncology, NICU, emergency room), or a combination of both location and medication type. At Baylor, a combination of both location and medication type is used. Most sections of the library are based on location (sometimes called clinical care areas [CCAs]); however, there are also sections for antibiotics and standard IV fluids. By creating antibiotic and standard fluid sections, the health system avoided duplication of the vast number of antibiotic IV piggyback (IVPB) drug items and simple fluids for each location. This creates a more manageable list of medications in each section, and it also reduces the amount of scrolling required on the pump display during IV selection by the nurse.

Before medications can be built into the library, there are some key decisions that must be made. One area that should be considered is the expectation for use regarding fluids. There are 2 thought processes regarding IV fluid administration. One idea is that all IVs are equal, so each must be administered via a smart pump using the library. A different perspective is that the library and subsequent pump safeguards typically are not needed for the administration of simple maintenance fluids, so they need not be included in the library.

Another key decision relates to IVPB antibiotics. An institution may require that all antibiotics be administered using the library or that only those that have strict infusion parameters be administered through the library. Considering the impact on compliance reporting is worthwhile when determining which of these methods is most appropriate for the health system. If certain antibiotics or plain IV fluids are administered on the pump without using the library, the data reported may not provide this differentiation. Thus, it may appear that the library is not being used for a large percentage of items, when in fact, it may be used for all other medications that do not fall into these 2 categories.

There are some additional practice area considerations that should be weighed. Dosing units may vary based on practice setting. For example, an ICU may use weight-based dosing and a medical-surgical unit may use volume-based dosing (eg, mL/h) for the same medication. The library entry accommodates all types of dosing parameters, which means that if multiple dosing units are used throughout the facility, then it would be necessary to program a line item for each dosing unit into the pump. Ideally, a library should contain as few line items as possible to facilitate ease of movement through the program and a user-friendly platform.

Another essential implementation requirement is the development of hard and soft limits. In many cases, the manufacturer of the pump will not provide these limits because of the potential liability involved. Some IV medications have specific upper and lower limits described in the package insert. For those medications that do not have this information, other published references or clinician experience must be considered. There also may be unit-specific limitations based on hospital policy that must be incorporated into the CCAs. Nursing and pharmacy consensus on upper and lower limits is recommended.

The rollout plan for smart pump installation must include time for building the library, user training, and any necessary operational changes (eg, implementation of standard concentrations and/or dosing units). Asking that pharmacists and nurses review the final library recommendations before their initial upload into the pump is also helpful. Policies should be developed that address library-use requirements and exceptions, such as medications used in emergent situations or pump utilization for medications that may not be in the library. Leadership commitment to these policies—by both nursing and pharmacy—is essential to ongoing compliance with library use.

Nursing and other user education is another essential piece of a successful implementation, and many vendors will provide significant assistance with this process. Developing a group of "super users" to assist with ongoing training is recommended. It is important that all trainers be aware of the key decisions that are made and that they teach to that accepted practice rather than to standard smart pump capabilities. This will help with policy compliance and will prevent users being overwhelmed. As with any new technology, training end users close to the "go-live" date to make their education more meaningful and keep it fresh in their minds is a prudent step.

On the day of the rollout, anticipation of patient flow and scheduling the rollout accordingly is crucial. For example, the operating room (OR) can start with the pumps on the go-live day, and the first units that convert to smart pumps would be the receiving postoperative units, followed by the remaining units. Furthermore, consideration would be needed for more self-contained units, such as the NICU or an oncology unit. These units may go live independent of the OR, ICU, and medical-surgical floors.

ONGOING MONITORING AND MAINTENANCE

After the smart pumps have been implemented, ongoing monitoring is essential to ensure appropriate polices are followed and to provide opportunities for continued improvement. Like the implementation, monitoring and maintenance also should be a multidisciplinary function. The reporting capabilities available are based on the functionality of the system provided by the vendor. Some vendors now provide Web-based reporting options, which make data-analysis tools readily accessible to nursing, pharmacy, biomedical engineering, and other users that may require access.

Typically, the vendor offers a variety of standard reports, and there are usually methods by which customized reports can be created. Standard reports are generally available for summarizing information on hard stops, soft stops, and overall library compliance. There are reports that can detail drug-specific minimum and maximum infusion rates used. In most cases, reports can be run globally or can be CCA or pump specific. Library utilization summaries are helpful for identifying possible drug concentrations that are minimally used. When suspected errors occur, retrieving a detailed history of pump use, including specific programming completed by the user, is possible.

Many systems also offer an asset-tracking feature. Depending on the structure of the facility's wireless network, location of specific areas where pumps are stored is often possible. Furthermore, this feature is helpful for locating pumps for regular maintenance, library updates, or pump recalls. Finally, reports can be generated that summarize the frequency of pump use to assist with possible changes in pump allocation by unit.

Patient safety is only enhanced if the smart pump library is utilized. At Baylor, ongoing manual audits are conducted to assess user practices after initial implementation. Visual audits can be conducted to review and document medications that are being infused with the pump but bypassing the library function. These types of audits allow identification of medications that are not in the library and whether specific infusions are in the library but are not being selected for use. Follow-up education is provided when instances of the latter occur.

The validity of the utilization reports may depend on how IVPB antibiotics and fluids are used and classified within the system. A second type of assessment focuses on high-risk medications (eg, anticoagulants, insulin, pressors), in which a target list of medications is identified and audited. Results from these studies are reviewed care fully by department leadership because the goal for library compliance with high-risk medications is 100%.

Additional ongoing library maintenance assessments should include monitoring the frequency of hard and soft limits and the use of individual line items. This information can be helpful to further improve library functionality. These types of assessments often can be done on a standardized schedule using the vendor's software. Library changes that result from these findings can be addressed as part of the planned library updates.

Library updates typically take between 10 to 20 minutes when completed over a wireless network. The pump is not functional during this time, so it may be difficult for users to accept the update when the prompt occurs. Monitoring the number and locations of pumps that have not been updated and working with nursing and biomedical engineering to complete the update is vital.

OTHER LESSONS LEARNED

Once the libraries have been developed and are in full use, creation of a small group or committee of pharmacists and nurses who can review acceptance and utilization of the library on an ongoing basis is helpful. Data and anecdotal experiences can be reviewed, and changes and improvements can be made as needed. Conversion of hard limits to soft limits or visa versa may be necessary. Unless specific patient safety issues must be addressed, minimizing the number of library edits that are made is helpful. Quarterly (or less frequent) updates are often all that is required, and using wireless capabilities significantly simplifies library updates.

Editing privileges for the system should be limited to a small group of individuals. These individuals must be trained thoroughly on the software and have a clear understanding of the pumps' capabilities and limitations. At Baylor, this task has been limited to a small group of pharmacists who verify the concentrations and alerts being programmed once the changes have been approved. Because the drug libraries in this health system are standardized across all 13 facilities, library updates must be carefully communicated in advance.

The library can be built in many ways, and another significant decision regarding naming conventions must be determined upfront. Most vendor libraries have a finite number of line item entries per CCA, as well as a limited number of characters that are visible on the pump screen. Therefore, limiting naming conventions to generic name only and not including medication trade names may be necessary. If trade name and generic name are both necessary, then 2 line items would be required in each CCA, which would reduce the CCA capacity by half. This may be feasible in some CCAs that use a limited number of medications; however, this may not be possible in larger CCAs (such as in the ICU setting).

Also of note, many vendor libraries require that the user scroll through the library rather than allowing the user to select a letter to "jump" to a specific item. Therefore, the more medication line items that are available, the more scrolling that is required. Thus, the library list of medications can easily become long and cumbersome. Health systems must continually work to streamline and standardize infusion concentrations. Initially, buy-in for standardization of concentrations across facilities, medical specialties, and practice settings may be overwhelming, but ongoing efforts are necessary to improve patient safety.

The management of bolus doses is another initial practice decision that should be made. To make the library more useful, determining which boluses will come from the infusion bag and which will be provided as separate infusions is essential. The library must reflect these decisions appropriately.

Providing regular feedback to pharmacy and nursing staff regarding library utilization and errors avoided is also important. This reinforces the advantages of using the pumps as intended and underscores the patient

safety benefits. Review of data by the pharmacy and therapeutics committee, patient safety committee, and other appropriate groups also can improve visibility to the project.

Finally, the use of failure mode and effects analysis (FMEA) has been described as a means for assisting with the implementation of smart pump technology.[18] This technique was found useful for identifying potential problems in the medication-use process related to pump implementation, but it was concluded that monitoring for system failures and errors after implementation remains necessary. FMEA helped with process redesign and also assisted in identifying potential new sources of error that could be introduced by the new technology.

SUMMARY

The patient safety data supporting the use of smart infusion pumps continually expands as the technology evolves. A multidisciplinary approach is essential during the initial implementation steps, as well as the continuing practice changes and technology enhancements of the facility moving forward. The pharmacy department can take a leadership role in the selection, planning, rollout, and ongoing maintenance of this important technology.

REFERENCES

1. Proceedings of a summit on preventing patient harm and death from I.V. medication errors. Am J Health Syst Pharm. 2008;65(24):2367-2379.

2. Pedersen CA, Schneider PJ, Scheckelhoff DJ. ASHP national survey of pharmacy practice in hospital settings: dispensing and administration—2005. Am J Health Syst Pharm. 2006;63(4):327-345.

3. Pedersen CA, Gumper KF. ASHP national survey on informatics: assessment of the adop-

tion and use of pharmacy informatics in U.S. hospitals—2007. *Am J Health Syst Pharm.* 2008; 65(23):2244-2264.

4. "Smart" infusion pumps join CPOE and bar coding as important ways to prevent medication errors. *ISMP Medication Safety Alert!* February 7, 2002. http://www.ismp.org/newsletters/acute care/articles/20020207.asp. Accessed March 2, 2009.

5. Larsen GY, Parker HB, Cash J, O'Connell M, Grant MC. Standard drug concentrations and smart-pump technology reduce continuous-medication-infusion errors in pediatric patients. *Pediatrics.* 2005;116(1):e21-e25.

6. Malashock CM, Shull SS, Gould DA. Effect of smart infusion pumps on medication errors related to infusion device programming. *Hosp Pharm.* 2004;39(5):460-469.

7. Rothschild JM, Keohane CA, Cook EF, et al. A controlled trial of smart infusion pumps to improve medication safety in critically ill patients. *Crit Care Med.* 2005;33(3):533-540.

8. Williams CK, Maddox RR. Implementation of an I.V. medication safety system. *Am J Health Syst Pharm.* 2005; 62(5):530-536.

9. Adachi W, Lodolce AE. Use of failure mode and effects analysis in improving the safety of I.V. drug administration. *Am J Health Syst Pharm.* 2005;62(9): 917-920.

10. Jacobs B. New intravenous pumps help increase safety measures and improve cost-effectiveness. *Nurse Manage.* 2005;36(12):40-44

11. Cassano AT. IV medication safety software implementation in a multihospital health sys-

tem. *Hosp Pharm.* 2006;41(2):151-156.

12. Williams CK, Maddox RR, Heape E, Richards HE, Griffiths DL, Crass RE. Application of the IV Medication Harm Index to assess the nature of harm averted by "smart" infusion safety systems. *J Patient Saf.* 2006;2(3):132-139.

13. Fanikos J, Fiumara K, Baroletti S, et al. Impact of smart infusion technology on administration of anticoagulant (unfractionated heparin, argatroban, lepirudin, and bivalirudin). *Am J Cardiol.* 2007;99(7):1002-1005.

14. Bates DW. Preventing medication errors: a summary. *Am J Health Syst Pharm.* 2007;64(14)(suppl 9):S3-S9.

15. Hess J, Whiting S. Making an intelligent smart pump purchase. *Materials Management in Health Care.* www.matmanmag.com. Published August 2007. Accessed February 7, 2009.

16. Smart pumps. KLAS Web site. http://www.klasresearch.com/Klas/Site/News/NewsLetters/2008-09/sp2008.aspx. Accessed February 7, 2009.

17. Siv-Lee L, Morgan L. Implementation of wireless "intelligent" pump IV infusion technology in a not-for-profit academic hospital setting. *Hosp Pharm.* 2007;42(9):832-840.

18. Wetterneck TB, Skibinski KA, Roberts TL, et al. Using failure mode and effects analysis to plan implementation of smart I.V. pump technology. *Am J Health Syst Pharm.* 2006;63(16):1528-1538.

19. Cohen MR, Smetzer JL. Lack of standard dosing methods contribute to IV errors. *Hosp Pharm.* 2007;42(12): 1100-1101. ■

Core Competencies in Hospital Pharmacy Practice

Core Competencies in Hospital Pharmacy: Regulatory Compliance

Michael Sanborn, MS, FASHP*

The focus of this *Director's Forum* is on regulatory compliance and it serves as the last in the small series of articles on core practices or competencies in hospital pharmacy practice. Future *Director's Forum* topics will include decentralized pharmacy services, medication safety, clinical program development, and automation. The goal of the *Director's Forum* throughout 2006 is to provide readers with information on all of the necessary core competencies of hospital pharmacy practice, comprising a "toolkit" in establishing a patient-centered pharmacy department.

Regulatory compliance is probably one of the most important, yet least exhilarating, aspects of pharmacy practice for many pharmacists. Nonetheless, the profession of pharmacy, like medicine in general, is surrounded by regulation and it is absolutely essential for every pharmacy director to be familiar with pharmacy rules, statutes, standards, and regulations to ensure compliance in all aspects of operations associated with medication use.

Regulations are an important part of practice from drug discovery and investigation to marketing, purchasing, and all aspects of hospital medication use (including dispensing). In some cases, regulatory bodies dictate law that is enforceable by the local, state, or federal government (eg, Drug Enforcement Administration [DEA]). In other situations, regulatory entities set minimum standards of practice required for accreditation or participation, such as the medication management standards set forth by the Joint Commission on Accreditation of Healthcare Organizations (JCAHO). While, it is impossible to summarize regulations in one article, the reference section will direct you to the most recent document or Web site available. Rather than review the regulations, this article will serve to provide an overview to regulatory agencies and their purpose. The various regulatory bodies are divided into three broad categories: federal agencies, state agencies, and accrediting organizations.

FEDERAL REGULATORY AGENCIES AND COMPLIANCE

Several US government agencies are responsible for both implementation and enforcement of statutes and regulations at the federal level. Most of these agencies focus on the maintaining high quality and safety standards for medications. For example, the FDA is responsible for the oversight of the Federal Food, Drug, and Cosmetic Act, which regulates the marketing, labeling, quality, use, and interstate commerce associated with drugs and devices in addition to food and cosmetics.[1] Originally passed by Congress on June 30, 1906, the Act also addresses misbranding, safety, efficacy, and inspection authority and has been completely rewritten and revised over the years; the current version was amended through December 31, 2004.

*Health System Pharmacy Director, Baylor Health Care System, Dallas, TX.

Another federal regulatory agency is the Centers for Medicare and Medicaid Services (CMS) (formerly known as the Health Care Financing Administration [HCFA]).[2] This agency is responsible for administering a number of federal programs, including Medicare and Medicaid. Specifically, the agency is responsible for setting participation requirements and details related to drug and procedure coding for reimbursement. CMS also administers several other programs, including the State Children's Health Insurance Program (SCHIP), the Health Insurance Portability and Accountability Act (HIPAA), Clinical Laboratory Improvement Amendments (CLIA), and advisory jurisdiction over Consolidated Omnibus Budget Reconciliation Act of 1985 (COBRA). Additionally, CMS is becoming more involved in the collection of hospital quality data and is currently in the midst of a 3-year experiment that ties hospital performance over 10 quality-of-care measures with enhanced inflation-based increases in Medicare payments.

HIPAA deserves special mention from a regulatory perspective. This 1996 act established national standards for electronic health care transactions and also addresses the security and privacy of health care data. Many aspects of this act are designed to protect patient privacy and the confidentiality of data which has both direct and indirect effects on daily pharmacy operations. As an example, patient-specific labels on used IV admixture preparations must be disposed of by a means that will protect patient confidentiality and privacy. Violations to HIPAA regulations can result in civil monetary penalties or imprisonment.

Two federal agencies that impact many of the physical aspects of pharmacy practice are the Occupational Safety and Health (OSHA) and the National Institute for Occupational Safety (NIOSH). OSHA operates under the US Department of Labor and is responsible for developing and enforcing workplace health and safety regulations. NIOSH, on the other hand, is geared towards preventing work-related injuries and illnesses and operates under the CDC.[3] In 2004, NIOSH issued an alert addressing the prevention of occupational exposure to antineoplastics and other hazardous drugs. The alert provides specific guidelines and recommendations for the safe handling of such hazardous drugs and addresses areas such as the use of personal protective equipment, ventilation, waste containment and disposal, and training.

The American Society of Health-System Pharmacists (ASHP) has recently published revised guidelines on the handling of hazardous drugs that incorporate the NIOSH, OSHA, and Resource Conservation and Recovery Act (RCRA) guidelines and will also produce a video training program addressing the same subject.[4] The article is well-referenced, and also contains many helpful appendices that list specific recommendations for various types of compounding environments and situations. Useful information on potential complications related to cytotoxic drug exposure has been published by Davis and Benner in 2003.[5] Also, Chapter <797> of the United States Pharmacopeia (USP) provides regulations for pharmaceutical compounding of sterile products and was addressed in the April *Director's Forum* article.[6,7] USP recently published revisions to the chapter (www.usp.org), and these revisions are open to public comment through August 15, 2006.

A final federal agency that deserves mention due to its influence on daily practice is the Drug Enforcement Administration (DEA) which operates under the US Department of Justice.[8] Part of the DEA's broad responsibilities includes the enforcement and control of products listed under the Controlled Substances Act. All health professionals entitled to dispense, administer, or prescribe controlled drugs, and all pharmacies entitled to dispense prescriptions or fill medication orders must register with the DEA. All pharmacies must comply with a series of regulatory requirements relating to drug security, records accountability, and adherence to standards. Most pharmacists are very familiar with DEA Form 222, which is required for the order and purchase of many scheduled drugs.

STATE REGULATORY AGENCIES AND COMPLIANCE

At the state level, two primary agencies provide legal and regulatory oversight for pharmacy; these are the state boards of pharmacy and the state Department of Health. Rules and regulations for each of these entities can vary dramatically from one state to another, so it is important for every pharmacy director to be keenly familiar with the conventions in the state in which they practice. For example, some states, such as Florida and Texas, have multiple types of pharmacy licenses and different regulations apply to each. Personnel and practice standards can also vary widely, such as with some states requiring licensure for pharmacy technicians and others requiring national certification.

State level agencies are also the most likely to provide on-site inspections that evaluate not only state law but federal compliance as well. In many cases, these inspections are relatively routine (annual or biennial), but unscheduled inspections are also quite common, especially in response to a patient complaint or to follow-up on a previous infraction. Fortunately, most states use a checklist for inspections that highlights required areas of compliance and a frequent review of this checklist can assist in maintaining the required level of conformity.

State boards of pharmacy serve to regulate pharmacy practice within a given state, and the mission of most boards involves the enforcement of uniform standards for the purpose of protecting the public health. The Web site for the National Association of Boards of Pharmacy (NABP) (www.nabp.net) has useful information for most state boards, including access to newsletters, links to individual board Web pages, and contact information for each state. NABP also publishes an electronic *Survey of Pharmacy Law* on CR-ROM that includes summary charts of legal differences from state to state.[9]

The state Department of Health (DOH) also provides regulatory oversight to hospitals and hospital pharmacies. Often these agencies are responsible for administering state Medicaid programs, facility licensing, state vaccination programs, and/or disaster preparedness. It is also common for the state board of pharmacy to exist under the umbrella of the state DOH. First and foremost, most states use the DOH to promote and protect the health and safety of its residents and visitors. As such, DOH interactions are commonly related to inspections or investigations due to patient complaints. However, it is important to be familiar with DOH regulations that may directly or indirectly affect the pharmacy. In one state, for instance, a DOH administrative code requires 30-day stop orders for medications to force a minimum monthly review of therapy.

COMPLIANCE WITH ACCREDITATION AGENCIES

Compliance with accreditation standards is not necessarily required by law, but demonstrates that a certain facility or program meets or exceeds standards set forth by the accrediting body. In hospitals, one of the most recognized accrediting bodies is the JCAHO, which evaluates and accredits more than 15,000 health care organizations and programs in the US.[10] Accreditation by JCAHO is voluntary; however, most institutions have opted to request the accreditation primarily, because it provides deeming authority for Medicare, Medicaid, and other third-party payor certification (for Conditions of Participation) and in some states, satisfies hospital licensing requirements.

The accreditation standards set forth by JCAHO are extensive, and most of the standards that are directly related to pharmacy can be found in the medication management standards (although pharmacy participation is critical in many of the other chapters, including management of human resources, information, and provision of care). A useful summary of JCAHO medication management standards was recently published in *Hospital Pharmacy*, and this publica-

tion has also provided helpful guidance with respect to JCAHO compliance in the *Ask the Joint Commission* column.[11] Finally, ASHP has recently revised their publication entitled *Preparing the Pharmacy for Continuous Compliance with Joint Commission Standards*, which is a comprehensive guide designed to assist pharmacy directors in their preparation for a JCAHO survey.[12] JCAHO has also developed a series of National Patient Safety Goals (NPSG) that includes goals and requirements for accreditation designed to improve patient safety. The 2006 NPSGs were approved in May of 2005 and can also be found on JCAHO's Web site (www.jcaho.org).

There are other organizations that are also involved in the accreditation of hospitals and hospital pharmacies. For example, ASHP, through its residency accreditation program, surveys hospital pharmacies against published standards and best practices. By participating in ASHP's residency accreditation process, a facility is accepting responsibility for meeting or exceeding the standards set forth by ASHP and in the accreditation guidelines. The American Osteopathic Association also serves as an accreditation body for many osteopathic hospitals, often in lieu of JCAHO accreditation. Other organizations such as the American Pharmacists Association, the American College of Clinical Pharmacy, and the American Society of Consultant Pharmacists have also developed best practices, guidelines, and/or standards that can influence pharmacy practice.

SUMMARY

In many cases, regulations and standards are developed to protect patients and improve the quality of care. Pharmacy directors must have a working understanding of all applicable regulatory and accreditation requirements at the federal, state, and local level and must ensure their implementation into the health system's medication use process. This can be an ongoing challenge but is an essential core competency to master.

REFERENCES

1. US Food and Drug Administration. Federal Food, Drug, and Cosmetic Act. Available at: http://www.fda.gov/opacom/laws/fdcact/fdctoc.htm. Accessed May 27, 2006.

2. US Department of Health and Human Services. Centers for Medicare and Medicaid Services. Available at: http://new.cms.hhs.gov/. Accessed May 27, 2006.

3. Department of Health and Human Services. Centers for Disease Control and Prevention. Available at: http://www.cdc.gov/niosh/homepage.html. Accessed May 27, 2006.

4. ASHP guidelines on handling hazardous drugs. *Am J Health-Syst Pharm.* 2006;63:1172-1193.

5. Davis KM, Benner KW. Potential complications of exposure to cytotoxic agents for caregivers. *Hosp Pharm.* 2003;38:1097-1102.

6. Pharmaceutical compounding—sterile preparations (general information chapter <797>). In: *The United States Pharmacopeia*, 27th rev., and *The National Formulary*, 22nd ed. Rockville, MD: The United States Pharmacopeial Convention; 2004:2350-2370.

7. Sanborn, MD. Core competencies in hospital pharmacy: intravenous admixtures. *Hosp Pharm.* 2006;41:377-380.

8. US Drug Enforcement Administration. Available at: http://www.usdoj.gov/dea/index.htm. Accessed May 27, 2006.

9. *Survey of Pharmacy Law* [CDROM]. Mount Prospect, IL: National Association of Boards of Pharmacy; 2006

10. Commission on Accreditation of Healthcare Organizations. Available at: http://www.jointcommission.org/. Accessed April 11, 2006.

11. May SK. Improving patient safety—one standard at a time. *Hosp Pharm.* 2005;40:921-924.

12. Coe CP, Uselton JP, eds. *Preparing the Pharmacy for Continuous Compliance with Joint Commission Standards.* 6th Ed. Bethesda, MD: American Society of Health-System Pharmacists; 2006. ∎

Core Competencies in Hospital Pharmacy: Drug Dispensing

Michael Sanborn, MS, FASHP

The next several *Director's Forum* articles will focus on core practices or competencies in hospital pharmacy practice. This series of articles will discuss the key fundamentals, resources, challenges, and opportunities associated with drug dispensing. Future core competency forums will include discussions on medication ordering, intravenous admixtures, data analysis, and regulatory requirements.

In *Director's Forum*, we hope to answer key questions that pharmacy directors face and provide others with information to foster growth in pharmacy leadership. The articles in this column will build on one another and, when put together, will serve as a "tool kit" to develop patient-centered pharmacy services in hospitals of all sizes. Examples of topics in future *Director's Forums* will include establishing clinical service priorities, justifying clinical pharmacist positions, implementing a patient safety program, and budgeting for patient-centered services.

Drug dispensing is a broad topic and arguably one of the most important competencies to master in hospital pharmacies. It truly is core. Right or wrong, it is the yardstick that most nurses and some physicians use to measure pharmacy effectiveness. Further, the most thorough and accurate vancomycin consult can be rendered meaningless if the drug is not available to administer at the appropriate time, or worse, if the incorrect dose is dispensed and administered. In many ways, medication dispensing within the realm of pharmacy practice is analogous to mastering a musical instrument—you need to be an expert in the fundamentals before you can be a maestro. Mastering dispensing fundamentals, however, is often less alluring than implementing new, high-level clinical programs and services.

WHAT IS THE BEST WAY TO DISPENSE?

One of the challenges in hospital pharmacy is that there is not one definitive way to dispense. A dispensing methodology is dependent upon a variety of factors that can include hospital logistics, patient census, department size, pharmacist to technician ratio, hours of operation, and the availability of hospital resources. Evidence of this fact can be seen in recent surveys of pharmacy directors on dispensing activities.[1] In this survey, 80% of hospitals employed a centralized dispensing methodology, whereas 20% had a decentralized system. The authors found that hospitals with greater than 400 beds tended to be decentralized more so than hospitals with fewer than 100 beds. Dispensing shortcomings were also identified, such as approximately 19% of intravenous admixture or solution doses were prepared by nursing personnel.

Patient safety is a critical benchmark by which to measure the effectiveness of a particular dispensing methodology. Studies have shown that dispensing error rates can comprise 8% or more of adverse drug events,[2] and this demonstrates an ongoing need for improvement of the dispensing process. Errors in medication selection and dispensing are the most common type of errors that the general public associates with pharmacies, and both lay and professional publications are full

*Health System Pharmacy Director, Baylor Healthcare System, Dallas, Texas

of examples where the incorrect medication has resulted in dire patient consequences.[3] Therefore, it is important that every hospital pharmacy monitor errors associated with dispensing and work to improve overall error rates.

Tools exist that can assist in developing safe and effective dispensing modalities. One of the best resources available is the annual publication from the American Society of Health-System pharmacists entitled *Best Practices for Hospital and Health-System Pharmacy*.[4] This resource includes position statements, guidelines, and technical assistance bulletins (TAB) on many of the critical elements associated with medication distribution and handling. The TAB associated with drug distribution and control provides moderately detailed information on the unit-dose system and dispensing fundamentals (procurement, preparation, packaging, labeling, and delivery). It also provides standards for unique circumstances, such as patients' own medications, emergency medications, and dispensing when the pharmacy is closed.

Published information on the advantages and disadvantages of different dispensing models is another helpful resource. The pharmacy literature is replete with information on various types of distribution methodologies and information on dispensing in various practice settings. *Hospital Pharmacy* has also published many useful bibliographies on subjects such as unit-dose dispensing, the role of pharmacy technicians, and automation in acute care pharmacies.[5-7]

The role of the pharmacy technician in the dispensing process cannot be overlooked. A significant majority of hospitals use pharmacy technicians to prepare unit doses for pharmacists to check prior to delivery.[1] Over the last several years, the role of the technician has continued to expand into areas that have improved departmental efficiencies and have enhanced the pharmacist's ability to provide patient care. For example, in some limited cases, technicians have been used to check unit doses prepared by other technicians (often referred to as a "tech-check-tech" program). The ability to deploy technician resources is different for every hospital and should be carefully considered as part of the overall dispensing plan.

There are some important elements necessary for any effective dispensing system in a hospital. These include:

1. Use of unit-dose dispensing where drugs are delivered in a dosage form that does not require further manipulation before administration to the patient.
2. A pharmacist check of all manually dispensed doses (or in some special circumstances, a "tech-check-tech" methodology can be employed).
3. Commercially available products should be used whenever possible.
4. Accurate and timely delivery of the product to the nurse or patient must be ensured.
5. Adherence to federal, state, and other regulatory requirements is essential.
6. The multidisciplinary impact of the dispensing system must be considered.
7. Dispensing technology, when used, must be validated and then implemented in a way that does not compromise patient safety or bypass important patient safeguards.

CENTRALIZED VS DECENTRALIZED DISPENSING

Years ago, a centralized unit-dose dispensing system was unquestionably the safest and most effective way to deliver medications to patients. Floor stock was generally minimized in an effort to improve drug-use control. In some hospitals, decentralized pharmacists were deployed with locked dispensing carts, and these pharmacists could dispense first doses and/or a 24-hour supply of medications to their assigned patients. With the advent of decentralized automation in the late 1980s and early 90s, floor-stock systems once again became popular, and these systems introduced electronic safeguards that improved the pharmacist's ability to control access to floor-based medications. Centralized dispensing automation has also gained wide acceptance, and now pharmacy directors must decide which type of system to hinge their dispensing philosophy upon.

There are advantages and disadvantages to each of the two systems, and in reality, there is not one perfect system that can meet the needs of every hospital. In fact, many hospitals have started using a hybrid approach (where both decentralized and centralized dispensing is used depending on the type of medication needed) to capitalize on the benefits of both methods. The use of fixed pharmacy dispensing satellites is also common, especially in areas with high-patient acuity such as in operating rooms, intensive care units, oncology units, and neonatal intensive care nurseries.

When deciding between a centralized vs decentralized approach, care should be given to the types of patients being served, the needs of hospital personnel caring for the patient, and whether the approach is complimentary to the short- and long-term goals of the hospital. For instance, if the hospital has a 3-year plan to implement computerized prescriber order entry (CPOE) and bedside medication scanning, consideration must be given to the dispensing approach that will best complement that new environment.

Hospital logistics and space availability can also play a pivotal role in the decision. If space is limited on the nursing unit, it may be impossible to implement a fixed satellite for decentralized dispensing. Many times, minor-to-moderate renovation is necessary to install decentralized automation. In contrast, limited pharmacy space, medication delivery challenges, and distant or off-site patient care areas may suggest the need for a more decentralized model.

TO AUTOMATE OR NOT TO AUTOMATE?

Automation has both satisfied and frustrated many pharmacy directors. Pharmacists today can choose from a wide variety of dispensing-related automation ranging from unit based cabinets (UBC), centralized robotic systems, automated high-capacity storage devices, and automated IV compounders. The first decision point associated with automation should be one of magnitude. While not always true, it is difficult to build a business case for automated dispensing, when a very small number of doses must be dispensed using the automation. Automated equipment can be very costly, and it is often necessary to cost justify any new automation in this era of limited hospital resources. High volume is often needed to build this justification.

Some facilities, on the other hand, have made the decision to automate based solely on improved regulatory compliance or other factors unrelated to dispensing volume. This is especially true in small hospitals where 24-hour services are not available, yet the ability to provide enhanced control of medications after hours can be handled more effectively with a UBC. Improved prevention of controlled substance diversion is another common justification for automation.

The decision between moving forward with automation or bypassing it entirely is difficult; however, it can be quite helpful to develop a summary of advantages and disadvantages for both scenarios by asking a series of key questions.

- Can manpower truly be redeployed with the proposed automation?
- What are the true costs of the technology vs the costs of the non-automated state?
- What processes will need to be redesigned prior to the implementation of the equipment?
- Which system provides the safest environment for the patient?
- What resources will be necessary to support the different systems on a 24-hour basis?
- Are there hospitals similar to ours that have effectively employed this technology?

All of these questions, and many others, must be evaluated during the decision-making process. Site visits can also prove to be extremely informative when weighing the benefits of various types of automation.

The integration of bar code technology within pharmacy automation has also been shown to improve dispensing accuracy and overall efficiency.[8] Much of the automation that is available today can utilize bar codes; however, not all systems are compat-

ible with one another, and the labor needed to prepare bar coded medications for dispensing can be considerable. The potential use of bar codes (or in the future, radio frequency identification) may be an additional decision point when evaluating automated devices.

SUMMARY

When considering the best way to dispense, there is not one "right" answer. Centralized vs decentralized dispensing, as well as the choice to incorporate automation, are decisions that must be made based on available resources, the strategic plans of the department and hospital, and the needs of the department in terms of enhancing patient safety and efficiency. Best practices and various publications are available for a variety of situations and can be very useful in evaluating specific methodologies. Assessment of the current drug dispensing process and the expected goals of a redesigned process must be carefully evaluated prior to moving forward with improvements. In any case, it is fundamentally important that every pharmacy director masters this core competency.

REFERENCES

1. Pedersen CA, Schneider PJ, Scheckelhoff DJ. ASHP national survey of pharmacy practice in hospital settings: dispensing and administration—2002. *Am J Health Syst Pharm.* 2003;60:52–68.

2. Leape LL, Bates DW, Cullen DJ, et al. Systems analysis of adverse drug events. *JAMA.* 1995;274:35–43.

3. Sanborn MD. What to focus on first—prioritizing safety improvement initiatives. In: Manasse Jr. HR, Thompson KK. *Medication Safety: A Guide for Healthcare Facilities.* Bethesda, MD: American Society of Health-System Pharmacists; 2005:57–72.

4. American Society of Health-System Pharmacists. *Best practices for hospital and health-system pharmacy.* Bethesda, MD: The Society; 2005.

5. Woods B. Bibliography: Pharmacy Technicians. *Hosp Pharm.* 2003; 38:1185.

6. Nelson SP. Bibliography: Unit Dose Drug Distribution. *Hosp Pharm.* 1998;33:1583.

7. Sanborn MD. Bibliography: Automation in Acute Care Pharmacies. *Hosp Pharm.* 2002;37:334–338.

8. Ragan R, Bond J, Major K, Kingsford T, Eidem L, Garrelts JC. Improved control of medication use with an integrated bar-code an packaging distribution system. *Am J Health Syst Pharm.* 2005;62:1075–1079. ∎

Core Competencies in Hospital Pharmacy: Department Financial Management

Robert J. Weber, MS, FASHP*

This series of articles in the *Director's Forum* continue to review key core competencies necessary for a pharmacy department to define their value in patient care. Competencies of medication order review, medication order dispensing, preparing intravenous admixtures, and data management provide a foundation in patient centered services. The goal of the *Director's Forum* throughout 2006 is to provide readers with information on all of the necessary core competencies of hospital pharmacy practice, comprising a "toolkit" in establishing a patient-centered pharmacy department.

Hospitals and health care organizations depend on data and information to manage clinical care and operations. For example, hospitals use information and data to project and track their revenue and expenses and to establish appropriate patient care programs. All hospitals have a financial responsibility to their respective governance to monitor both costs and quality, and publish information internally and externally. Importantly, the yearly budgeting process in hospitals is solely dependent on information on financial performance from the previous year along with projected expenses for additional programs for the upcoming budget year.

Managing the finances of a pharmacy department is not a static process of calculating the yearly budget and writing variance reports to explain budget discrepancies. Financial management of a pharmacy department is a dynamic process that adapts to changing environments within the organization. The pharmacy director must be able to quickly and effectively assess and use financial information to maintain the department's ability to meet the strategic goals of their organization.

Every hospital pharmacy director must have the ability to analyze and measure the financial performance of a pharmacy department on a daily, weekly, monthly, and yearly basis. In fact, a less experienced or new pharmacy director may have little or no experience in the financial management of a department. Their thorough understanding of financial details of a pharmacy may determine their success as a department head.[1]

Close monitoring of a department's finances may seem like a daunting task; the key to this close monitoring is to use information from various sources in the hospital and develop a system for consistently reviewing and acting upon information. An analogy that applies to managing a hospital pharmacy's finances in real-time is how most hospitals respond to sentinel events. All hospitals have access to specific information through their reporting systems that provides them with data to make decisions and improvements in care to prevent serious errors. This same philosophy should

*Associate Professor and Department Chair, University of Pittsburgh School of Pharmacy, Executive Director of Pharmacy, University of Pittsburgh Medical Center, Pittsburgh, PA.

apply to the finances of the pharmacy department, with information being readily accessible and easily analyzed to promote effective decision making.

This article reviews fundamental concepts in managing the financial aspects of a hospital pharmacy department. The goal of this article is to provide hospital pharmacy directors with a summary and explanation of steps and strategies in hospital pharmacy financial management. The specific aims of this article are to (1) describe a dynamic approach to financial management that promotes patient-centered services; (2) review specific information and steps to monitor the financial performance of the department; (3) describe a proactive approach used by the University of Pittsburgh Medical Center (UPMC) to manage drug expenses. Hopefully, the lessons learned from this article can be applied to establish a system for financial management that promotes a patient-centered pharmacy service.

DYNAMIC APPROACH TO DEPARTMENT FINANCIAL MANAGEMENT

The pharmacy director is responsible for the quality and costs of the hospital's medication use process. Inherent in that responsibility is a thorough understanding of the financial aspects of the pharmacy service. Routinely, pharmacy directors are often asked the following questions regarding the finances of a hospital pharmacy: How much is the pharmacy budget, specifically, how much do we spend on drugs, and which drugs account for the highest expense? How many full-time equivalencies (FTEs) are budgeted in the pharmacy, and what is the mix of pharmacists and technicians? How do our expenses compare to what we have predicted for the budgetary cycle? What is the yearly inventory turnover rate? What is the revenue generated by the Pharmacy Department? How do our operational expenses compare to other hospitals similar in size?

As stated in a previous article in the *Director's Forum*, the answers to these questions are often referred to as "metrics" and every pharmacy director should be comfortable with articulating how these metrics apply to the patient care services of the pharmacy. These "metrics" however, are used as part of an overall philosophy of financial management that involves a dynamic process of managing departmental expenses. The pharmacy budgeting process is an initial place for a pharmacy director to begin taking a more dynamic approach to department financial management.

The Pharmacy Budget as a Dynamic Process

Many hospitals pressure the pharmacy director to "meet budget" since almost 7% of a hospitals' operating expense involves the Pharmacy Department.[2] The pharmacy budgeting process projects the costs of providing services based on historical information and an assessment of future programs and hospital strategies. Since many hospitals experience unexpected changes in their programs in a given budgetary cycle, the pharmacy's budget must adapt to these changes. Reporting the reasons for a monthly budget variance and actions to reduce the variance is a very static process that does not promote effective analysis of pharmacy programs. The pharmacy budgeting process becomes dynamic when the pharmacy director uses the monthly budget variance as a continuous quality improvement tool. The following case demonstrates this concept.

A pharmacy director of a 300-bed community hospital is asked to explain a 12% monthly variance in drug expense in spite of an expected number of admissions and types of patients treated. During that month, the pharmacy director made a conscious decision, in the interest of patient safety, to eliminate the extemporaneous compounding of a drug product and purchase the same drug produced by the manufacturer. The pharmacy director took the opportunity, in explaining the variance, to review this change with the Pharmacy & Therapeutics (P&T) Committee and Patient Safety Committee stressing the fact that the expense was a commitment to the safest patient care, despite an increased cost. The pharmacy director also explained how resources necessary to extemporaneously compound the drug product could be allocated to direct patient care. Finally, the director of pharmacy showed the potential cost savings to the organization by eliminating the possibility of an adverse event with the extemporaneously prepared drug.

The case demonstrates that, instead of a one-sentence static variance explanation (ie, "Expense due to availability of new drug product from the manufacturer"), a more dynamic approach was taken. This approach indicated the pharmacy director's willingness to be adaptable in managing the pharmacy budget in a way that supports the hospital's core mission of providing patient-centered services. Specifically, the pharmacy director took the opportunity to use the budget variance to promote the department's mission of safe and effective medica-

tion use. This dynamic approach can be applied to most responses to budget variances.

MONITORING FINANCIAL PERFORMANCE

There are essential financial data that the director of pharmacy must review to assure for the effective financial performance of the department. To accomplish this, the pharmacy director must determine the financial goals for the Pharmacy Department.

Financial goals of the Pharmacy Department are determined by aligning with the financial goals of the organization. Typically, the focus of the Inpatient Pharmacy Department is to control expenses, since the revenues generated from dispensing medication to hospitalized patients are not relevant to most reimbursement models (eg, Center for Medicare and Medicaid Services, private insurers). The most important expense to monitor in a hospital pharmacy is overall drug cost, representing 70% to 75% of the pharmacy budget. Other important expenses include personnel and supplies. As a result, the major financial focus of a pharmacy director must be on controlling the department's drug and personnel expense. **Table 1** lists an example of a pharmacy department's financial goals.

Table 2 lists the expense items that comprise over 90% of the pharmacy budget at the UPMC. This list may be helpful to focus the pharmacy director on important areas of expense within the pharmacy operations. For example, a director of pharmacy with limited resources may want to develop an intensive monitoring system for drugs, pharmacist and technician salaries, equipment and space rental, office supplies, and printing that may

Table 1. Sample Financial Goals for a Pharmacy Department

Goal	Measure
Pharmacy expenses within the control of the director of pharmacy are within 0% to 2% of volume-adjusted projection	• Total pharmacy costs per patient day • Required full-time equivalents based on productivity measures • Drug expense per patient day • Salaries per patient day
Yearly pharmacy inventory turn rate at 18 or greater	• Monthly drug expense/physical pharmacy inventory value
Difference in drug purchases amount vs drug charges amount is between 0% to 1%	• Compare the amount purchased and the amount charged to determine lost charges or system issues related charging for medications
New drug technology expense does not exceed projected ranges established by the American Society of Health System Pharmacists (usual ranges are 6% to 9%)	• Identify new drug technology expense on proactive basis, and develop evidence-based assessment of new drug usage to control costs and promote quality prescribing
Hospital-based retail pharmacy margin is between 4% to 6%	• Total expense compared to total revenue
Accounts receivable for a hospital-based retail pharmacy is no longer than 60 days	• Measures ability to be reimbursed in timely manner for prescription adjudication

control a large portion of the pharmacy's expenses.

For those pharmacy departments that operate a clinic-based or hospital-owned retail pharmacy, the focus is on maintaining an adequate margin to support the operations and growth of the outpatient pharmacy. Financial goals include developing strategies to increase prescription volume, maintain the accounts receivable balance within 30 to 60 days, effectively manage prescription claim adjudication, and 100% collection of prescription copayments.

A PROACTIVE APPROACH TO MONITORING DRUG EXPENSES

Pharmaceutical costs are an important area for hospital financial admin-

Table 2. Hospital Pharmacy Expenses as a Percentage of Total

Expense	% of Total Pharmacy Expense	Comment
Drugs	72.2	Includes inpatient and hospital-based clinic expense
Pharmacist salaries	13.3	All levels of pharmacists included
Technician salaries	3.5	All levels of technicians
Rental of equipment	2.2	Rental for pharmacy automation
Office supplies, space rental, printing	1.5	
IV solutions	0.75	All IV solutions including solutions prepared by the manufacturer
Medical surgical supplies	0.38	Personal protective equipment
Recruitment, travel, telephone	< 1	

*Based on analysis of the University of Pittsburgh Medical Center Budget

istrators. The national costs of pharmaceuticals, for example, have risen by 6% to 15% yearly since 1997; 70% of those costs are associated with new drug approvals.[3] The director of pharmacy must have an excellent handle on the purchasing trends of pharmaceuticals, even to the granular detail of understanding the daily purchases of drugs. Hospital patient days, or the number of patients that spend a 24-hour period in a hospital bed, predict use of pharmaceuticals. The pharmacy director should track and analyze the pharmaceutical costs per patient day to detect any trends in costs that indicate a change in patient diagnosis or physician prescribing patterns. Others ways to examine drug costs include the following: (1) drug cost per hospital admission or discharge; (2) "Top 30" Report that highlights the top 30 drugs by expense; (3) velocity report that lists drug use by volume (units dispensed); and (4) monthly expenses of drugs compared to a historical average of drug expense (establishes rapidly changing drug expense).

The UPMC employs a proactive Drug Expense Review Team (team) for managing the hospital's drug expense. The goal of this process is to track drug purchases to promote the rational use of drugs while maintaining adequate inventory control. This goal is accomplished by the following aims: (1) establish a collaborative team; (2) design a daily process and tool for monitoring drug expense; and (3) establish a communication system for drug expense management.

Establish a Collaborative Team

The team consists of the Pharmacy Director of Finance, Drug Buyers, Operations Manager, Drug Use and Disease State Management Pharmacists,

and UPMC's Drug Purchasing Agent (HC Pharmacy Central, Inc.). These individuals have direct responsibility for processing the daily drug order, managing the inventory, and interfacing with physicians on evidence-based prescribing. Others may be included on the team on an "as needed" basis and include the Executive Director of Pharmacy, the Chief Financial and Operating Officers of the UPMC.

Design a Daily Process and Tool for Monitoring Drug Expense

The team meets daily (around 8:30 to 9:00 AM) after the drug buyers have formulated the drug order for the day to review purchasing needs. The team meets in a conference room that has computer and projection capabilities allowing the team to access data from the hospital's information system, the purchasing agent, and individual reports established for monitoring drug expense. Conference phone capabilities are also available in the room.

The team uses a spreadsheet to monitor and discuss the trends in drug purchases; a sample of this spreadsheet is included in **Table 3**. Specific drug products that show erratic purchasing patterns or costly medications are added as separate line items on the spread sheet, and tracked by the team as needed.

Purchasing patterns are segregated by area of the department (eg, IV room, refrigerators). The software from the UPMC purchasing agents is tailored to order by the specific area of the pharmacy to facilitate the drug ordering and tracking process. Each area has an expense budget, which is based on the historical drug expense for that area during the past 6 to 12 months. If there is a budget variance in a given area, then a more detailed list-

Table 3. Daily Drug Expense Tracking Spreadsheet—University of Pittsburgh Medical Center

Monthly Drug Expense Tracking			*Purchase Day-1*			*Purchase Day-2*	*Purchase Day-3*
Actual Variance to date:	Budget Month	Budget Daily	Friday	Saturday	Sunday	Monday	Tuesday
Presbyterian cases Presbyterian main pharmacy							
Refrigerator							
Presbyterian IV room							
Presbyterian pharmacy automation area							
Factor concentrate purchases							
Presbyterian unit dose area							
Presbyterian department stock							
Bar-code packaging - Presbyterian							
Bar-code packaging - Southside							
Bar-code packaging - Magee							
Adjustments							
Montefiore operating room pharmacy							
Presbyterian operating room pharmacy							
Narcotic room Presbyterian main							
Prismasate							
Pre-packaging area							
Total daily purchases							
Daily budget							
Actual (purchases less dept. issues)							
Operational target							

ing of drug expense is generated and analyzed for variations. The amount of drug expense is entered into the spreadsheet on a daily basis, with a monthly running total of expenses displayed and compared against the budget number for that month. The team uses this spreadsheet to update (wk-2 and -4 of the mo) the hospital executive management and pharmacy administration on the status of the monthly drug expenses.

The team identifies a variety of issues that explain changes in drug purchases and use. These include, but are not limited to, the following: order entry and patient charging errors, pharmacy processes for handling stock-outs and shortages, pharmacy dispensing issues, "off-label" drug use, potential medication safety problems (drug product packaging and labeling), and bar-code packaging and labeling concerns related to the hospital's bar-code medication administration system.

Establishing a Communication System for Managing Drug Expenses

The most important function of the team is to communicate changes in drug purchasing trends to various organizational decision-makers to promote rational drug therapy. For example, the team identified a purchasing trend (within 24 h) of a medication, investigated the patient's medical record and determined the drug was being prescribed for an "off label" indication restricted by the P&T Committee. The chair of the P&T Committee notified the prescriber of the variance, and suggested a therapeutically equivalent alternative. As a result, the prescriber discontinued use of the medication and change to the alternative suggestion.

This process is particularly effective in handling drug shortages, as a daily review of patients needing a drug experiencing a shortage helps to assure that only qualified patients (eg, those where the drug is necessary) are treated during the shortage. In addition, the members of the team serve as the point of contact for staff that need information on drug product availability. This was particularly important several years ago, when there was a shortage of influenza vaccine. The team developed a process for screening patients and was able to effectively distribute medication to only high-risk patients.

The team has generated impressive outcomes, documented cost savings in excess of $1 million dollars from intercepted purchasing, inventory control, and prescribing errors. The team has also reduced the number of inventory "stockouts" while maintaining an inventory turn ratio of 19.3.

SUMMARY AND CONCLUSION

Effective financial management is essential for establishing and maintaining patient-centered hospital pharmacy services. The director of pharmacy must use a dynamic approach to budgetary management combined with a proactive system for identifying and resolving the pharmacy's financial needs.

REFERENCES

1. Nold EG, Sander WT. Role of the director of pharmacy: the first six months. *Am J Health Syst Pharm.* 2004;61:2297-2310.

2. Pierpaoli PG. The rising cost of pharmaceuticals: a director of pharmacy's perspective. *Am J Hosp Pharm.* 1993;50:S6-S8.

3. Shah ND, Vermeulen LC, Santell JP, Hunkler RJ, Hontz K. Projecting future drug expenditures-2002. *Am J Health Syst Pharm.* 2002;59:131-142. ∎

Core Competencies in Hospital Pharmacy: Essential Department Data

*Robert J. Weber, MS, FASHP **

The initial installments of the *Director's Forum* reviewed key core competencies necessary for a pharmacy department to define their value in patient care. Core competencies include medication order review, medication order dispensing, and preparing intravenous (IV) admixtures. The next article will review the final core competency: compliance with regulatory standards. Additional pharmacy department programs such as medication therapy management and patient safety are also critical in establishing a patient-centered focus, and will be discussed in future articles.

Information and data have been a vital component in understanding and managing health care. These data address health care management on a national, regional, and local level. An example is Pennsylvania's Healthcare Cost Containment Council (PHC4).[1] PHC4 is an independent agency that uses interactive databases to report the costs and quality of health care in Pennsylvania. PHC4 publishes information for the public on costs and outcomes associated with a variety of disease states and medical procedures, including diabetes care, and coronary artery and orthopedic surgery outcomes. In order to distinguish problems and issues in providing health care in a given area of the Commonwealth, hospitals, patients, and insurers use data from PHC4. The data from PHC4 are used in research to examine the epidemiology of certain outcomes based on different variables of the patient population in Pennsylvania.

Hospitals and health care organizations depend on data and information to manage their clinical care and operations. For example, hospitals use information and data to project and track their revenue and expenses and to establish indicators of quality improvement. All hospitals have a financial responsibility to their respective governance to monitor both costs and quality, and publish information internally and externally. Importantly, the yearly budgeting process in hospitals is solely dependent on information on financial performance from the previous year along with projected expenses for additional programs for the upcoming budget year.

Every hospital pharmacy director must have the ability to analyze and measure all key operational and clinical activities. In fact, it is recommended that pharmacy directors, new in their position, place a high priority on data management and reporting.[2] Essential information is responsible not only to run the daily patient care service of a pharmacy, but vital in strategic planning of patient-centered services.

This article reviews the important data that every pharmacy director must be able to access and understand to operate an efficient department and to establish patient-centered pharmacy services. The goal of this article is to provide hospital pharmacy directors with a summary and explanation of important financial, operational, and

*Associate Professor and Department Chair, University of Pittsburgh School of Pharmacy, Executive Director of Pharmacy, University of Pittsburgh Medical Center, Pittsburgh, PA.

quality data for their departments. The specific aims of this article are to (1) describe the importance of the pharmacy directors' understanding and managing of departmental data and information; (2) describe specific information that monitors the financial, operational, and clinical performance of the department; (3) present steps that the hospital pharmacy director can take to obtain and monitor key departmental information. Hopefully, the lessons learned from this article can be applied to establish a system for data collection, management, and interpretation in a patient-centered pharmacy service.

IMPORTANCE OF ESSENTIAL DATA

The pharmacy director is responsible for the quality of the medication use process in the organization. Inherent in that responsibility is a thorough under standing of the operational, clinical, and financial aspects of the pharmacy service. As a result, pharmacy directors are often asked the following question by hospital board members, executives, and staff:

- How many doses does the pharmacy dispense?
- What is the average salary of a pharmacist or technician?
- How many medication errors are reported on a monthly basis, and what medications are associated with serious outcomes?
- How much is the pharmacy budget, specifically, how much do we spend on drugs and which drugs account for the highest expense?
- How many FTEs are budgeted in the pharmacy, and what is the mix of pharmacists and technicians?
- What is the yearly inventory turn rate?

- What is the order processing time for a routine medication?
- What is the order processing time for "STAT" or urgently needed medication?

These are just examples of the questions posed to most pharmacy directors in their institutions. Often these data used to answer the above questions are referred to as "metrics" by accounting and quality improvement departments. Firmly grasping the financial, clinical, and operational information in the department is vital to a pharmacy director's success for a variety of reasons. First, most hospital administrators expect the pharmacy director to have a firm understanding of data related to the department. The pharmacy director's ability to effectively articulate basic information regarding the department, and its role in patient care, promotes a confidence in the director's focus of necessary services for patient care. Secondly, the director's understanding of information demonstrates an involvement in the pharmacy that is fundamental to leading a department.

ESSENTIAL DATA FOR THE PHARMACY DIRECTOR

Essential data for the pharmacy director are classified into three general areas: financial, operational, and quality. Financial data encompass information related to department expenses and revenues; operational data describe the efficiency of the medication use system—specifically drug distribution and clinical operations; quality information tracks the outcomes of the pharmacy service and the **Tables 1, 2,** and **3** provide a comprehensive list of essential data for a hospital pharmacy director. Some key

Table 1. Essential Financial Data for the Pharmacy Director

Essential Data	Comment
Drug expense	Daily, monthly, quarterly, and yearly drug expense with detail of top 20% of purchases and other metrics (eg, expense/patient day)
Drug rebates/credits	Indicates effectiveness of buying contracts
IV solution expenses	Daily, monthly, quarterly, and yearly expenses with detail of specialty solutions purchased
Personnel expense	Regular and overtime hours paid based on position (pharmacists, etc)
Billing and crediting	Returned medications for credit (a sign of possible dispensing and report administration issues); captured charging errors (high or low charges)
Supply expenses	Miscellaneous supplies that impact pharmacy operations

IV = intravenous

Table 2. Essential Operational Data for the Pharmacy Director

Essential Data	Comment
Doses dispensed	Daily, monthly, quarterly, and yearly dispensing activity categorized by type (unit dose, IV admixtures, compounded items)
Medication order	Quarterly review of pharmacy processing time for routine and "STAT" processing time medications
Required FTEs	Indicates the mix of personnel (pharmacist vs technician) necessary to meet patient medication needs, defines optimal staffing patterns
Medication waste	Usually expressed as a percentage of prepared medications and most critical for IV admixtures
Pharmacist medication	Includes interventions (changed or discontinued orders); medication order review activities order entry volume
Inventory turnover rate	Calculated by dividing the yearly supply expense by the measured inventory value; indicates the efficiency of the purchasing process
List of medication storage areas	This list guides fundamental medication safety efforts
Facility and employee licensure, orientation, and training	Pharmacy facility license information along with required original copies of pharmacist's licenses; training and competency required at least yearly

Table 3. Essential Quality Data for the Pharmacy Director

Essential Data	Comment
Reported medication errors	Daily, monthly, quarterly, and yearly reported medication errors by type, cause, severity, and drug class
Patient and staff satisfaction	Yearly surveys of nursing, pharmacy, and medical staff gives indication of service quality
Quality control records	Includes nursing unit medication inspections, laminar flow hood inspection records and certification, end-product testing results, extemporaneous compounding and packaging records, and expiration-date tracking processes

essential data are described in this section.

Financial Information
Drug and Personnel Expenses

Pharmaceutical costs are an important area for hospital financial administrators. The national costs of pharmaceuticals, for example, have risen by 6% to 15% yearly since 1997, with over 70% of those costs being associated with new drug approvals.[3] Pharmaceuticals represent 4% to 7% of the yearly operating expense of most hospitals.[4] The director of pharmacy must have an excellent handle on the purchasing trends of pharmaceuticals, even to the granular detail of understanding the daily purchases of drugs. Hospital patient days, or the number of patients that spend a 24-hour period in a hospital bed, predict use of pharmaceuticals. The pharmacy director should track and analyze the pharmaceutical costs per patient day to detect any trends in costs that indicate a change in patient diagnoses or physician prescribing patterns. Other ways to examine drug costs include the following: (1) drug cost per hospital admission or discharge; (2) "Top 30" report that highlights the top 30 drugs by expense; (3) velocity report that lists drug use by volume (units dispensed); and (4) monthly expenses of drugs compared to a historical average of drug expense (establishes rapidly changing drug expense).

Personnel costs are the next highest expense in a department and must be managed effectively. Importantly, the pharmacy director must understand the required staffing for the department; that is, what number and mix of pharmacists, technicians, and other staff are necessary to meet the patient needs in a timely manner? The answer to this question requires the pharmacy director to establish a productivity and workload process that captures and measures all vital functions.

Operational Information
Doses Dispensed, Medication Order Processing Times, and Staff Satisfaction

The pharmacy director must understand information related to the daily dispensing operation of the pharmacy. In most hospitals, primary staffing and budget depends on the types and numbers of doses dispensed. As a result, it is important for the director to understand drug-dispensing volume in several ways. First, drug-dispensing patterns that reflect the periods of busiest activity should be measured and analyzed. Secondly, information on the mix of medications (IV admixtures, oral, liquid doses) dispensed is vital in predicting staffing and other services.

Medication order processing time (turn-around-time [TAT]) is the most significant pharmacy operational concern of physicians, nurses, and other staff and is also the largest source of complaints to the pharmacy director. As a result, the pharmacy director must develop a process for systematically monitoring TAT and develop agreed-upon standards for acceptable times through the Pharmacy & Therapeutics Committee. This monitoring can be done by collecting data by observation and also electronically from the pharmacy's information system. The pharmacy director should also track TAT by type of drug order and entity. For example, the pharmacy director may want to track the TAT for IV medication, chemotherapy preparations, medication for intensive care units, or for "STAT" and urgently needed medication.

Pharmacy and nursing satisfaction is another important piece of information for the pharmacy director to understand. Most hospital pharmacies survey their staff on a regular basis to determine areas where human resources management and operational processes can be improved, with survey questions ranging from the timeliness of drug delivery to the perceived quality of the service.[5]

Quality Information
Medication Safety Data

The pharmacy plays a key role in patient safety and is a key collaborator in collecting, analyzing, and managing information related to medication errors and adverse drug events. Understanding reported medication errors is critical to improving the safety of medication use. Specifically, the pharmacy director must know the rate of reported medication errors and be able to analyze how the voluntary reporting of errors reflects actual medication errors. Medication errors should be analyzed by type (eg, wrong dose or route), cause (eg, communication error, procedure not followed), and severity (eg, no harm, treatment required, death). The most common drugs associated with serious errors should be identified in order to focus medication safety efforts. Medication errors that occur in the pharmacy and intercepted by the pharmacist or other staff must be reported and tracked to determine system changes in drug dispensing to improve safety. The United States Pharmacopeia (USP) MED-MARX voluntary medication error reporting system published its 5-year analysis of reported medication er-

rors.[6] Their analysis of errors may serve as a template for your institution's approach to analyzing medication error reports.

Adverse drug reactions (ADRs) are reactions not related to medication errors, but are important to track for quality purposes. Specifically, the FDA's voluntary recall of the COX-2 inhibitors seriously questions the rigor of post-marketing drug safety monitoring. As a result, the pharmacy director must collect ADR data and classify them in the same format as medication error information.

OBTAINING AND MONITORING ESSENTIAL DATA

The pharmacy director must develop a mechanism for collecting data and information on the medication system and the pharmacy service. Information can be gathered from informational audits, from the pharmacy information system, and the hospital's financial and clinical repository. In addition, medication error and ADR data can be most easily analyzed using proprietary reporting systems.

An important first step to monitoring essential data is to develop a report that summarizes and analyzes the daily, monthly, quarterly, and yearly results. This is often referred to as a "report card" or "dashboard" and can be used in a variety of venues throughout the organization. These data can be presented in chart format, color coded for easy reading (eg, red indicates need for improvement, green indicating the indicator has met goal), or presented as a one-page executive summary. Importantly, the information must be presented in a manner that provides a clear message and plan to the organization on the pharmacy's role in patient-centered services.

SUMMARY AND CONCLUSION

Data on the efficiency and quality of the medication system are essential for establishing and maintaining patient-centered services. The director of pharmacy must understand and promote this information through the organization as it is critical to the department's success and future growth.

REFERENCES

1. PHC4 Pennsylvania Healthcare Cost Containment Council. Available at: http://www.phc4.org/. Accessed February 28, 2006.

2. Nold EG and Sander WT: Role of the director of pharmacy: The first six months. *Am J Health Syst Pharm.* 2004;61:2297-2310.

3. Shah ND, Vermeulen LC, Santell JP, Hunkler RJ, Hontz K. Projecting future drug expenditures-2002. *Am J Health Syst Pharm.* 2002;59:131-142.

4. Pierpaoli PG. The rising cost of pharmaceuticals: a director of pharmacy's perspective. *Am J Hosp Pharm.* 1993;50:S6-S8.

5. Weber RJ, Skledar SJ, Sirianni CR, Frank S, Yourich B, Martinelli B. The impact of hospital pharmacist and technician teams on mediation process quality and nurse satisfaction. *Hosp Pharm.* 2004;39:1169-1176.

6. Hicks RW, Santell JP, Cousins DD, Williams RL. *MEDMARX 5th Anniversary Data Report: A Chartbook of 2003 Findings and Trends,* 1999-2003. Rockville, MD: USP Center for Patient Safety; 2004. ∎

Core Competencies in Hospital Pharmacy: Medication Order Review

Robert W. Weber, MS, FASHP*

The next several *Director's Forum* articles will focus on core practices or competencies in hospital pharmacy practice. This series of articles will discuss the key fundamentals, resources, challenges, and opportunities associated with drug dispensing. Future core competency forums will include discussions on medication ordering, intravenous admixtures, data analysis, and regulatory requirements.

In *Director's Forum*, we hope to answer key questions that pharmacy directors face and provide others with information to foster growth in pharmacy leadership. The articles in this column will build on one another and, when put together, will serve as a "tool kit" to develop patient-centered pharmacy services in hospitals of all sizes. Examples of topics in future *Director's Forums* will include establishing clinical service priorities, justifying clinical pharmacist positions, implementing a patient safety program, and budgeting for patient-centered services.

The February *Director's Forum* in *Hospital Pharmacy* reviewed drug dispensing as the first core competency in establishing a patient-centered pharmacy service within hospitals. Core competencies of a health professional are those skill(s) that define their value in patient care. Medication order review by a licensed pharmacist is the second of the core competencies that are necessary in developing a patient-centered pharmacy service. The medication management standards from the Joint Commission on Accreditation of Healthcare Organizations (JCAHO) recommend that all hospitals develop a comprehensive system for medication order review by a licensed pharmacist (Standard MM.4.10).[1] In addition, the American Society of Health-System Pharmacists (ASHP) recommends medication or-

der review by a licensed pharmacist as a best practice in health-system pharmacy.[2]

Medication order review is a specific activity that involves a pharmacist comparing and evaluating a patient's medication order against certain guidelines to ensure that the medication order meets the standards of medical practice and therapeutic goals for the patient. This activity differs greatly from medication dispensing, and medication electronic order entry. Medication dispensing refers to a system of tracking and accountability of medication distribution within a hospital; medication electronic order entry is the activity of placing an order for a medication in a computerized prescriber order entry (CPOE) system, by a technician, pharmacist, physician, or other provider. While each of these activities are critical to the medication use process, medication order review is the initial quality check in providing for safe and effective medication use. The primary difference between these two functions is that medication order review requires pharmacists to practice evidence-based medicine, which is thought by most to be the application of the medical literature and specific patient characteristics to the overall care of a patient.[3]

Importantly, establishing your department as a patient-centered service requires that medication order

*Associate Professor and Department Chair, University of Pittsburgh School of Pharmacy, Executive Director of Pharmacy, University of Pittsburgh Medical Center, Pittsburgh, PA

review be conducted in a systematic and consistent manner, and viewed as an essential part of the pharmacy operations. For example, transcribing a patient's medication order into your pharmacy computer system without regard for specific patient characteristics and concurrent medications may result in a serious medication error, or less then optimal pharmacotherapy.

This article reviews the process of medication order review by hospital pharmacists. The goal of this article is to provide hospital pharmacists with an approach to effectively review medication orders to assure for optimal pharmacotherapy. The specific aims of this article are to: (1) describe the importance of the medication order review process; (2) describe specific medication order review activities; (3) present steps that hospital pharmacists can use when reviewing a medication order; and (4) describe a successful program that facilitates an effective medication order review process. Hopefully, the lessons learned from this article can be applied to make an immediate positive impact on striving for a patient-centered pharmacy service.

MEDICATION ORDER REVIEW AND PATIENT CARE

Medication order review has been identified as an important function since the early days of hospital pharmacy practice. Researchers have investigated the nature and type of pharmacist interventions as a result of medication order review—demonstrating the value of this process. In one of the earliest and more significant of studies, Lesar and colleagues analyzed prescribing errors in a teaching hospital.[4] Their review of medication orders showed that serious errors

in prescribing occurred in approximately two out of every 1,000 orders. These errors related to drug dosing, frequency, duration, and indication. If you extrapolate these findings to a busy hospital pharmacy department, which may process 2,000 to 3,000 medication orders daily, there is a risk of at least six serious errors occurring in the absence of pharmacist medication order review on a daily basis.

Pharmacy medication order review and intervention serves as an effective safety check.[5] Medication override is an example of a potentially unsafe practice, where a pharmacist dispenses medications prior to medication order review. Serious medication errors have resulted when drugs are inadvertently ordered and administered to a patient with a known allergy, and over sedation from higher-then-required opiate agonists in high-risk patients.

MEDICATION ORDER REVIEW ACTIVITIES

There are a variety of medication order review activities that have been shown to be successful in improving medication use. The fundamental steps in reviewing a medication order involve the following: (1) patient and physician identification; (2) drug selection; (3) dose, route, frequency, and duration; (4) monitoring and evaluating therapeutic outcomes and side effects. Importantly, hospital pharmacy departments have employed a variety of successful programs that use these key steps and include pharmacy coordinated dosing programs, therapeutic interchange, intravenous (IV)-to-oral route conversion, dosing in renal disease, standard IV fluid concentrations, electronically generated or pre-printed order sets, and physician order entry.

Fundamental Steps in Medication Order Review

Patient and Physician Identification

Proper patient identification is an important first step to reduce the incidence of medical errors. Examples of hospital-wide patient identification processes include "surgical pauses" to prevent wrong-side surgery, barcode medication administration, and administration of donated blood. Verifying that the medication order is written for the intended patient is as equally important as these safety programs. For example, there may be situations where patients have the same last name, or even the same name. Most hospitals use an addressograph plate to stamp blank medication order forms with a patient's name, room number, physician name, and insurance information. When medication orders are not stamped with an addressograph name and are instead written by the nursing and medical staff, illegible and incorrect information can be transmitted. Using an addressograph system or a computer program that downloads the patient's name and other information to a medication order sheet can prevent patient identification errors. A critical system break down in hospitals is the quality of the patient's name on the addressograph plate; medication errors can result from improper or illegible addressograph information. Hospitals are encouraged to review the quality of their addressograph information and provide for regular maintenance of addressograph equipment to prevent illegible patient information.

Identifying the physician that writes an order for a patient is also important in helping to effectively facilitate medication order processing time, particularly if the physician needs to be contacted to clarify information on the medication order. Illegible or unclear signatures of physicians contribute to this problem. To prevent unclear physician names, it is recommended that physicians print their names in block format and clearly print their contact number (eg, pager or phone number).

Drug Selection

The next fundamental step in medication order review is evaluating drug selection. The pharmacist can assess the proper drug selection by asking questions as follows: Is the drug product on the hospital's formulary of approved drugs? Is the use of the drug product restricted to specific medical specialty areas? Is the drug product approved for the indication for which it is prescribed? Is the drug product appropriate to treat the patient's medical condition? Are there cost considerations associated with a drug product? Does the drug interact with any other ordered medications or food?

Dose, Route, Frequency, and Duration

After the pharmacist has determined that drug product selection is appropriate for a patient, the next step is to determine whether the dose, frequency, and duration of therapy meets the needs of the patient. An example is a medication order for the surgical prophylactic use of antibiotics. An order that reads, "cefazolin 500 mg IV every 12 hours" in a patient with normal organ function is suspect, since the dose is lower than expected for surgical prophylaxis, and should always be prescribed with a stop date, usually 24 to 48 hours. Additionally, an order for "gentamicin 80 mg IV every 8 hours" in a frail 80-year-old female patient to treat a gram-negative urinary tract infection should be questioned since aminoglycosides in older patients may be toxic in dosing intervals less than 12 hours.

An important assessment of an ordered medication dosage is whether the ordered dosage form is available from the manufacturer. This can serve as an important safety check to prevent inadvertent overdosing. For example, It may be an indicator of a potential error, if an ordered dose involves using five vials of a given drug, when one vial is normally used. A simple review of the ordered medication route can involve assuring the medication is able to be administered by the prescribed route. For example, ordering a sustained-release drug product in a patient that cannot take medications orally should be a signal for pharmacist intervention. A final question to consider is whether the duration of the medication order is appropriate for a patient's medical condition.

Monitoring and Evaluating Therapeutic Outcomes and Side Effects

In some hospital pharmacies, after the drug is verified in the pharmacy's computer system and dispensed to the patient, the time and resources necessary to follow the outcomes of each patient's therapy are not available. However, given that limitation, hospital pharmacists can consider some simple activities that may provide for the effectiveness of pharmacotherapy. Analysis of returned regularly scheduled medications or the use of as needed medications (PRN), for example, is a simple way to assess outcomes and side effects. Medications may be returned for reasons to include lack of patient tolerance of the medication or

the dosage form. The excessive use of "as needed" medications may indicate treating a side effect (eg, PRN antiemetics or stool softeners) in response to drug therapy.

PROGRAMS THAT ENHANCE MEDICATION ORDER REVIEW

Detecting problems with drug selection, drug dosing, frequency and duration during medication order review can seem overwhelming for hospital pharmacists taking care of many patients in a hospital or nursing unit. There are tools available to assist pharmacists in the medication order review process, and these will be briefly reviewed here. However, these tools are no substitute for the application of basic pharmacy practice and principles of therapeutics by pharmacists to each medication order. A simple, proactive technique involves establishing a mental "checklist" that can be used when reviewing a medication order. Table 1 suggests items in the mental checklist and can be used to detect medication order problems.

Another example of tools for medication review is a comprehensive program developed at the University of Pittsburgh medical Center (UPMC), which combines evidence-based medicine with pharmacy operations to provide support to hospital pharmacists during the medication order review process.

UPMC Drug-Use and Disease-State Management Program

The Drug-Use and Disease-State Management (DUDSM) Program of UPMC applies a systematic approach to design multidisciplinary, evidence-based guidelines for drug use and the role of pharmacotherapy in disease management.[6] The DUDSM program

Table 1. Mental Checklist for the Medication Order Review Process

Can I clearly read the patient's name and other identifying information?
Does the patient have a "look alike" or "sound alike" name to my other patients?
Can I clearly read the physician's name and contact information?
Can I clearly read the drug name, strength, frequency, and duration?
Is the ordered medication available on our formulary? If not, what is the formulary alternative?
Is the medication order appropriate for the patient's medical condition?
Is the dosage, frequency, and duration appropriate, given the patient's medical condition and organ function?
Is the dosage available from the manufacturer, or does the dosage need to be compounded from multiple doses?
Can the prescribed route be administered safely by the nurse?
Are there side effects that I should tell the nurse and patient?

identifies therapeutic opportunities for optimizing drug use from analysis of high-volume drug use, cost, disease state, and resource utilization. Additionally, opportunities are identified from recently published literature, national and local adverse event, and medication error data. Guidelines for new therapeutic entities are created to set practice patterns as agents are approved for general marketing vs after practice patterns are established. Continuous quality improvement methods are used to design specific, directed plans of action for implementation of guidelines and monitoring of clinical, process, and economic outcomes. The DUDSM Program outcomes have been significant, improving drug-therapy prescribing and promoting medication safety.

The structure of the DUDSM program provides the pharmacy staff with guidelines for medication order review, with over 50 initiatives approved by the UPMC Pharmacy & Therapeutics Committee. Examples of these guidelines include therapeutic interchange, renal drug dosing, drug dosing in the elderly, antibiotic management, vaccination, patient-controlled analgesia therapy, anemia

management, sepsis treatment, blood factor product prescribing, and handling of non-FDA-approved indication for medications. **Table 2** lists examples of medication order review initiatives implemented through the DUDSM program.

The success of this program depends on the active involvement of the medical staff in reviewing and approving the evidence-based guidelines. The progress of the program is reported regularly at the UPMC medical staff executive committee as a strategy for continued emphasis of the pharmacy's patient-centered service. As discussed in the first article of the *Director's Forum* titled "Establishing a Patient-Centered Pharmacy Service" the pharmacy director's active participation with the hospital's medical executive committee is critical in establishing these key programs.

The DUDSM program applies a systematic approach to implementation of medication order review guidelines. First, an approved initiative is reviewed to determine the most effective way for implementation in the pharmacy staff. For example, identifying ways to alert the pharmacist of a specific initiative on order review

Table 2. Examples of Order Review Initiatives at the University of Pittsburgh Medical Center

Medication Order Review Activity (Drug or Disease State)	Type	Rationale
Meperidine	Patient safety	Meperidine neurotoxic metabolite
Promethazine	Patient safety	Over-sedation
Diphenhydramine (in the elderly)	Patient safety	Anticholinergic side effects, delirium, falls
Ketorolac (duration of therapy)	Patient safety	Gastrointestinal bleeding
Intravenous immune globulin	Drug shortage	National shortage; need to reserve for approved indications
Clostridium difficile management	Infection control	Identify proper treatment and reduce unnecessary antibiotic usage
Community-acquired pneumonia	Disease management	Center for Medicare and Medicaid Services and JCAHO indicator
Cefazolin	Therapeutic interchange	Automatic dosing at every 8 h (vs every 6 h)
Factor concentrate medication	Patient safety	Patient-specific dosing; high cost; high-error risk; potential for "off -label" usage

may be handled by adding information to the pharmacy computer system. Second, an educational program is developed to teach the pharmacists about the medication order review initiative, along with a "Frequently asked questions" sheet to assist the pharmacists during the course of their work. Third, the DUDSM program establishes a monitoring process that tracks the outcome of each initiative, and provides the pharmacy staff with feedback on the medication order review initiative. Importantly, this process solicits feedback from the pharmacy staff to improve the efficiency of implementing these initiatives.

Information Systems

The pharmacy computer system can be a tool to effective medication order review by providing a series of "alerts" or "rules" when certain medications are transcribed into the system. In addition, the pharmacy computer system can also link to other aspects of a patient's medical care (eg, lab, radiology, and microbiology reports) to provide the pharmacist with additional information for medication order review.

CPOE systems allow for physicians and authorized health professionals to electronically transcribe medication orders. While these systems have potential to improve patient safety and process efficiency, the pharmacist's role in medication order review is not clear. Most likely, the review of the order will require a greater knowledge by the pharmacist of therapeutic goals for the patient, requiring pharmacists to fundamentally change their roles in hospitals.

SUMMARY AND CONCLUSION

Medication order review is an important core competency for hospital pharmacists to apply in a comprehensive and systematic manner. Hospital pharmacy departments can implement an effective medication order review program through applying pharmacy best practices, and using tools including, but not limited to, the pharmacy information system, CPOE systems, and an evidence-based drug-use model.

REFERENCES

1. Joint Commission Resources: Medication Management. In: *2006 Hospital Accreditation Standards*. Oakbrook Terrace, IL: Joint Commission on Accreditation of Healthcare Organizations; 2006:217–236.

2. American Society of Health-System Pharmacists. *Best practices for hospital and health-system pharmacy.* Bethesda, MD: American Society of Health-System Pharmacists; 2005.

3. Sackett DL, Rosenberg WM, Gray JA, et al. Evidence-based medicine: what it is and what it isn't. *BMJ.* 1996;312:71–72.

4. Lesar TS, Briceland LL, Delcoure K, et al. Medication prescribing errors in a teaching hospital. *JAMA.* 1990; 263:2329–2334.

5. Cohen M. Pharmacists should review all nonurgent drug orders before administration. *Hosp Pharm.* 2000;35:1178–1179.

6. Skledar SJ, Hess MM. Implementation of a drug use and disease state management program. *Am J Health Syst Pharm.* 2000;57:S23–S29. ■

Drug Policy

Pharmacist Involvement in Order Set and Protocol Development

Tammy Cohen BS, PharmD, MS* and Michael Sanborn, MS, FASHP†

The *Director's Forum* series is written and edited by Michael Sanborn and Robert Weber and is designed to guide pharmacy leaders in establishing patient-centered services in hospitals and health systems. Another specific goal of this column is to address many of the key challenges that pharmacy directors face today while providing information to foster growth in pharmacy leadership and patient safety. This *Director's Forum* will highlight opportunities for the pharmacist to participate in standardized order set and protocol development.

Order sets are not a new concept and have been used for many years to simplify and standardize complex treatment regimens such as those used for chemotherapy and transplant patients.[1] The traditional goal behind their development is to standardize best practices and optimize patient care. Developed in the 1990s, disease-specific order sets were known by many names, including critical pathways and care maps. In 1995, Shane defined the purpose of these detailed treatment protocols as a means to "delineate the pharmacologic and nonpharmacologic therapies, interventions, activities, and outcomes expected throughout the patient's hospitalization, from before admission through discharge and, in some cases, afterward."[2]

Since that time, the benefits of standardized order set development have continued to gain recognition within hospitals and other health care organizations. Drivers such as The Joint Commission's Surgical Care Improvement Project (SCIP) core measure set have challenged hospitals to develop standardized methods to ensure high quality and efficient patient care for every hospitalized patient. Most hospitals currently have formalized, automatic treatment protocols for glucose control, pneumonia, ventilator management, and many other patient conditions. Detailed protocols that initiate treatment and monitoring parameters from preadmission through discharge have become commonplace in most hospitals. They allow hospitals to meet or exceed national standards for care, often achieving 100% compliance with requirements such as surgical site infection prevention, congestive heart failure guidelines, acute myocardial infarction core measures, and medication reconciliation. Order sets also facilitate the national effort to move towards an electronic health record—driven by computerized prescriber order entry (CPOE)—by simplifying the ordering process and allowing the quick and easy initiation of multiple evidence-based patient orders.

THE CASE FOR STANDARDIZED ORDER SETS

The implementation of order sets can be a polarizing issue among practicing clinicians. Some clinicians say that order sets encourage "cookbook" medicine, while other clinicians say that order sets are essential to keep up

*System Director of Clinical Pharmacy Services, Baylor Health Care System, Dallas, Texas; †Corporate Vice President, Baylor Health Care System, Dallas, Texas.

with the changing demands of practicing medicine and evidence-based care in the 21st century. While no 2 patients are exactly alike, the use of predetermined, standardized protocols and order sets can be valuable if developed and used appropriately.[3]

Order sets can be helpful in minimizing clinician reliance on memory for such tasks as dosing calculations, selecting the correct combination of agents (eg, antibiotics) and including tangential therapies such as venous thromboembolism (VTE) prophylaxis. Preprinted or computerized order sets help minimize transcription error that could result from poor handwriting. They are also helpful in highlighting deviations from the standard orders since alterations to the standard pre-approved orders would need to be crossed out and the nonstandard order would be manually entered. Even without CPOE, the use of preprinted order sets minimizes handwriting and draws attention to deviations from the general order set (eg, writing in a dosage adjustment for renal insufficiency).

Order sets encourage routines among clinicians that ensure all patients received the necessary treatment, at the right time. This can also ensure a consistent standard of care across the institution for the targeted patient population. Order sets can serve to help the prescriber include all necessary components of treatment while allowing the nurse, pharmacist, and other care providers to anticipate which treatments will be needed.

Additionally, order sets often include necessary treatments that are not considered as part of the core disease state. For example, a pneumonia order set can include orders for VTE prophylaxis and glucose control. They can also include various "as needed" (PRN) orders (such as medications for indigestion, insomnia, fever, or pain) that tend to be standard for most patients. Order sets can also invoke standing delegated medical orders (SDMOs) for anticipated episodic treatments such as electrolyte management or influenza immunization.

Formulary adherence can also be a benefit of order set development. Designing order sets to include only formulary agents not only supports the formulary process but also makes it easier for prescribers who must remain familiar with formularies at multiple facilities. Updating order sets as formulary items change ensures ongoing formulary adherence as well as serves as a real-time communication method for prescribers.

The Institute for Safe Medication Practices encourages the use of order sets to enhance patient safety for high-risk treatment areas/types such as patient controlled analgesia (PCA).[4] There are other opportunities for patient safety enhancements. For example, a nurse can utilize a preprinted hyperkalemia order set, contact the physician who initiates the order, and check the correct therapy option after reading it back. The availability of a preprinted form reduces the likelihood of inaccurately transcribing a dose or overlooking a portion of the order. These types of order sets can also include detailed monitoring parameters that set expectations for all clinicians involved in the patient's care.

Finally, order sets can serve to initiate comprehensive pharmacy services.[5] As an example, during the early phases of the order set development process within our health system, it became clear that some physicians assumed certain pharmacist interventions were automatic and others routinely ordered pharmacist monitoring to make sure that it occurred. At the time, pharmacists did not have approval for automatic adjustment of drug dosages based on renal insufficiency; it required a specific physician order or a call to the physician for approval. The order sets streamlined this process and formalized the pharmacist's role in monitoring patients and adjusting therapies. An order was included on the pneumonia order set for a pharmacist to adjust antibiotic doses as needed for renal function and routinely manage any medications needing pharmacokinetic monitoring. Subsequent order sets now have standing orders for pharmacists to make dosage adjustments to all medications as needed.

VALUE OF INVOLVING A PHARMACIST

Order sets can originate from a variety of sources. Some institutions subscribe to order set libraries provided by health care companies that develop standardized protocols based on available research (eg, ProVation order sets). Many hospitals use internal resources and multidisciplinary teams to create their own customized order sets. In either case, pharmacists are an essential part of the development process, due to their knowledge of medication therapy and detailed understanding of drug delivery. Beyond appropriate drug therapy selection, pharmacists can also offer a unique perspective over other health care providers. For example, pharmacists typically transcribe or verify orders in the pharmacy information system and, despite what may be initially ordered, convert the order to the appropriate product that is ultimately dispensed to the patient. Pharmacists,

therefore, can offer input on how the order should be written to ensure that it is complete, accurate, clinically appropriate, and complies with all the necessary standards, such as those from The Joint Commission. Pharmacists can also recommend necessary laboratory tests and appropriate monitoring parameters.

Including a pharmacist in the order set development process also allows for the upfront incorporation of regulatory and operational interventions, such as documenting the route of administration on all orders or including appropriate parameters and indications for PRN orders. Simple suggestions regarding this type of operational change can lead to significant efficiency improvements. As an example, the inclusion of saline flushes on an order set results in a specific order to be processed, which then allows the nurse to select the necessary flush from the patient's profile on the automated dispensing cabinet. This ultimately reduces over-ride transactions, which then makes the override reporting and analysis process less cumbersome. Pharmacists can also ensure that the doses and dosage forms on any type of order set are available and meet the required storage requirements. If it is a product that would need to be compounded in the pharmacy or if it requires refrigeration, this can be noted on the order set so that the nurse does not waste time looking for the product.

Pharmacists can also play a valuable role in helping an organization achieve the required core measures from the Centers of Medicare and Medicaid Services (CMS). For example, the pharmacist can offer antibiotic suggestions for patients that are undergoing surgery and are allergic to the preferred medication. They can also ensure that medications are ordered for the correct time and operationally allow the medication to be given over the correct amount of time (eg, allowing for a 60-minute infusion of a prophylactic dose of vancomycin prior to surgery). A pharmacist working on a multidisciplinary order set development team can help to determine which orders should be on the preoperative order set and which should be given in the operating room.

Pharmacists can also suggest which alerts can be hard coded on order sets to remind the prescriber or the nurse of various warnings such as "not to exceed 4 grams of acetaminophen in 24 hours" and "use with caution in patients with creatinine clearance less than 30 mL/min."

A central element of order set success is a focus on ongoing improvement. Whenever possible, collect patient data to measure patient outcomes. Pharmacists can play an integral role in determining appropriate data elements to be included in this evaluation, can assist in the data collection process, and should be involved in the analysis, education, and planning for subsequent protocol improvements.

For all of these reasons, pharmacy leadership is a critical element in any order set development effort. The pharmacy director must be focused and involved in all hospital initiatives that involve practice standardization. The participant in the order set development process may be the director or another pharmacist appointed to address a specialized area. Regardless, it is the director's responsibility to evaluate and identify appropriate membership and allocate any resources necessary for effective participation in the process. Active involvement in the development of protocols and order sets ensures that day-to-day pharmacist activities, the formulary process, and other department initiatives and priorities are progressively addressed.

ORDER SET DEVELOPMENT FOR THE BAYLOR HEALTH CARE SYSTEM (BHCS)

Several years ago, BHCS initiated a focused, multidisciplinary effort to standardize best care and focus on evidence-based practice. There are currently 28 standardized, comprehensive order sets in place across 13 hospitals; in total, there are over 60 sets developed and implemented. They include a variety of procedures and disease states such as labor and delivery, cesarean section, total hip and knee surgeries, ischemic stroke, hemorrhagic stroke, heart failure, and gastrointestinal hemorrhage. In some cases, order sets are in place for specific medications or drug classes, including drotrecogin alfa, heparin, insulin, and thrombolytics.

A critical element to the success of the program has been the team structure itself. The approval body consists of a steering committee that is primarily composed of physicians but also includes pharmacists, nurses, and other disciplines. Initial order set development is typically completed by a subgroup of experts in a particular specialty that is also multidisciplinary. Early on, it was readily apparent that one of the most valuable pieces of this process was the collaboration among health care professionals. For many of the specialty order set teams, this process was the first time that the physicians discussed differences in daily practices. Getting physicians together to discuss the differentiation among their own individual order sets allowed an exchange of ideas that resulted in a final product that was superior to any pre-existing document. Each order set required the inclusion of evidence-based medicine when literature was available and also incorporated operational practices to further support patient centered care.

As the system-wide standardization effort commenced, the terms "order set," "protocol," and "standing delegated medical order (SDMO)" were defined. For our health system, an order set is defined as a list of orders from a prescriber that requires a signature to implement. A protocol on the other hand, is a practitioner-approved defined practice that guides health care providers (eg, nurse, pharmacist) through a process such as managing electrolyte imbalance, glucose control, or pain management via a PCA device. Therefore, protocols can be ordered and initiated within an order set; for example, "Implement glucose control protocol" can be a line item on a postsurgical order set rather than requiring the entire protocol to be written out within every order set.

An SDMO is an order that can be initiated without a physician order in predefined urgent situations (eg, hyperkalemia, hypoglycemia). SDMOs require advance approval by the medical staff and apply to all patients and therefore, do not need to be written for each patient. For example, the nurse can order glucose-related labs and begin treatment as outlined in the SDMO for hypoglycemia prior to contacting the physician. This process has multiple benefits, the most important of which is that evidence-based treatment is initiated quickly and patient data are immediately collected to provide to the prescriber at the time of notification.

We found significant value in having pharmacists involved in the process to address operational concerns early on in the order set development process. We proactively addressed issues such as how orders for multiple pain medications should be handled and required standard concentrations for intravenous infusions. For our labor and delivery order sets, our group defined a standard concentration and fluid for oxytocin drips for all of our facilities based on literature and product stability. By working together, we were able to educate the physicians and nurses regarding oxytocin stability limitations. This project ultimately resulted in standardized oxytocin drip concentrations and diluents, which then allowed the product to be stocked on the unit making it readily available to the clinicians for urgent situations. The physicians have been supportive of pharmacist involvement in the process and the resulting collaboration. Since the process is being addressed through input from all disciplines, the focus is always on the patient.

One of the initial order sets implemented at BHCS was for community and hospital-acquired pneumonia. The order set is comprehensive and includes VTE prophylaxis, an antibiotic-selection algorithm, and patient education requirements, in addition to detailed orders for nursing, pharmacy laboratory, and respiratory care. Initially, pneumonia order set adoption across the system was slow and only 39% of patients were placed on the order set during the first 6 months of availability.

This slow adoption rate was frustrating but also provided our organization with an opportunity to compare patient outcomes between patients that were treated with the BHCS order set versus those who were not as well as those who used prescriber specific order sets. The results were compelling. Mortality, length of stay, readmission rates, and treatment costs were significantly reduced for patients in whom the BHCS order set was utilized. Performance on The Joint Commission's pneumonia core measures was also statistically higher in patients who received the BHCS order set.

Paradoxically, order set use across the system was lowest for patients with the highest risk of mortality, yet the documented mortality benefit was greatest for patients with the highest risk of mortality. The general perception was that sicker patients required more customized (non-standardized) treatment, when in fact, those high-risk patients actually experienced the most benefit from the pneumonia order set. As education and communication with the medical staff regarding these patient outcomes increased, more physicians began using the order set. Currently, over 85% of pneumonia patients throughout the Baylor system are now on the BHCS order set. Based on data from nearly 4,000 patients, it is estimated that for every 31 patients treated with BHCS order set, one patient death is prevented.

CONCLUSION

Order sets have many potential benefits if correctly developed and implemented. A multidisciplinary approach is essential to ensure incorporation of evidence-based care in a manner that is operationally feasible. The pharmacist provides a unique and important perspective in this process and is an essential contributor to effective order set development that improves patient outcomes. Every pharmacy director should ensure their department is well represented in all order standardization efforts.

REFERENCES

1. Beckwith MC, Tyler LS. Preventing Medication Errors with Antineoplastic Agents, Part 2. *Hosp Pharm.* 2000; 35(7):732-749.

2. Shane R. Critical pathways. Take the first step on the critical pathway. *Am J Health Syst Pharm.* 1995;52(10): 1051–1053.

3. Bobb AM, Payne TH, Gross PA. *J Am Med Inform Assoc.* 2007;14(1):41-47.

4. Medication Safety Alert. Institute for Safe Medication Practices Newsletter, July 24, 2003.

5. Robke JT, Woods M, Heitz S. Pharmacist impact on pneumococcal vaccination rates through incorporation of immunization assessment into critical pathways in an acute care setting. *Hosp Pharm.* 2002;37(10):1050-1054. ∎

Strategies for Effective Medication Use Evaluations

Nickie D. Greer, PharmD, BCPS* and Michael Sanborn, MS, FASHP†

The *Director's Forum* series is written and edited by Michael Sanborn and Robert Weber and is designed to guide pharmacy leaders in establishing patient-centered services in hospitals and health systems. Another specific goal of this column is to address many of the key challenges that pharmacy directors face today, while providing information to foster growth in pharmacy leadership and patient safety. This month's *Forum* focuses on specific ways to improve the medication-use evaluation process.

As mentioned in previous *Director's Forum* articles, the medication use evaluation (MUE) process is an essential type of surveillance program designed to analyze and improve medication use throughout the hospital and, ultimately, improve patient care.[1,2] MUE initiatives are typically under the purview of the Pharmacy and Therapeutics (P&T) Committee, but are almost always initiated, designed, and conducted by the department of pharmacy. Most hospital pharmacies have ongoing therapeutic drug monitoring programs in place[3]; however, the role of the MUE allows for a more detailed analysis of medication use within hospitals.

MUEs should be strategic in nature and focus on medication use issues within the organization that may require improvement. At least annually, it is important to develop and update a list of proposed evaluations that can be used as a working document to guide MUE efforts. Because an MUE is an observational analysis, it is typically only the initial step in medication use improvement. Occasionally, an MUE will demonstrate complete and appropriate use and monitoring of a particular agent. Typically, however, an MUE will uncover multiple areas for improvement, which can lead to the further development of guidelines, protocols, restrictions, educational programs, or other techniques to improve the medication use process.

An MUE can be prospective, concurrent, or retrospective in nature.[4,5] A prospective MUE evaluates a patient's new or proposed drug therapy prior to the drug reaching the patient. This is most often accomplished via a drug regimen review performed by a pharmacist during their daily activities. A concurrent MUE evaluates and monitors drug therapy during the treatment course and allows the pharmacist to modify the treatment course if necessary. A retrospective MUE evaluates drug therapy after a patient has already completed treatment and is most often accomplished by a pharmacist review of charts or electronic records. This type of MUE is the more traditional form that is reported to the P&T Committee.

MEDICATION SELECTION

A medication may be selected for MUE for a myriad of reasons.[4,5] Some medications, such as antibiotics, are chosen because they are prescribed for a large number of patients in the institution. Others, such as warfarin

*Clinical Pharmacist—Internal Medicine/Drug Information, Baylor University Medical Center, Dallas, TX; †Corporate Director Pharmacy, Baylor Health Care System, example, Rudisill and colleagues Dallas, TX.

or other anticoagulants, are chosen because of potential or reported adverse reactions or drug interactions. Medications may be chosen because of their narrow therapeutic index or when prescribing requirements are complex (such as agents requiring a loading dose). Medications are also selected when appropriate use of the drug is necessary for optimal patient care and inappropriate use could have a negative impact on outcomes. An example of this would be an evaluation of certain antibiotics to ensure that the agents are used appropriately to avoid the development of resistant organisms. Finally, medications may be chosen for evaluation due to their high cost to the institution. Table 1 summarizes the rationale and measurement parameters for several recent MUEs conducted at Baylor University Medical Center.

It is important to match the appropriate type of MUE to the medication(s) being evaluated. For example, Rudisill and colleagues (2006) recently published the results of a prospective MUE that studied the use of factor VIIa (recombinant).[6] The stated goal of their analysis was to maximize clinical benefits while minimizing risks and expenditures in order to prepare guidelines for use and develop an implementation process for these guidelines. The prospective design allowed the authors to critically evaluate the prescribing, monitoring, and outcome for each patient during therapy, which potentially allowed for the ongoing collection of parameters that may not otherwise be documented in the patient's chart.

DEVISING AN EFFECTIVE MUE

The objective of the MUE must first be defined before an effective evaluation can be performed.[5] Some evaluations focus on identifying or preventing adverse events and other medication-related problems, whereas some are designed to identify over-or under-utilization of an agent in the institution. Others may focus on evaluating the appropriateness of drug therapy when used for a particular disease process or drug protocol. Finally, an MUE may be developed to evaluate the appropriateness of the overall treatment of a particular disease state, patient population, or guideline adherence. From these types of evaluations, opportunities for education, standardization, and cost-minimization can then be identified.

Once the objective of the MUE is determined, criteria for optimal use of the medication or optimal treatment of the disease state must be established.[4,5,7] These criteria should be evi-

Table 1. Recent Medication Use Evaluations at Baylor University Medical Center

Drug/Class/Disease State	Parameter(s) Measured	Rationale
Insulin infusion	Efficacy, adherence	New protocol
Fondaparinux	Indications, patient safety, monitoring	High risk, low use
Broad-spectrum antibiotics	Empiric use, streamlining	High use
Pharmacokinetics protocol	Labs, consistency, outcomes	Policy adherence
HCAP/VAP[a]	Guideline adherence, outcomes	High antibiotic use
Naloxone	Indications, dosing, safety	High risk
Modafinil	Indications, dosing, monitoring	Off-label use

[a]HCAP/VAP = health care-associated pneumonia/ventilator-associated pneumonia.

dence based and should also include safety, monitoring, and patient outcome data. For example, if a particular antibiotic is being evaluated, the criteria might include the following: appropriate indications for use, including recommendations from treatment guidelines and Food and Drug Administration (FDA)-approved indications; appropriate dosages based on indication; appropriate dosage adjustments for organ dysfunction; monitoring parameters such as white blood cell count with differential, temperature, and other laboratory tests that are recommended by the manufacturer; adverse effect data; and outcome measures such as organism eradication or lack of efficacy. On the other hand, if the treatment of pneumonia is being evaluated, the criteria should be based on compliance with recommended treatment guidelines rather than focused on one particular medication.

The next step in the MUE process is the collection of data.[5,7] Once criteria are developed, a data collection form can be designed. These forms should include all the information stated in the predetermined criteria formatted in an easy-to-document manner. They may include checklists, "yes/no" questions, and tables to prompt entry of certain information. Once a data collection form is created, patients receiving the target medication or who are being treated for the studied disease can be identified via computer-generated lists. If the MUE is prospective or concurrent, the data collection form is filled out when a patient is initiated on a certain agent or diagnosed with a disease state as well as followed throughout the treatment course. If the MUE is retrospective, charts or electronic medical records

are pulled and the data collection form is completed after the patient is discharged (or no longer on the medication). When a retrospective MUE is performed, data may often be incomplete in the chart; for this reason, a prospective or concurrent MUE is generally preferred.

Once the data are collected, they must be analyzed.[5,7] The actual usage of the agent or treatment of the disease state must be compared with the approved criteria for use. If the criteria are not followed, it must be determined if the deviations are logical and expected based on the particular situations. Once this is determined, patterns of inappropriate use or treatment may be determined. Dosing, adverse events, monitoring, and outcomes are also compared with the criteria and opportunities for improvement are noted. Additional external data can also be included to augment the analysis, such as a summary of common prescribers by service line, comparison data published from outside sources, and/or a detailed purchase history for the studied agent. These results should be shared with the most common prescribers, as well as the P&T committee.

Because an MUE is merely an observation, the next important step is to intervene where areas for improvement are identified.[4,5,7] Drug-use guidelines may be developed to assist physicians and others in using the agent more appropriately. Guidelines generally outline the appropriate indications for use of an agent as well as appropriate dosing and monitoring parameters. Education may be done one-on-one with the prescriber or per presentations or newsletters. Pharmacists should also be educated on the appropriate use of the agent so interventions can be made when guidelines or prescribing recommendations are not being followed. Pharmacy information systems may be altered to notify pharmacists when a drug interaction exists or when an inappropriate dose has been prescribed. Agents may also be restricted to particular groups of physicians with more experience using the agent. Protocols and order sets may also be developed to assist health care workers with following treatment guidelines for particular disease states.

Once changes are implemented, a repeat evaluation should be done to evaluate the success of the interventions.[5,7] Steps should be taken to intervene when new areas for improvement are identified. Previously implemented interventions should be evaluated when improvements are not seen and new interventions should be made when necessary. For complex or high-risk medication-use issues, it may be necessary to conduct an MUE on a repeated basis to ensure continuous adherence to established guidelines and appropriate use.

In a recent example of MUE application and reassessment, Williams (2007) analyzed the use of parenteral nutrition (PN) in a 324-bed facility that did not have a formal nutritional support team.[8] The MUE found significant opportunities for improvement with serum electrolyte management, managing the frequency of hyperglycemia, meeting daily protein and caloric needs, as well as other patient monitoring requirements. PN waste was also monitored and found to be significant, primarily due to issues surrounding the standard cut-off order-time requirement. In addition to prescriber education, numerous enhancements to the prescribing, compounding and PN procedures were made. A follow-up analysis indicated an increase in the use of the pharmacist PN consult service, an improvement in the deficiencies identified, and a decrease in PN waste. Further opportunities were identified—such as compliance with safe practice guidelines—and efforts are underway to further improve PN practices.

ADDITIONAL CONSIDERATIONS

The MUE process is essential but may require a considerable amount of time, clinical expertise, and resources to be effective. There are several strategies that can be employed to improve the effectiveness and efficiency of the MUE process. For example, once an appropriate data collection form is devised, pharmacy students or technicians can be used to assist with data collection. Involving pharmacist staff and residents in the drug selection and MUE process is an effective means to complete multiple projects throughout the year. If clinical opinions and analysis are required beyond the scope of available pharmacy resources, it can be helpful to enlist physician specialists within the organization to assist with the evaluation. This can also add credibility to the MUE results.

There is some limited evidence to suggest that the reliability of MUE results can be negatively affected by the use of multiple individuals performing collection and analysis of on these data.[9] During the MUE design process, it is important to consider opportunities where subjective data collection can occur and to develop objective criteria that do not require interpretation by the person collecting data. When this level of objectivity is not possible, consideration should be given to using a single person to collect data or, ideally, using 2 separate evaluators whose findings are compared and then adjudicated by a third reviewer.

As electronic health records become more common, it is feasible to conduct large portions of an evaluation (or at least a preliminary analysis) without the traditional individual-chart review requirement. Examples of specific types of data and their potential use in the MUE process have been described.[10,11] For this type of analysis to be effective, the same process for drug selection, criteria development, and data analysis must be followed. For example, medication use summaries can be electronically generated and then analyzed against All Patient-Refined Diagnosis-Related Group (APR-DRG) information and their subclasses. Combined with other parameters documented in the patient's electronic record, this information can be used to construct a detailed analysis of the types and risk levels of patients in which the target medication is prescribed.

Finally, many hospitals have implemented critical pathways or detailed disease state algorithms to engender evidence-based treatment, improve patient outcomes, and promote multidisciplinary care. Oftentimes, an ongoing MUE and monitoring program can easily be incorporated into such pathways. The American Society of Health-System Pharmacists has developed guidelines on the pharmacist's role in such efforts.[12]

CONCLUSION

In summary, MUE is a performance improvement methodology that should focus on evaluating and improving medication-use processes with the goal of optimal patient outcomes.[5] Strategic selection of medications to be evaluated, as well as effective MUE design, data analysis, and follow-through are essential to achieving this goal.

REFERENCES

1. Weber RJ. Strategies for developing clinical services—advanced practice programs. *Hosp Pharm.* 2006;41(10):986-992.

2. Sanborn MD. Getting the most out of your pharmacy and therapeutics committee. *Hosp Pharm.* 2007;42:1077-1080.

3. Pedersen CA, Schneider PJ, Scheckelhoff DJ. ASHP national survey of pharmacy practice in hospital settings: monitoring and patient education—2003. *Am J Health Syst Pharm.* 2004;61:457-471.

4. Academy of Managed Care Pharmacy. *Concepts in Managed Care Pharmacy Series: Drug Use Evaluation.* http://www.amcp.org/amcp.ark?p=AAAC630C. Accessed October 17, 2007.

5. Phillips MS, Gayman JE, Todd MW. ASHP guidelines on medication-use evaluation. *Am J Health Syst Pharm.* 1996;53(16):1953-1955.

6. Rudisill CN, Hockman RH, DeGregory KA, Mutnick AH, Macik BG. Implementing guidelines for the institutional use of factor VIIa (recombinant): a multidisciplinary solution. *Am J Health Syst Pharm.* 2006; 63(17):1641-1646.

7. American Society of Hospital Pharmacists. ASHP guidelines on formulary system management. *Am J Hosp Pharm.* 1992;49(3):648-652.

8. Williams NT. Evaluation of parenteral nutrition management in a hospital without a formal nutrition support team. *Hosp Pharm.* 2007;42(10):921-930.

9. Shelton PS, Hanlon JT, Landsman PB, et al. Reliability of drug utilization evaluation as an assessment of medication appropriateness. *Ann Pharmacother.* 1997;31(5):533-540.

10. Pizzi LT, Howell JB, Deshmukh A, Cohen H, Nash DB. Clinical information management systems: an emerging data technology for inpatient pharmacies. *Am J Health Syst Pharm.* 2004;61(1):76-81.

11. Sanchez LA, Lee JT. Applied pharmacoeconomics: modeling data from internal and external sources. *Am J Health Syst Pharm.* 2000;57(2):146-155.

12. American Society of Health-System Pharmacists. ASHP guidelines on the pharmacist's role in the development, implementation, and assessment of critical pathways. *Am J Health Syst Pharm.* 2004;61(9):939-945. ∎

Getting the Most Out of Your Pharmacy and Therapeutics Committee

Michael Sanborn, MS, FASHP[*]

The *Director's Forum* series is written and edited by Michael Sanborn and Robert Weber and is designed to guide pharmacy leaders in establishing patient-centered services in hospitals and health systems. Another specific goal of this column is to address many of the key challenges that pharmacy directors face today, while providing information to foster growth in pharmacy leadership and patient safety. This month's *Forum* focuses on the Pharmacy and Therapeutics Committee and discusses essential functions and ways to maximize committee effectiveness.

A proactive Pharmacy and Therapeutics (P&T) Committee is essential to the goal of providing patients with the safest and most effective medication therapy possible. Nearly all hospitals (almost 98%)[1] in the United States have a functioning P&T Committee, and this institution is fundamental to hospital governance. Despite the universal acceptance of the P&T Committee, it is important for pharmacy directors to regularly reassess the overall structure, function, and membership of this influential committee—at least on an annual basis.

For the purposes of this article, a good working definition of a P&T Committee is: a body of individuals consisting of physicians, pharmacists, nurses, and other health care professionals appointed by the health care organization to oversee issues related to medication use. The P&T Committee develops and approves policies regarding the evaluation, selection, procurement, distribution, and use of pharmaceuticals with an emphasis on efficacy, safety, and cost effectiveness. This article will review the important functions of the committee, structure, membership, and strategies for a successful meeting.

IMPORTANT FUNCTIONS OF THE P&T

When asked to describe the purpose of a hospital P&T Committee, many pharmacists initially think of establishing and maintaining a drug formulary as the main role. In fact, the Conditions of Participation for Hospitals, established by the Centers for Medicare and Medicaid Services' (CMS) Department of Health and Human Services, states that "a formulary system must be established by the medical staff to assure quality pharmaceuticals at reasonable costs."[2] While not specifically required by CMS, in most hospitals, it is the P&T Committee that fulfills this requirement. Formulary management is an extensive, complex process beyond the scope of this article; however, 3 instructive references on this topic are the guidelines and technical assistance bulletins published by the American Society of Health-System Pharmacists.[3–5]

While formulary management is a critical element of any effective P&T Committee, there are many other important responsibilities that are typically charged to this group. A signifi-

[*]Health System Pharmacy Director, Baylor Health Care System, Dallas, TX.

cant portion of many P&T meetings often encompasses development and discussion of medication-use policy. Because the membership of the committee is diverse and intentionally represents health care professionals involved in the medication-use process, the P&T Committee is typically the best suited group to fulfill this role. A primary committee charge should be to review and approve all policies and procedures relating to the appropriate use of drugs. Additionally, existing policies associated with medication use should be reviewed periodically by the P&T Committee.

Patient safety, especially as it relates to medication safety, is another central responsibility of an effective P&T Committee. The committee (or a subcommittee that reports directly to the P&T Committee) should be responsible for the review and analysis of all medication errors, errors associated with devices that deliver medications, pharmacist interventions, and adverse drug reactions.

Trends should be scrutinized in an effort to develop and implement safe practices. These efforts should be part of a larger medication-use quality improvement initiative monitored by the P&T Committee and designed to ensure safe and appropriate prescribing, distribution, and administration of medications throughout the facility.

Other important functions of the P&T Committee, beyond the traditional formulary role, include medication-use evaluations focused on analyzing and improving medication use with a particular agent or class of drugs. Another key role is education of other health care professionals regarding the use of medications as well as associated policies and procedures. Many P&T Committees also review

investigational drug studies after they have been approved by the Institutional Review Board. The committee can also be quite effective in the endorsement, design, and promotion of hospital-wide technology efforts, such as: bar-code medication administration, computerized provider order entry, pharmacy automation initiatives, or the selection of "smart" infusion pumps. Finally, the promotion of evidence-based medicine, clinical practice guidelines, and protocol development should be a fundamental function of the P&T Committee.

COMMITTEE STRUCTURE AND MEMBERSHIP

The medical staff structure within health systems can vary significantly from one organization to another. The P&T Committee should be a recognized medical staff committee, reporting directly to the Medical Board or Executive Committee of the Medical Staff. In some cases, the P&T Committee functions are encompassed by a broader medical staff committee that is focused upon patient care issues (often called a Policy and Quality Review Committee or Patient Care Monitoring Committee), and this type of structure can be equally effective as a separate committee. Regardless of the specific configuration of the committee, it is important that the P&T function be sanctioned as a medical-staff quality entity to assure that the information discussed is considered privileged and confidential.

With all of the functions typically assigned to the P&T Committee, meetings can easily become lengthy and overwhelming. To resolve this, many institutions employ subcommittees as a structural element to improve efficiency. These groups can meet in advance of the actual P&T meeting and are often focused on areas such as antimicrobials, medication safety, drug-use evaluation, pharmacoeconomics, or adverse drug reactions. Because they have a more focused agenda, these subcommittees have ample time to consider issues in more detail and can then present summaries and recommendations to the P&T Committee. This type of P&T substructure can be very effective in streamlining the actual P&T meeting, especially in large facilities.

Membership on the P&T Committee is critical to overall success, with the goal of assembling participative, knowledgeable, and influential members for each meeting. At a minimum, the physician membership should be representative of each of the major medical specialties within the hospital. Other important physician appointments to consider include an infectious disease physician, hospitalist, radiologist, and pathologist or microbiologist. Non-physician members should include a hospital administrator, at least 1 nursing representative, and of course, pharmacists. The pharmacy director most often serves as the secretary of the committee, and this role can be a voting or non-voting position. Additional health care professionals, such as respiratory therapists, can add significant value to the committee, and these individuals can either be standing members or can be asked to attend on an ad hoc basis. In some facilities, nutrition support is also part of the committee's charge, and appropriate representation for this function is essential.

In 1999, Mannebach and colleagues published the results of a survey regarding P&T Committee structure in large, academic, teaching facilities.[6]
While not applicable to all hospitals, their findings did include some interesting results. The committees met an average of 9.7 times per year, and consisted of an average of 20 members, more than 70% of whom were physicians. In 98.9% of the hospitals surveyed, the chair of the committee was a physician, and a pharmacist served as secretary on nearly 95% of the committees. Roughly 91% of members had voting privileges. Pharmacy responsibilities for the committee were significant and included preparation of the meeting agenda and supporting documents, generating meeting minutes, and monitoring formulary-control activities outside of the meetings. In this survey, 69% of hospitals had a formal therapeutic interchange program, which was substantially lower than the nearly 91% of hospitals reporting interchange programs in a more recent survey.[1]

Another consideration for large, multihospital systems is that of an overarching system P&T Committee. These types of committees can be very effective in setting the overall direction of system-wide medication-use initiatives. The structure and role of such a group can differ depending on the structure of the health system, the organization of the system's medical staff boards, and even legal issues surrounding facility ownership. At the most consolidated level, a system P&T Committee consists of representative membership from each of the system's facilities. Some systems have developed a model, wherein the system committee serves more of an advisory role to each of the system's individual facility P&T Committees.

Over the last 2 years, the Baylor Health Care System (BHCS) has developed this concept of a P&T Advisory Board, which meets quarterly to discuss system programs and issues. The BHCS Board membership is made up of the physician P&T chairs and directors of pharmacy from each facility as well as administrative and nursing representatives. This structure has been successful because it allows each facility to maintain its own autonomy at the hospital level, yet it aligns efforts and pools resources for major initiatives (eg, formulary selection, protocol development, patient safety efforts, technology evaluation).

STRATEGIES FOR A SUCCESSFUL P&T MEETING

There are a variety of methods that pharmacy directors can use to improve the effectiveness of the overall P&T Committee function. Many of these tactics apply to any prominent hospital committee meeting, but some are specific to the P&T role. These strategies can have a significant impact on attendance, meeting efficiency, and ultimately the outcome of committee decisions.

Member attendance at each meeting is always important. A quorum is necessary to conduct committee business, and poor participation can lead to committee actions that are not completely vetted or are poorly received. One of the most effective ways to encourage consistent member participation is to make sure committee activities are substantial and influential to patient care. Agenda management and advance planning is very important. There are always agenda items that may seem rather mundane to some members, but an essential part of agenda planning is to balance these topics with other subjects that are challenging, controversial, or might otherwise elicit more passionate

responses from the membership. The meeting time should also match times that are convenient for the majority of members, and it is often helpful to provide a meal—especially if the meeting time corresponds with breakfast, lunch, or dinner.

The committee should be run formally, following *Robert's Revised Rules of Order*.[7] Agendas should be sent out well in advance, and members should be contacted 1 or 2 days prior to the meeting to confirm attendance. The attendance of each member should be monitored, and those who do not attend regularly should be replaced by members who will commit to regular participation. Oftentimes, meeting attendance by physician members must be reported to the Executive Committee of the medical staff and may even be used in physician credentialing. Agendas should be well organized and follow major thematic headings, such as formulary review, drug-use evaluation, and medication safety. Significant effort should be placed on including necessary background information and data for each agenda item in the meeting packet.

Meeting with the P&T Chair in advance of the meeting is also a good practice. Any controversial or divisive topics should be thoroughly discussed. Goals for each agenda item should be reviewed, and it should be clear which agenda items require a vote and which are for informational purposes or discussion only. It is often helpful to identify members who might not support a particular initiative in advance of the meeting and schedule a discussion with them to review concerns. This type of meeting "prework" can prevent surprises and improve opportunities for program success.

Choosing P&T members should be a judicious process. Typically, membership is appointed by the medical staff leadership, and the chairperson and secretary should review and submit a list of recommended participants annually. The ideal members are those who are recognized and influential within their respective discipline and who are also willing to be a participative member of the group. Physician members should generally have an active practice within the hospital. Incorporating nonmember physicians on an ad hoc basis is also worth consideration, especially for issues where the committee is lacking expertise. A number of P&T committees also require guest attendance of physicians that request items for formulary consideration.

Many institutions now encourage some level of voluntary or mandatory disclosure statements and ask members to recuse themselves from voting when a conflict of interest may exist. As many as 50% of facilities require some level of reporting of industry relationships, such as research funding from outside companies, participation in advisory boards, speakers bureaus, or stock ownership beyond that of traditional mutual funds.[6]

SUMMARY

The P&T Committee can be described as the engine that drives safe and effective medication use throughout the institution. Progressive P&T action can have a major impact on patient care, health care delivery, cost of care, as well as breadth of services provided by the pharmacy department. Leadership on behalf of the pharmacy director is critical to maximize the productivity and efficiency of the P&T Committee.

REFERENCES

1. Pedersen CA, Schneider PJ, Scheckelhoff DJ. ASHP national survey of pharmacy practice in hospital settings: prescribing and transcribing—2004. *Am J Health Syst Pharm.* 2005; 62(4):378-390.

2. Conditions of participation: Pharmaceutical services. Code of Federal Regulations, Title 42, Volume 3, Section 482.25. Revised as of October 1, 2004. http://a257.g.akamaitech.net/7/257/2422/12feb20041500/edocket.access.gpo.gov/cfr_2004/octqtr/pdf/42cfr482.25.pdf. Accessed September 11, 2007.

3. American Society of Hospital Pharmacists. ASHP guidelines on formulary system management. *Am J Hosp Pharm.* 1992;49(3):648–652.

4. American Society of Hospital Pharmacists. ASHP technical assistance bulletin on drug formularies. *Am J Hosp Pharm.* 1991;48:791–793.

5. American Society of Hospital Pharmacists. ASHP technical assistance bulletin on the evaluation of drugs for formularies. *Am J Hosp Pharm.* 1988;45:386–387.

6. Mannebach MA, Ascione FJ, Gaither CA, Bagozzi RP, Cohen IA, Ryan ML. Activities, functions, and structure of pharmacy and therapeutics committees in large teaching hospitals. *Am J Health Syst Pharm.* 1999; 56(7):622-628.

7. Robert HM. *Robert's Rules of Order: Newly Revised.* 10th ed. Uhrichsville, OH: Barbour and Company; 1989. ∎

Human Resources Management

Human Resources Management for the Pharmacy Director

Robert J. Weber, MS, FASHP*

This article of the *Director's Forum* provides hospital pharmacy directors with an introduction to the essential human resources skills of behavioral interviewing and performance management. While patients are a pharmacy department's most valued asset, the staff that care for those patients are critical to a patient-centered pharmacy service. Hospital pharmacy directors must practice effective human resource management to effectively recruit and retain a highly qualified and professionally satisfied staff.

The *Director's Forum* provides hospital pharmacy directors and managers with practical tips and suggestions in developing a patient-centered pharmacy service. Past articles of the *Director's Forum* stressed that a hospital pharmacy's most important assets are patients, with all focus and programs centered on meeting patient needs and providing optimal pharmaceutical care.

Central to meeting patient needs are the employees of the pharmacy. Their functions are critical to providing the necessary patient-centered care. Every member of the pharmacy plays a vital role in providing patient-centered care; these include, for example, the IV room technician who prepares the life-saving chemotherapy; the inventory pharmacist who assures there are no shortages and "stock outs;" the director who develops a strategy to keep the department vital and functioning, and the clinical pharmacist who adjusts a patient's pain medication to prevent a medication error. The efforts of these staff and others must function collaboratively and without disruption to provide a comprehensive patient-centered pharmacy services. Maintaining a satisfied and professionally fulfilled staff requires knowledge and expertise in human resources management as well as the ability to apply this knowledge to solving problems in employee relations.

Failing to effectively manage human resources may impact the operations, quality, and finances of the pharmacy department. Excessive employee turnover results in poor continuity of services and increased costs of training new employees. New employees usually require additional time to develop workplace relationships to integrate themselves into the patient care team, particularly with the nursing staff. As a result, a communication gap may exist between pharmacy and nursing in departments with a high turnover rate that can disrupt the efficient processing of care. The University of Pittsburgh Medical Center estimates that it costs the institution approximately $65,000 to hire and train a pharmacist, regardless of their experience. These facts, combined with a continued pharmacist shortage places greater importance on effective management of human resources.[1]

Most employees change jobs due to their perception of how they are treated by their supervisor; particularly if their supervisor does not provide

*Associate Professor and Chair, University of Pittsburgh School of Pharmacy, Executive Director of Pharmacy, University of Pittsburgh Medical Center, Pittsburgh, PA.

them with opportunities for professional satisfaction. Specifically, employee satisfaction is directly related to the supervisor's performance management skills including the manager's ability to consistently and effectively manage daily workflow.

Despite the best efforts of managers, employees may become frustrated with their positions as the job may not be the "right fit" for them. This is most likely due to a poor interviewing process; one that does not assess the employee skills and attitudes that affect their job performance. The following case example illustrates this concept.

A 27-year-old male pharmacist is hired to work the night shift (7 day on and 7 day off schedule) in a busy academic medical center. The pharmacist was hired from a smaller hospital where he worked "solo" on the evening shift. The pharmacist interviewed for 1 hour with the director of pharmacy, the pharmacy manager and the human resources liaison to the pharmacy. After an acceptable orientation period, the pharmacist is placed in the night shift rotation; within 2 to 3 weeks of their starting the rotation, coworkers begin to complain about the pharmacist, bringing these complaints to the pharmacy manager. Coworkers report the pharmacist "snapping" at nurses and coworkers, complaining about the volume of work, and not communicating general workflow processes. These reports prompt a meeting with the night pharmacist and the pharmacy manager. During that discussion, the pharmacist is anxious, states that there are "too many things going on" in the pharmacy during his shift, and he is not comfortable with his ability to perform his job. He also describes that coworkers are "not patient" with

him, and he has become frustrated with the work group. The pharmacy manager implements a performance development plan that includes additional training and follow-up on a daily basis with the night pharmacist. Despite this, the employee's ability to deal with the stressful workload causes him to return to his previous employer just 4 months after accepting the night pharmacist position.

This scenario is relatively common, and it is obvious that the pharmacist's ability to deal with stress was not a good "fit" for his night pharmacist position. The question should then be asked: how could this situation have been prevented? The answer: conducting an effective interview process. For example, the manager could have asked the following questions during the interview that may have signaled concern: Describe for me a situation where you could not keep up with the workload? How did you handle the situation? The night pharmacist position at our hospital requires you to enter approximately 400 orders into our computer system during the 12 hour shift. How many orders do you enter in your current job? How do you ask for help when the pharmacy gets busy? Gathering data from these answers in an effective way would have most likely uncovered this pharmacist's weakness in tolerating stressful and fast-paced work environments.

Most pharmacy directors do not have formal training in the principles and practices of human resources management. In fact, most learn "on the job" or through educational programs offered through their hospital's human resources department. This results in most directors failing to use effective communication styles nor to provide clear expectations and follow-up on performance issues with their employees.

Based on the previous case scenario and the author's personal experience, the two most critical human resource skills for a hospital pharmacy director to refine are behavioral interviewing and performance management. Behavioral interviewing chooses the right person for the job and performance management gets effective results from the pharmacy staff.

Behavioral interviewing is a technique that determines an employee's "approach" to their job, or behaviors they exhibit regularly in the workplace. These behaviors are often guided by the employee's personal style and abilities, and can positively and negatively influence the workgroup. Using the interview process to assess professional behaviors provides the pharmacy director with valuable information on predicting employee performance in the department.

Performance management involves establishing clear standards of performance and measurement for the workgroup, as well as a system for mutual feedback between the manager and the employer. The fundamental principle of effective performance management is that the leader of the workgroup must have a clear vision and strategy of department goals. These goals then must be translated into job functions that have established performance standards. Importantly, the performance standards should be applied consistently by the pharmacy director within the department.

The goal of this article is to provide hospital pharmacy directors with an introduction to the essential human resources skills of behavioral interviewing and performance manage-

ment. The specific aims of this article are to (1) describe how to properly interview a potential hospital pharmacist; (2) review the fundamentals of establishing a performance management system and process; and (3) describe how these two systems are interrelated to improve the operations of the pharmacy department. In addition to this article, references on interviewing and performance management may be used as a resource for the hospital pharmacy director.[2,3]

CONDUCTING A HOSPITAL PHARMACIST INTERVIEW

As stated in the introduction, the interview process is extremely valuable in helping the pharmacy director select a person who is the right "fit" for the organization's strategic plan. As stated earlier, an effective pharmacy interviewing process will always select the right person for the job. Interviewing a pharmacist involves (1) establishing a clear job description; (2) developing effective interview questions; (3) planning for and conducting the interview and (4) selecting the employee who meets the organization's needs.

Review and Update the Pharmacist Job Description and Performance Standards

A critical first step in the interview process is to update the pharmacist job description and performance standards to the current practice in the department. Pharmacists interviewing for a job expect the most current description on a desired position; a current description also demonstrates that the department continually assesses its services and performance. This may be done by reviewing the job description with the current pharmacy staff, and considering organizational changes that have impacted the pharmacist job function. A sample job description for a hospital pharmacist is included in **Table 1**. In addition, any performance standards related to the job functions should be updated as well. **Table 2** lists a sample of performance standards for a hospital pharmacist.

Establish the Interview Questions

The interview questions should be geared to assessing a pharmacist's technical proficiency and their professional behaviors. Technical proficiency is assessed by reviewing the resume, documenting licensure and certification, and directing questions regarding

Table 1. Sample Job Description for a Hospital Pharmacist

Job Function

Reviews medication orders and assures for safe and effective indication, dose, route, and scheduled administration.

Manages drug therapy and administers injectable medications according to protocol.

Prepares and dispenses medications in accordance with professional practice guidelines, state pharmacy laws, and regulatory standards.

Actively participates in medication safety programs. Active participation means identifying opportunities to improve safety (reporting errors and adverse drug events), and implementing system-based changes as a result of those opportunities.

Educates health care professionals and patients on the safe and effective use of medication. This education may be informal (eg, patient care rounds) as a staff development educational program, or as part of the hospital's interdisciplinary education program.

Mentors pharmacy students in applicable educational experiential training programs.

Serves as a role model of customer service by responding constructively to the needs of hospital staff. Responding constructively means using a respectful communication style that is consistent with professional collaboration.

Table 2. Example of Performance Standards for a Hospital Pharmacist

Job Function	Performance Standard	Measure
Actively participates in medication patient safety programs	Completes nursing unit medication control checks for assigned unit by the 15th of each month	Meet standard = One to two exceptions
	Identifies medication errors and error-prone situations	Meet standard = Medication error reports are within ± 8% to 12% of the pharmacist departmental average
Reviews medication orders and assures for safe and effective indication, dose, route, and scheduled administration	Actively contacts physicians for problem medication orders and documents interventions as "near miss" medication errors	Meet standard = "Near miss" medication error reports are within ± 8% to 12% of the pharmacist departmental average
	Screens all patient orders for potential adverse drug reactions	Meet standard = Reported adverse drug reactions are within ± 8% to 12% of pharmacist departmental average
Provides health professional and patient education	Conducts nursing inservice education programs	Meet standard = Two to four nursing education programs presented yearly

experiences. To determine workplace behaviors, a series of questions that present case scenarios can elicit valuable information. The behaviors that predict a hospital pharmacists' success include (1) use of effective communication styles; (2) ability to effectively plan and organize work tasks; (3) high tolerance for dealing with work stress; and (4) sound judgment and decision-making skills. **Table 3** lists some sample questions to determine a potential candidate's display of these workplace behaviors. Importantly, all interview questions should be "open-ended" allowing the interviewer to gather as much information as possible from potential candidates. Questions that prompt only "Yes" and "No" answers are referred to as "closed" and do not offer valuable information on a potential job candidate.

Prepare for the Interview

Managers often do not adequately prepare for the interview and are not able to establish the "best picture" of the potential candidate. Minimum preparation time for an interview is approximately 60 minutes. The manager should review the resume and employment application very carefully, noting employment history and job references. The manager should prepare a file for each candidate that includes the resume and preinterview notes and questions. Adequately preparing for an interview also shows potential candidates that hiring decisions are very important to the department's success. The manager should also meet with staff involved in the interview to review the candidate's resume and to clarify interview questions. Finally, the manager should prepare an evaluation grid to be used by all involved in the interview. An example of an interview grid is included in **Table 4**.

Conduct the Interview and Take Detailed Notes

The interview should be conducted in a quiet place, with adequate time allowed for the interview. Effectively interviewing a pharmacist candidate often takes 3 to 4 hours; interviews of less then 1 hour are often not effective.

Table 3. Sample Interview Questions

Professional Behavior	Interview Question
Communication	How do you communicate medication order problems before your shift ends? Describe a scenario where a physician did not accept your medication recommendation. How did you handle it? How do you make your supervisor aware of potential improvements to the pharmacy service?
Planning and Organizing	Describe your typical day in the pharmacy? Describe a situation where you had more than one urgent patient medication issue? How did you prioritize your activities? Describe how you plan and organize the activities of technicians?
Stress Tolerance	How do you ask for help when you need it on the job? An ICU nurse "yells" at you when a medication is not available for one of her patients. How would you handle the situation?
Judgment and Decision-making	You receive an order for chemotherapy that is not written in accordance with a specific protocol. How would you handle the situation?

Table 4. Sample Interview Evaluation Form

Interview Candidates	#1	#2	#3
Technical Skills			
Medication order review, dispensing			
Medication patient safety			
Pharmacy operations			
Medication therapy management			
License/certification			
Behavioral Skills			
Communication			
Planning and Organizing			
Judgment			
Decision-making			
Stress tolerance			
Adaptability			

Rate both technical and behavioral components as follows:
1 = Below standards and expectations
2 = Meets standards and expectations
3 = Exceeds standards and expectations

Specific notes and/or comments:

Interviewers taking notes during an interview may alarm the interviewee. The interviewer should be clear with candidates they will be taking detailed notes in the interview in an effort to gain as much information about the potential candidate.

The goal of the interview is to elicit as much information from the candidate; as a result, the interviewer should not monopolize the interview conversation and allow the candidate adequate time to answer questions. In addition, the candidate should meet with a variety of staff including the pharmacy staff and other managers. It is important that all staff involved in the interview complete the interview evaluation grid. In most hospitals, the Human Resources department will require a copy of interview notes to comply with equal opportunity employment rules and regulations; the manager should provide the notes in an organized manner in order to provide easy reference in the future.

Select the Employee that Meets the Organization's Needs

After the interview, it is important to collect these data and information about the candidate as soon as possible and summarize the evaluation within 24 to 48 hours of the interview. This provides a "fresh" assessment of the candidate, and improves the efficiency of the interview process. When all of the candidates are interviewed, the manager should meet with the interview team to review the evaluation grids, and to make a final selection of the best candidate. The rating system as shown in **Table 4** can be used easily and allows for an effective comparison of potential candidates. The manager should rank the candidates from highest to lowest preference making the job offer in that order.

As an employee is selected, the manager should review the summary of the interview notes in detail to identify the pharmacist's strengths and weaknesses. As the pharmacist begins their employment, the manager should review these findings from the interview with the pharmacist and implement the necessary development plans to help the pharmacist to be successful in the department.

FUNDAMENTALS OF PERFORMANCE MANAGEMENT

This section describes some fundamental steps in developing a performance management system. Examples of job functions and performance standards are included in **Table 2**. This system involves establishing clear and measurable performance standards and a data collection system to track performance. An effective performance management system involves (1) clearly defining and communicating performance expectations; (2) developing a system for collecting measures of performance; and (3) providing frequent performance feedback. If performance management is done correctly, the yearly performance review is not a "surprise" to the employee since they are well aware of his or her performance throughout the evaluation year.

Defining and Communicating Performance Measures

As stated previously, effective interviewing requires defining job expectations. In a performance management system, clear and easily understood job functions and standards are essential. The pharmacy director should evaluate, on a yearly basis, the performance standards of their positions to assure they are still consistent with the pharmacy practice standards and the organization's strategic plan. The pharmacy staff should also be involved in this review to empower the staff to define

job functions. The pharmacy director should communicate the job functions and standards to staff; staff should be required to sign the job function and standard form to document their review. As newly hired employees begin their orientation, the job expectations and performance standards should be reviewed in detail with the employee to clearly understand the department's expectations.

Developing a Data Collection System for Performance Standards

The performance measures for jobs should be easily gathered from departmental essential data. For example, data on reported medication errors, pharmacy interventions, and adverse drug reactions can be collected from certain voluntary reporting systems. Additional data can be collected from department quality assurance systems, or by conducting observational audits of work processes.

Providing Frequent Feedback on Performance

The results of the employee's performance should be reviewed on a regular basis, and at a minimum of twice a year (during the annual review and in the middle of the review cycle). The review of performance information with employees may be more frequent if issues are identified. For example, frequent review of pharmacist interventions by the manager may demonstrate a need for review of specific concepts (eg, monitoring drugs for proper dosing in renal failure) to improve competency in various areas of practice. Performance data may also be used in a peer-review process to improve skills.

SUMMARY AND CONCLUSION

Behavioral interviewing and performance management systems should be designed as dynamic and interrelated systems. For example, as the job functions and standards of the pharmacy change, the technical and behavior skills necessary to achieve the organizations' mission will also change. As a result, the interview process must change accordingly to select candidates that best meet the mission of the organization.

Hospital pharmacy directors must practice effective human resources management as they recruit and retain a professionally motivated pharmacist staff. Behavioral interviewing chooses the right person for the job and performance management gets effective results from the pharmacy staff to meet the pharmacy's mission of developing patient-centered services.

REFERENCES

1. Knapp KK, Quist RM, Walton SM, Miller LM. Update on the pharmacist shortage: national and state data through 2003. *Am J Health Syst Pharm.* 2005;62:492-499.

2. Schmidt RA, West DJ Jr. Interviewing pharmacists for patient-focused health care organizations. *Pharm Pract Manag Q.* 1996;16:42-51.

3. Schumock GT, Leister KA, Edwards D, Wareham PS, Burkhart VD. Method for evaluating performance of clinical pharmacists. *Am J Hosp Pharm.* 1990;47:127-131. ∎

Innovative Roles for Pharmacy Technicians: Developing and Implementing a Unit-Based Clinical Support Pharmacy Technician Model

Scott M. Mark, PharmD, MS, MEd, FASHP, FACHE, FABC*;
Rafael Saenz, PharmD, MS†; Bryan E. Yourich, PharmD‡; and
Robert J. Weber, MS, FASHP§

The *Director's Forum* series is written and edited by Michael Sanborn and Robert Weber and is designed for guiding pharmacy leaders in establishing patient-centered services in hospitals and health systems. Another specific goal of this column is addressing many of the key challenges that pharmacy directors currently face while providing information that will foster growth in pharmacy leadership and patient safety. Developing innovative roles for pharmacy technicians promotes job growth, as well as staff satisfaction and retention. This *Director's Forum* article describes how patient-centered roles for technicians can be developed and implemented.

INTRODUCTION

The role of the pharmacy technician is vital in developing a patient-centered pharmacy service. In a pharmacy department, each member of the staff plays a role in promoting quality and efficiency. Examples of this include processing missing doses, providing patient medication education, and preparing life-saving chemotherapy. In previous *Director's Forum* columns, focus was placed on pharmaceutical care programs and their development, as well as on real-life examples of how these programs can be started. This article focuses on an innovative role for pharmacy techni-

cians in supporting a unit-based pharmaceutical care model.

Changing the role of the pharmacy technician is critical for a variety of reasons.[1] As a result, training programs for pharmacy technicians are becoming more sophisticated, with many community colleges offering an associate degree program in this field.[2] The focus of these programs is more patient centered; technician students are taught that their roles directly impact the quality of patient care. Subsequently, pharmacy technicians entering the workforce are motivated to obtain employment in pharmacy departments that provide a more patient-centered focus, and they have expectations for advancement and challenge. Failure to provide these progressive, challenging environments may decrease employee retention and satisfaction. Thus, changing the role of the pharmacy technician to one that is more patient centered will ultimately improve technician satisfaction.[3]

The goal of this article is to provide an overview of how the role of

---

*Director of Pharmacy, University of Pittsburgh Medical Center; Assistant Professor and Vice Chair, University of Pittsburgh School of Pharmacy; †Manager, Pharmacy, University of Pittsburgh Medical Center Presbyterian; ‡Director of Pharmacy, University of Pittsburgh Medical Center Shadyside; §Associate Professor and Chair, University of Pittsburgh School of Pharmacy; Chief Pharmacy Officer, University of Pittsburgh Medical Center, Pittsburgh, Pennsylvania.

a pharmacy technician can be incorporated into the pharmaceutical care process. Throughout the text, the patient care model at the University of Pittsburgh Medical Center (UPMC) is used as a guide for pharmacy directors in changing the role of the pharmacy technician.

BACKGROUND

The UPMC is a regional health system comprised of 19 unique hospitals covering a broad range of clinical care from pediatrics to geriatrics. The flagship institution of the system, UPMC Presbyterian Shadyside Hospital (UPMC PUH-SHY), is a 1,093-bed, tertiary-care academic medical center. It is consistently ranked among the best hospitals in the United States for its progressive clinical programs. The hospital is closely affiliated with the University of Pittsburgh, further strengthening the clinical and translational mission of both organizations.

The department of pharmacy at UPMC PUH-SHY provides pharmacy services to patient care departments throughout the hospital. The mission and vision of the pharmacy department is to provide patient-centered services to all patients. Historically, the department used a centralized pharmacy practice model to provide services. Orders for medications were transcribed onto an order form and sent to the central pharmacy for processing. Medication orders were subsequently manually entered into the computer information system (CIS) by pharmacists. Once processed through the CIS, a label was generated and a technician filled the medication order. Medications were then delivered on a routine schedule to medication cassettes on the nursing units. These functions were supported in part by

automation provided from a dispensing robot, a medication carousel, and automated dispensing cabinets located on the units.

Although efficient, the centralized model of pharmacy practice presents a unique set of challenges. In high-volume pharmacies, overall turnaround time (TAT) can be less than optimal. At UPMC Presbyterian, 12,000 doses are dispensed daily. With the centralized model, internal audits frequently demonstrated prolonged TAT during peak volumes, which, at times, would approach 4 hours. As a result, pharmacists were rushing to input orders and felt pressure when trying to fulfill patient care needs. The resulting stress manifested as failure in several critical service areas, such as poor telephone customer service, poor follow-through with drug-use-policy enforcement, and poor compliance with established medication-use safety practices, which resulted in errors.

In fall 2004, a unit-based practice model was developed and implemented to increase pharmacist presence on the units. The implementation followed an initial pilot study conducted in 2003 that showed promising results in terms of TAT and overall nursing satisfaction.[4] The outcome measures for the practice model included reducing TAT for medication orders; increasing visibility and responsiveness of staff pharmacists; and increasing nurse, patient, and physician satisfaction with pharmacy services. Full deployment of pharmacists to the nursing units began in a stepwise fashion in 2005. During the initial deployment, pharmacists were sent to the units without technician support. Although medication-order input time began decreasing on units that had pharmacists present, the program did

Table 1. Impact of Model on Turnaround Time

	PreModel[a]	Post-RPh– Only Model[a]	Post-RPh and Technician Model[a]
Order entry time (min)	76.9	63.4	15.4
Order fill time (min)	50.5	27.5	30
Total TAT	127	90.9	45.4

[a]All times are means; RPh = registered pharmacist; TAT = turnaround time.

not meet the intended targets, which included an initial entry into the computer in 15 minutes and an overall medication TAT of less than 60 minutes (see **Table 1**). Analysis revealed that although pharmacists were on the units, they often were called away from their offices to answer medication questions or to review charts. It was believed that the addition of a pharmacy technician who could partner with the pharmacist to ensure a constant presence in the unit-based office and to maintain order entry during the pharmacist's absence would further decrease TAT.

INITIAL BARRIERS TO IMPLEMENTING A UNIT-BASED PHARMACY MODEL: STAFFING

The solution to TAT issues at UPMC PUH-SHY seemed clear. The deployment of pharmacy technicians to the units would solve several of the order entry, fulfillment, and delivery issues, as well as assist pharmacists in providing patient-centered cognitive services. Given the significant changes in job duties that were being proposed, there were concerns regarding the organization's ability to recruit and train new staff. At the time, the department had a technician vacancy factor of 10 full-time equivalents (FTEs), and the initially proposed, unit-based rollout would require 5 FTEs to sufficiently support the units. As a result, the first major barrier to the development

and implementation of the unit-based pharmacy technician program was the challenge of balancing the implementation requirements with the existing operational needs.

DEVELOPING THE INFRASTRUCTURE FOR A UNIT-BASED PHARMACY MODEL
Workload Analysis

To determine the placement of the unit-based technicians, a workload and workflow analysis was conducted. The proper placement of technicians was critical for ensuring that the resulting outcome measures would improve. In addition, the proper distribution of personnel was vital for guaranteeing that support was provided to pharmacists in the areas most needed, which would result in the greatest patient-centered care. As a result of the assessment, one critical parameter implemented to ensure that personnel remained balanced—and therefore able to complete the expected tasks—was maintenance of ratios. Personnel assigned to critical care areas or intensive care units were given responsibility for 25 beds (25:1), and those assigned to general medicine units were given responsibility for 45 beds (45:1).

Defining Technician Responsibilities

To standardize responsibilities, all unit-based pharmacy teams performed the same basic functions regardless of the types of units on which they were based (critical care or general medicine). It was required that technicians process all orders at the start of their shifts and then prepare for patient care rounds by collecting predetermined patient information. While pharmacists were on rounds, it was their responsibility to process all oral medication orders that may have been received. Pharmacists would be alerted by phone or pager to any orders requiring immediate action. After rounding, pharmacists would verify any medication orders already entered, process any intravenous (IV) medication orders, or enter any new admissions and transferred patients. Furthermore, technicians would perform predetermined profile reviews and conduct medication reconciliations on new and transferred patients. If a medication was needed urgently and could not be sent via pneumatic tube, the expectation was that a technician would go to the central pharmacy, fill the medication, have it checked by the pharmacist, and deliver it to the nurse for administration.

To develop a proper infrastructure for technicians working in the new pharmacy model, a focus group of 8 pharmacists and 3 technicians was formed to develop the list of responsibilities and the workflow for the unit-based technicians. It was anticipated that all technicians based out of units would have the same basic work functions so that assignments would be standardized. The intent was establishment of a standardized workflow that would allow for the creation of a single training module for the technicians staffing these units. The focus group determined that the unit-based technician responsibilities should include the following:

- Perform regular hourly deliveries of medications from central pharmacy to the units
- Establish working relationships with nurses to increase pharmacy department presence on the unit
- Carry and maintain contact with nurses and the unit pharmacist throughout the shift through use of a wireless telephone on the medical center network (*SpectraLink* telephone)
- Answer any and all phone calls from patient care providers and resolve missing medication doses
- Maintain cleanliness and labeling of patient medication bins

The list was simplified, and it was anticipated that the responsibilities would largely impact the outcome measures for the unit-based program. In addition, the pharmacist and technician work group identified a separate list of responsibilities that could be rolled out over the course of several months once technicians and pharmacists became acclimated to the new workflow, workload, and each other. This list included the following:

- Technician medication reconciliation (admission and/or transfer)
- Technician order entry
- Discharge medication counseling preparation
- Clinical data collection
- Medication drip rounds
- Patient medication bin updating
- Emergency and/or code support

It was recognized that the items on this extended list would require institution-wide acceptance and planning. The implementation of these tasks is discussed later in this article.

Prioritizing Technician Functions

Once the primary and secondary responsibilities of the unit-based technicians were determined, the goal of the focus group was determining the order in which the soon-to-be-identified unit-based technician would need to perform them. The work group determined that the primary goals of the unit-based program were decreasing TAT and increasing the departmental presence and visibility on the unit. Furthermore, the pharmacist's ability to provide cognitive services to the unit was expected to increase as a result of the new technician role. Therefore, the focus group determined the order in which the responsibilities would be performed as follows:

- Establish working relationships with nurses to increase pharmacy department presence on the unit
- Perform regular hourly deliveries of medications from central pharmacy to the units
- Carry and maintain contact with nurses and the unit pharmacist throughout the shift through use of a wireless *SpectraLink* telephone, answer any and all phone calls from patient care providers, and assist with the procurement of missing medication doses
- Maintain cleanliness and labeling of patient medication bins

The belief was that if each unit-based technician could perform the responsibilities in this order, the unit-based pharmacist program would make significant strides in achieving favorable outcomes.

TECHNICIAN STAFF SELECTION: CHOOSING THE RIGHT PEOPLE

The unit-based pharmacy technician would be considered a higher-level technician from inception as a result of the foreseeable evolution of the role. Because the role required establishment and maintenance of re-

lationships with nonpharmacy health care providers, it was essential that each candidate have excellent customer service skills. The work group nominated several technicians from the current staff to fill this role. Other requirements of candidacy included pharmacy technician certification (Pharmacy Technician Certification Board [PTCB]), an acceptable customer service rating on previous evaluations, and training in at least 4 of the existing 6 pharmacy department areas.

The criteria did not include any limitations or specifications on the candidates' seniority, nor emphasis on any other aspect of performance or behavior such as teamwork, accountability, or initiative. These criteria, although valuable, were typically observed to an acceptable degree in all candidates nominated by the work group, as well as in individuals who met the required criteria. An interview of all candidates nominated for this process was conducted, and a candidate was chosen.

TRAINING AND IMPLEMENTATION

The initial training of the unit-based technicians was critical to the success of the program.[5] Although the inaugural technicians were hired internally, completion of a structured standardized training program with the pharmacist on the unit was deemed necessary by the work group; this included extensive training on order entry. Furthermore, it was required that technicians spend a predetermined amount of time with pharmacists in the units on which they were expected to deploy. This was essential to clarify any nuances regarding the specific unit and to determine the best way of accomplishing the responsibilities of the position. The pharmacists were also expected to teach the technicians how to perform their new responsibilities in a manner that would best meet the pharmacists' needs. Further changes were made to enhance the intended program effects as discoveries were made. One such change required that pharmacists and technicians switch *SpectraLink* telephones. Because the pharmacists had entered the program first, the nurses had memorized their phone numbers, and transitioning to calling the technician phones was difficult for the nurses. This simple adjustment allowed that calls be triaged by the technicians as intended. In addition, pharmacists on the units determined that technicians would provide better TAT if they made as-needed (PRN) trips to central pharmacy to retrieve medications rather than scheduled hourly runs.

As the program matured and the model expanded, training on the core responsibilities of the unit-based positions was incorporated into the internal UPMC pharmacy technician school curriculum. Thus, assigning the responsibility of training future unit-based technicians to a dedicated trainer in the school became necessary.

Currently, each new technician selected for a unit also receives 2 additional weeks of unit-based training. The first week is spent with an existing unit-based technician, followed by a week of training with the unit-based pharmacist. As part of the first week of training, a comprehensive customer service program is administered. This includes an observational component that consists of telephone call monitoring and a review of the technician's interaction with nurses on the units. The goal of this additional training is firm establishment of the higher expectations of the role.

After the technicians were established on the units during the initial rollout, the program's TAT performance measures began improving (see **Table 1**). Furthermore, significant improvements in nursing satisfaction scores (the nursing department's level of satisfaction with pharmacy services) increased dramatically (see **Table 2**).

Once a partnership was formed with nursing services and the medical staff through the support of the technicians, the unit-based pharmacists wanted to begin expanding the technicians' scope of clinical responsibility. As part of this reinvention process, the roles that technicians could play in the extension was examined. In particular, focus was placed on the roles of pharmacy technicians with regard to patient safety on the units. New responsibilities were subsequently added, which included the following:
- Follow-up on *eRecord* charting omissions
- Drip rounds (monitoring IV administration rates)
- Investigation of duplicate re quests for PRN medications
- Investigation of multiple re quests for missing medications
- Narcotic surveillance and utilization of automated dispensing cabinets
- Discharge medication counseling preparation
- Drug utilization reporting and compliance reporting
- Adverse drug reaction surveillance (as triggered by select medication orders, such as diphenhydramine)
- Medication error trending for the unit

The focus group determined through consensus that these activities would be the most helpful to the

Table 2. Results of Nursing Satisfaction Survey

	PreModel	Post-RPh–Only Model	Post-RPh and Technician Model	Percentage of Improvement	
				Post-RPh–Only Model	Post-RPh and Technician Model
R$_x$-RN communication is effective	2	4	5	100	150
RN understands medication policy	3	4.7	5	57	67
R$_x$ shows service excellence	2	3	4	50	100
R$_x$ responds in timely manner	2	4	5	100	150
New and/or stat doses arrive in a timely manner	2	3	4	50	100
Missing doses are replaced in a timely manner	2	3.5	4	75	100
R$_x$ quality improved	3	4	5	33	67

RN = nursing; RPh = registered pharmacist; R$_x$ = pharmacy; stat = highest priority.

program and its ability to meet and exceed performance measure expectations.

ADVANCED TECHNICAL FUNCTIONS FOR UNIT-BASED TECHNICIANS
Medication Reconciliation

Medication reconciliation on discharge at UPMC PUH-SHY had historically been performed by nurses. However, pharmacists were largely responsible for medication reconciliation on transfer because all a patient's orders had to be discontinued and reordered on transfer. The pharmacists on the units saw this as an opportunity for expansion of the technicians' roles. A single pharmacist with a particular interest for medication reconciliation was responsible for training all of the technicians on the proper process of reviewing profiled, discontinued orders and comparing them to new, transfer orders. Any discrepancies were noted by the technicians, and

the technicians were also responsible for communicating with the provider.

Medication Computer Order Entry

The functionality for performance of order entry by technicians was built into the pharmacy's CIS (Cerner). Because this functionality had not been used at any of the UPMC hospitals, some system testing was required, and adjustments were made regarding how nonverified orders (entered by pharmacy technicians) would be viewed by nursing staff on the electronic medical record. Once completed, all unit-based pharmacy technicians received training from corporate information technology services on the basics of order entry through the CIS. Unit-based pharmacists subsequently trained their respective technicians on processing unit-or service-specific orders. Unit-based pharmacists also received training on verification of technician-entered orders. This particular initiative has been proven the most valuable responsibility of unit-based technicians. Not only was TAT significantly decreased through use of this process, but pharmacists were freed from their order entry responsibilities, thus becoming available for providing more direct patient care at bedside.

Discharge Medication Counseling Screening

In 2005, UPMC began participating in a medication education program sponsored by the Agency for Health Research and Quality; the program was called EPITOME: Enhanced Patient Safety Intervention to Optimize Medication Education. EPITOME was focused on measuring patient outcomes after receiving discharge counseling from pharmacists. The program, which centers on patients at risk for poor medication adherence and/or compliance, has been successful in improving patient education on drug dosing, adverse effects, and administration.[6] Because technicians are not allowed to provide medication information to patients, the unit-based technicians were trained to screen patients for counseling before discharge. Specifically, technicians asked patients for information regarding their lifestyle habits and any barriers to compliance. This information was collected for the pharmacist, who then counseled patients before discharge. Currently, this study is ongoing, and plans have been formed regarding further discharge screening once the study is complete.

Patient Medication Bin Updates

In an effort to reduce medication errors, the unit-based technicians have been trained to identify discontinued medication orders and to immediately pull the discontinued orders from patients' medication bins. This step is intended for prevention of accidental medication administration by nursing staff. The patients' medication bins are now accurate, real-time reflections of patients' active and intended medications.

Despite continuing expansion of their role, the unit-based technicians' core responsibilities remain a priority. The accurate and timely delivery of medications to the units in an effort to decrease TAT is tantamount. Although nursing and medical services have provided the institution with valuable input on the implementation and expansion of unit-based technician services, their primary concern is—likely always will be—the timely processing of medications for administration.

EXCEPTIONS TO DEVELOPING A STANDARD TECHNICIAN JOB RESPONSIBILITY

Although every effort was made to standardize the technician workflow throughout the various units, it was determined during implementation that each unit had certain unique nuances that would prevent a complete standardization. The core responsibilities of the technician role were fixed as much as possible, but as a result of these subtle differences, some of the clinical programs were not fully executed. For example, on units that had older versions of the electronic medical record, it was not possible for orders entered by nonlicensed personnel to remain in an unverified queue. Thus, orders entered by technicians were immediately available for administration by nursing staff. It was not possible to implement technician order entry under these circumstances.

Similarly, the EPITOME study is ongoing only on certain units, preventing across-the-board adaptation by unit-based technicians. For this reason, the basis of the study is being used for piloting discharge medication screening by technicians for future implementation of a pharmacy-based, discharge medication education program. It is hoped that a standardized workflow—or at least standardized set of responsibilities—can be achieved in this model as the unit-based pharmacy expansion continues through 2008.

THE FUTURE OF THE MODEL: COMPUTERIZED PRESCRIBER ORDER ENTRY AND BEYOND

As UPMC prepares for the eventual implementation of computerized prescriber order entry, changes in the unit-based pharmacy technician model will be required because physicians will be performing medication order entry. Replacement of the critical, order-entry role the technicians currently play by an equally meaningful and robust role will become necessary. A working group consisting of the 18 unit-based pharmacists and 10 technicians will be assembled to determine the course of the program. Current responsibilities, such as entered-order clean-up, clinical data collection, and drug-use-policy enforcement, will certainly increase. In addition, emerging responsibilities will play a greater part. These will include extended roles in medication reconciliation, anticoagulation, patient education, and medication charting oversight.

CONCLUSION

The demand for pharmacy departments to provide clinically oriented, patient care services will undoubtedly continually exceed supply in the future. As a result, the pharmacy field will be constantly challenged to invent new ways of providing services in efficient and cost-effective ways. Pharmacy technicians represent a critical element to the solution.

Through the creation of unit-based partnerships with pharmacists at UPMC, pharmacy technicians were integrated into patient-centered teams that allowed the expansion of services. In the UPMC model, these partnerships clearly demonstrated a decrease in TAT, improved satisfaction with pharmacy services by other health care professions, and a resulting increase in positive relationships. With increasing demands for pharmacy involvement, the expansion of the role of the pharmacy technician represents the future direction of the profession.

REFERENCES
1. Wick JY. Using pharmacy technicians to enhance clinical and operational capabilities. *Consult Pharm.* 2008;23(6):447-458.

2. Keresztes JM. Role of pharmacy technicians in the development of clinical pharmacy. *Ann Pharmacother.* 2006; 40(11):2015-2019.

3. Koch KE, Weeks A. Clinically oriented pharmacy technicians to augment clinical services. *Am J Health Syst Pharm.* 1998;55(13):1375-1381.

4. Weber RJ, Skledar SJ, Sirianni CR, Frank S, Yourich B, Martinelli B. The impact of hospital pharmacists and technician teams on medication-process quality and nurse satisfaction. *Hosp Pharm.* 2004;39(12):1169-1176.

5. Kuschinsky D, Touchette M. Preparing pharmacy technicians for patient-focused care. *Am J Health Syst Pharm.* 1999;56(4):324-325.

6. Donihi AC, Yang E, Mark SM, Sirio CA, Weber RJ. Scheduling of pharmacist-provided medication education for hospitalized patients. *Hosp Pharm.* 2007; 43(2):121-126. ∎

Progressive Discipline Skills for the Pharmacy Director

Michael Sanborn, MS, FASHP*

The *Director's Forum* series is written and edited by Michael Sanborn and Robert Weber and is designed for guiding pharmacy leaders in establishing patient-centered services in hospitals and health systems. Another specific goal of this column is addressing many of the key challenges that pharmacy directors currently face, while also providing information that will foster growth in pharmacy leadership and patient safety. Previous *Director's Forum* articles have discussed various aspects of personnel management. This feature addresses methods for improving employee performance and working through the progressive discipline process.

INTRODUCTION

Effective human resource management of the pharmacy enterprise is one of the most rewarding, yet challenging, aspects of being a pharmacy leader. Several *Director's Forum* articles have addressed various aspects of human resource management and leadership, focusing on reduction of employee turnover, effective performance management, staff development, and interviewing.[1-3] One subject that has not been covered is the topic of correcting negative employee behavior through effective discipline.

Virtually all employees come to work with the goal of performing well in the tasks needed to get their jobs done. Employees want to do their best every day, and this is especially true in departments in which patient-centered care is a foundation. Each employee understands the mission, vision, and values of the organization. At times, however, an employee may take a shortcut, act on an impulse, or otherwise violate a hospital policy, requiring that disciplinary action be taken. The goal of discipline is not to punish but to make the employee aware of the violation, to share managerial expectations surrounding the violation, and, ultimately, to ensure that the violations are not repeated.

BACKGROUND

Some may wonder why a comprehensive knowledge of employee discipline is required of pharmacy directors. First, disciplining an employee is one of the most difficult aspects of pharmacy practice management. In fact, in a recent pharmacy survey on leadership, pharmacy managers identified employee recruitment evaluation and discipline as one of the least favorable parts of their jobs.[4] Furthermore, according to that same survey, directing and supervising others is one of the least desirable facets of pharmacy management for students considering a leadership position. There are, however, methods for minimizing the undesirable aspects of this process that focus on staff improvement.

Second, when handled effectively, the disciplinary process corrects inappropriate behavior in a constructive way. Employees can knowingly or inadvertently put themselves, their co-workers, or their patients at risk by violating policies and procedures. Making sure that these violations are

*Corporate Vice President, Baylor Health Care System, Dallas, Texas.

not repeated and that safety in patient care is preserved is the director's responsibility. Situations in which discipline is necessary may be uncomfortable and complicated, but they require prompt action by the director or manager of the pharmacy. The goal of discipline is assurance that appropriate steps are followed and that the employee and the manager can learn from the process and minimize the negative consequences (eg, harm to patients, termination of employment).

Third, the fair application of corrective action can ultimately improve department morale. If continuous violation of policies, procedures, or guidelines by employees is allowed, co-workers who abide by the rules of the institution may become frustrated. Tolerating such behavior also can generate significant risk and possible patient-safety issues by establishing de facto procedures that are contrary to those that are intended. For example, allowing certain employees to occasionally subvert a pharmacist double-check for chemotherapy may create a situation in which all employees feel that this is an acceptable practice. Immediately bringing the problem to the employee's attention in a constructive way can ensure consistency and fairness in the practices of the organization. In a well-managed department, there are rewards for good performance and consequences for poor conduct.

Finally, there can be legal implications associated with employee discipline or with not applying corrective action when it is required. Knowing and following the rules for disciplinary action are essential for minimizing legal risk. For instance, inappropriate application of the disciplinary process can result in a wrongful termination lawsuit, but continuously overlooking poor behavior can result in legal action brought forth by another staff member. If pharmacy directors are viewed by their employees as managers who apply discipline fairly and in an appropriate timeframe, few employees will be motivated to take, or have recourse for, legal action.

RESOURCES FOR UNDERSTANDING THE DISCIPLINE PROCESS

There are many terms for the employee discipline process, including *performance management, corrective action, performance improvement planning*, and, the more common term, *progressive discipline*. The pharmacy literature contains few articles on employee discipline, however there are numerous general resources that discuss principles that can be applied to the pharmacy workplace. In 1984, White and Scott published a primer summarizing the application of the progressive discipline process to the pharmacy department.[5] A more comprehensive, nonpharmacy reference is the recently published book *The Progressive Discipline Handbook: Smart Strategies for Coaching Employees*. This handbook also addresses the legal implications associated with this aspect of management.[6] A third reference that may be helpful is *The Heart of Coaching: Using Transformational Coaching to Create a High-Performance Coaching Culture*, a book that reviews the fundamentals of effective coaching.[7] Finally, although it does not deal entirely with employee discipline, the popular book *Crucial Conversations: Tools for Talking When the Stakes Are High* is an excellent resource for tactics that make the most of difficult interactions with others.[8]

PREVENTING DISCIPLINE PROBLEMS

The best way to avoid disciplinary problems is through creation of a departmental environment in which staff are well trained, knowledgeable of policies and procedures, and engaged in the mission of helping patients. Assuring that all staff members are well trained and that they understand the duties and expectations of their jobs is vital. Periodically reviewing important or complex policies at staff meetings reinforces understanding and clarity of these guidelines.

Making sure that the department has the right complement of staff and that each pharmacist and technician is highly qualified in performing their duties is also essential. This starts with comprehensive recruiting and hiring practices. Always use behavioral interviewing during the candidate selection process, as well as using examples that are specific to the role for which the applicant is being considered. Meet with new staff members periodically to ensure that they are making appropriate progress and have the resources they need for functioning efficiently and effectively.

Another good practice is promoting a culture of direct communication within the pharmacy. Always be straightforward and honest with staff, and encourage them to do the same. If staff members come to the pharmacy director with minor issues regarding coworkers, ask them if they have addressed the issue directly with the other employee. Use coaching skills to help employees work through such problems. Of course, this is not an appropriate response if disciplinary action is required.

Often, the hallmark of a highly functional department is a good performance management system. Performance management should not be an event that occurs only during an annual performance review. Managers must meet with staff members regularly so that staff always have an accurate view of their performance, whether good or bad. Implementing and communicating with staff about a department "dashboard" or "report card" can set additional expectations of performance metrics and create opportunities for shared learning.

"Rounding" on employees is another tool that can improve performance and correct issues before they become serious problems. This concept was originally developed by Quint Studer and is essentially a more focused form of "management by walking around."[9] This method is analogous to physicians rounding on their patients to identify progress and to monitor patient status. The key with rounding is using it as a means of gathering information regarding staff activities and operational performance in a proactive (rather than a reactive) way. Spend a couple of structured hours each week communicating with employees to find out what processes are working well and where improvements can be made. This is also a great method for recognizing good performance and for correcting employees whose work habits may need some adjustment.

USING THE HEALTH SYSTEM AS A RESOURCE

Every health system has specific policies that detail important steps in employee discipline. It is essential that department managers are familiar with these policies at all times, and especially prior to initiating any employee response. Some facilities have required forms or processes that must be followed in every case. If employees are members of a union, there are typically specific steps that must be followed when addressing employee performance issues.

A necessary step before taking action regarding any employee problem is consultation with the facility's human resources (HR) department. HR representatives can provide valuable insight into the process and can serve as objective outside counsel. They also can contrast the specific circumstances to similar occurrences in other departments, ensuring that the planned response is fair and effective. In addition, they may assist with particular verbiage or coaching associated with the pending employee interaction. In most cases, HR approval is required before suspending or terminating any employee.

At times, HR may recommend a response that is more or less serious than what the pharmacy director or manager had intended. Directors should feel comfortable challenging HR regarding this response, with the goal of understanding why there may be a difference in the recommended action. Reaching a consensus on how to proceed is essential because a response that is not in accordance with HR recommendations may be problematic.

Depending on the situation, confidentially discussing the matter with respected peers inside or outside of the organization may be helpful. Without identifying the individual or individuals involved, review the details of the problem and ask for advice on how they would address the situation. Oftentimes, they may have dealt with a similar challenge and may have helpful feedback and advice on how to handle the situation. Any suggestion that is contrary to or different from the course of action recommended by the local HR representative should be reviewed with HR before moving forward. Hospital policies, state regulations, union contracts, or other situational caveats may prevent a manager from taking action that is identical to what was recommended.

THE PROGRESSIVE DISCIPLINE PROCESS

The progressive discipline process consists of 4 steps that can be adapted for addressing the specific situation: verbal counseling, written warning, suspension, and termination of employment. The goal of this process is the fair and methodical increase of the level of severity of employee counseling with the aim of correcting inappropriate behavior and improving performance. This process is also designed for generating appropriate documentation that will legally protect the managers involved, as well as the organization, should termination be required.

These steps can be modified depending on the nature and severity of the situation; however, there are many nuances associated with this process. For example, an employee who violates the department dress code may receive verbal counseling and be asked to return home to change into appropriate attire. Conversely, if an employee willfully omits using cleanroom garb, a written warning may be more appropriate. Certain hospital-defined violations, such as inappropriate disclosure of patient information, theft, violence, inappropriate use of electronic resources, or sexual harassment, may result in immediate suspension or termination.

Aside from the director or manager who is extending the disciplinary action, another manager should be present during the employee discussion. This is not essential for verbal counseling, but any steps that are higher in the process should include a witness. This can be an HR representative or another department manager, but it must never be another staff member. Before the actual discussion with the employee, a director may wish to act the situation out through role-playing with another manager, especially if this is the director's first experience with employee counseling or if the director would like to better prepare for the meeting.

Verbal Counseling

When conducted effectively, a verbal warning is typically the first and last step in the discipline process because the result is improved employee performance. Verbal counseling should always be held privately, and it should never be held in front of other staff members. Be friendly and direct, but not informal or excessively complimentary to "soften the blow." Inform employees of the reason for the meeting, and clearly identify the problem. Ask employees for input, and then specifically state the desired behavior or performance that is required. Ensure that employees understand the expectations, and review the consequences if those expectations are not met. At the end of the discussion, schedule an appropriate follow-up meeting with employees and ask for their commitment to improving their performance.

Pharmacy directors and managers rarely should impose disciplinary action if they do not have proof that a problem has occurred. However, if they suspect a problem, it is incumbent on them as managers to investigate and then to speak to the employees in question. Providing employees with an opportunity for response allows managers to hear the employees' perspectives on the situation and may or may not affect the outcome of the counseling.

Written Warning

The steps of a written warning are similar to those of verbal counseling. Clearly summarize the problem in writing, using the approved form or format if applicable. Also, state the expected future behavior and the consequences if that behavior is not achieved. Ask that the employee sign the written warning at the end of the meeting. Inform the employee that their signature is evidence that the issue was discussed and not necessarily an admission of guilt. If the staff member refuses to sign the document, ask that the witness sign and note that the employee refused. Always provide the employee with a copy of the document.

Once a decision to give a written warning has been made, the director or manager should consider whether a formal performance improvement plan is warranted. When structured correctly, such plans can be helpful in achieving the desired performance. An effective plan should be specific, with clear objectives and measurable end points. Providing the staff member with specific examples of desirable behavior is also helpful. As part of the plan, describe any resources or additional training that will be made available, and specify meeting times for ongoing assessment of performance.

Suspension

A suspension can be with or without pay, depending on the circumstances. Typically, a paid suspension is permitted when the offense is significant and supports suspending the employee but more time is needed for investigating the situation. Consult with HR to determine the appropriate length of the suspension and the employee's pay status. In some cases, such as excessive absenteeism, a final warning letter is provided to the employee in lieu of a suspension.

Develop a written document outlining the details of the suspension and the circumstances that necessitated the action. Include a brief summary of previous efforts to correct behavior when applicable. Many hospitals require a written notice of suspension for which an employee's signature is needed. Review this information with the affected staff member and answer any questions that he or she may have. In most cases, the next step beyond suspension is termination; make sure that the employee clearly understands this consequence if his or her behavior does not improve.

Furthermore, make certain employees understand the details of their suspension and when they are expected to return to work. On the day that the employee returns, it is a good idea to meet with the employee before his or her shift to review expectations, as well as follow-up on any needed communication.

Termination

This step takes place, according to hospital policy, when a severe offense occurs or when any or all of the steps listed previously do not correct inappropriate behavior. Pharmacy directors and managers must always ensure that they follow and document all of the necessary steps and procedures before ending a staff member's employment.

In every case, obtain HR approval before termination and have a detailed discussion with the HR representative regarding the specifics of how the termination will be handled. Never terminate an employee without following this step. For situations in which there is concern that employees may be dangerous to themselves or others as a result of the termination, considering assistance from security or notification of the police if an illegal act has taken place is necessary.

When terminating employees, be straightforward and direct, explain clearly that the decision to terminate employment has been made, and give a brief review of the reasons for the decision. Employees may become angry, but do not retaliate or argue. An HR representative should be present to serve as a witness and to explain the grievance process and other end-of-employment circumstances that might apply (continuation of benefits, disposition of vacation pay, unemployment application, 401k status, etc). Often employees will have questions regarding these issues.

Most hospitals have a checklist that may be helpful when conducting an employee's termination. The list can include required steps such as collecting all hospital property from terminated staff members, including pagers, name badge, keys, and so on. Allow time so that employees can collect their personal possessions, if applicable, under direct supervision. Make sure that they understand that any other personal items found after they leave will be mailed to them. Ensure that all department and technology access and passwords are disabled. Escort employees from the hospital, and make sure that they understand that they are no longer permitted in the department.

EFFECTIVE IMPLEMENTATION

Although the steps associated with progressive discipline are fairly straightforward, success is derived through how the steps are implemented.

Always research the problem as thoroughly and as confidentially as possible. There are a variety of questions that pharmacy directors and managers can ask themselves during the investigative process. Following are some of those questions:

- Do they have firsthand knowledge of the problem or did they hear about it from another source?
- How credible is that source?
- Is there a possibility that the assumptions could be incorrect?
- Was the employee provoked or encouraged in any way?
- How long has this problem been occurring?
- Are there any other circumstances that should be considered?

In almost every case, getting the employee's perspective during the investigative phase is also helpful.

Once the investigation is complete, identify the appropriate disciplinary action step. An HR representative can be very helpful during this part of the process. Do not associate the disciplinary measure with the employee; always tie it objectively to the offense. For instance, the disciplinary response to excessive tardiness should be the same for an employee who historically has had mediocre performance versus a staff member who traditionally has been an exemplary performer.

Schedule and conduct the discussion with the employee. Regardless of the level of discipline, following are some key elements that can improve the quality of this communication:

- Do not assume that the employee is aware of the problem.
- Clearly and concisely explain the unacceptable behavior using specific examples and then describe acceptable performance.
- Provide the employee with an opportunity to respond.
- Inform the employee of the consequences of failing to comply.
- Discuss a time frame for follow-up and reevaluation and make sure that this is followed precisely as detailed to the employee.
- Make sure the employee understands what was communicated and the ramifications if the behavior is not corrected.

Document all conversations carefully. For example, after a verbal counseling, jot down a written note summarizing the discussion with the employee, including the date and time, and place it in the employee's file. This is not part of the employee's permanent record, but it serves as a valuable reminder if follow-up or future action is needed. Pharmacy directors and managers also should document any follow-up meetings. They should speak with their HR representatives in advance of any disciplinary meetings regarding the appropriate use of e-mail to document any part of the process.

Copies of any supporting documentation should be included with the counseling material. Any supporting documents that include patient-care information should be appropriately deidentified.

If an employee improves after disciplinary action has been taken, tell them. Positive reinforcement is easier to deliver (and often more effective) than disciplinary action, and it highlights recognition of the desired behavior. Keep in mind that the goal of the entire process is not to punish but to make sure all employees are performing at the highest level possible.

The length and frequency of follow-up depends on the situation. If the offense is related to excessive absences, a 3- to 6-month review period may be appropriate. Conversely, if the behavior put a patient or co-worker at risk, then a shorter, more focused follow-up period should occur. In instances similar to the latter example, conducting multiple review meetings to ensure the behavior has been corrected may be helpful.

If the process is unsuccessful and termination results, inform the remaining staff that the employee has left the organization but do not provide any additional details. This may cause some level of gossip within the department, but protecting the departing employee's right to confidentiality is crucial. If it is suspected that other staff members may be involved in the same type of behavior or if a valuable learning experience is identified for all employees as a result of the process, schedule and conduct a staff meeting or educational session that addresses department and/or hospital policy, as well as each employee's responsibilities.

CONCLUSION

The best method for addressing employee performance issues is through ensuring that the pharmacy department is a highly functioning, patient-focused team in which employees clearly understand their expectations. If disciplinary action is warranted, pharmacy directors and managers must make sure that they are knowledgeable regarding hospital and department policies. The focus of performance management should always be improvement of employee behavior, as well as following the necessary steps to uphold the pharmacy's patient-care mission.

REFERENCES

1. Weber RJ. Human resources management for the pharmacy director. *Hosp Pharm.* 2006;41(12):1206-1214.

2. White SJ. Effective pharmacy department leadership. *Hosp Pharm.* 2007;42(1):77-79.

3. Sanborn MS. Tactics to reduce pharmacy staff turnover and increase job satisfaction. *Hosp Pharm.* 2008;43(8):670-675.

4. White SJ. Will there be a pharmacy leadership crisis? An ASHP Foundation scholar-in-residence report. *Am J Health Syst Pharm.* 2005;62(8):845-855.

5. White SJ, Scott BE. Progressive discipline. *Am J Hosp Pharm.* 1984;41(9):1824-1828.

6. Mader-Clark M, Guerin L. *The Progressive Discipline Handbook: Smart Strategies for Coaching Employees.* Berkley, CA: Nolo Publishing; 2007.

7. Crane TG, Patrick LN. *The Heart of Coaching: Using Transformational Coaching to Create a High-Performance Coaching Culture.* 3rd ed. San Diego, CA: FTA Press; 2005.

8. Patterson K, Grenny J, McMillan R, Switzler A, Covey SR. *Crucial Conversations: Tools for Talking When the Stakes Are High.* New York, NY: McGraw-Hill Company; 2002.

9. Studer Q. *Hardwiring Excellence: Purpose, Worthwhile Work, Making a Difference.* Gulf Breeze, FL: Fire Starter Publishing; 2004. ∎

Tactics to Reduce Pharmacy Staff Turnover and Increase Job Satisfaction

Michael Sanborn, MS, FASHP*

The *Director's Forum* series is written and edited by Michael Sanborn and Robert Weber and is designed to guide pharmacy leaders in establishing patient-centered services in hospitals and health systems. Another specific goal of this column is to address many of the key challenges that pharmacy directors currently face while providing information that will foster growth in pharmacy leadership and patient safety. Pharmacist turnover is a significant challenge for pharmacy directors today, and this *Director's Forum* article will focus on specific elements and tactics that can reduce staff turnover and improve pharmacist and technician job satisfaction.

One of the more challenging aspects of department leadership is the creation and ongoing development of a pharmacy team that is consistently engaged, motivated, and focused on core departmental goals. Previous *Director's Forum* articles have addressed the fundamentals of human resource management and leadership, with a focus on performance management, interviewing skills, staff development, and accountability.[1,2] Health care worker shortages abound in today's environment, and improving pharmacist and technician job satisfaction and the resulting reduction in staff turnover are topics that deserve additional discussion. Pharmacy directors must always be mindful of one of the most important maxims of human resource management: The best recruiting strategy is a strong retention strategy.

BACKGROUND

All pharmacy departments will experience staff turnover from time to time, but there is a big difference between turnover that is controllable and that which is uncontrollable. For example, it is generally very difficult to control turnover that occurs when a staff member moves out of state because of the relocation of a spouse. On the other hand, the loss of a staff member to a competitor hospital in the same city is almost always preventable. Developing a comprehensive strategy for employee satisfaction and retention can dramatically reduce such controllable turnover.

The cost of employee turnover is high and, by some estimates, exceeds the total cost of a position's annual compensation. Loss in department productivity, subsequent knowledge and experience deficits, overtime expenditures, recruitment costs, and training expenses can all factor into the cost of losing 1 staff member. There are other departmental costs as well because employee turnover can lead to a precarious downward spiral. More specifically, staff turnover is typically influenced by poor department morale, and departments with high turnover typically experience significant morale reductions as a result of the turnover itself.

Overall, turnover in health system pharmacies in the United States tends to be lower than the national combined average for all health care

*Corporate Vice President, Baylor Health Care System, Dallas, Texas.

workers, yet the range of turnover from one hospital to another is quite variable. In the most recent survey by the American Society of Health-System Pharmacists (ASHP) that evaluated pharmacist and technician turnover, mean turnover was 7.7% (range 6.7% to 13.4%) and 13.6% (range 9.2% to 14.7%), respectively.[3] Over the last several years, pharmacist and technician turnover has been relatively constant (see **Figure 1**), with minimal fluctuations year over year. The 2-fold difference between the hospitals with the lowest pharmacist turnover versus those with the highest turnover merits careful consideration. It is wise to establish a turnover target. Moving from a turnover rate that exceeds 13% to one that is less than 7% is entirely possible, and reducing annual turnover to less than 6% is not an unreasonable goal. The key is creating a positive professional culture and work environment.

There are "best practices" associated with staff job satisfaction and turnover reduction, and many of them will be covered in the following sections. In the innovative book

First Break All the Rules, the results of Gallup research involving over a million employees are analyzed; and this extensive survey pool consistently suggests that, by far, the main reason an employee becomes frustrated and leaves a current position is because of the immediate supervisor.[5] If staff are satisfied with their manager, then other factors—such as job expectations, work environment, co-worker relationships, feedback, salary, and professional growth—can all fuel long-term employee loyalty and engagement. This article will evaluate specific retention strategies based on 3 key areas: manager tactics, department-level strategies, and health system retention factors. When dutifully employed, these strategies can dramatically reduce department turnover and have a considerable impact on department morale.

MANAGER TACTICS FOR EMPLOYEE RETENTION

This section addresses some of the many strategies that any person with direct reports should contemplate. The use of these techniques is essen-

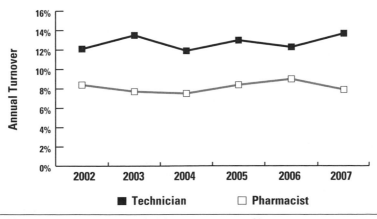

Figure 1. National pharmacist and technician turnover rates.[3,4]

tial because the relationship between employees and their immediate supervisor is the most important element to consider when focusing on reducing employee turnover. A good manager realizes that there is no "textbook" method to motivate every employee. Employees respond differently to recognition and rewards and also have varying degrees of tolerance for workplace frustrations. What is valuable to one employee may not be as meaningful to another. Most importantly, every employee wants to know that their job is worthwhile and that they make a difference, so efforts to implement retention strategies must be sincere. For these reasons, tactics used to improve staff morale and reduce turnover should be individualized whenever possible.

Good leaders also recognize the importance of a good professional relationship with their direct reports. Employees want a supervisor who is approachable, understands the work that must be done, sets clear expectations, holds people accountable, and is appreciative of their efforts. Good managers also ensure staff members have the necessary resources to do their jobs with a focus on improving department operations. Last, but not least, effective managers care about each employee as a person, value their employees' opinions, and provide staff with regular feedback on their performance.

An excellent reference that summarizes some of these recommendations is the ASHP guideline on recruitment, selection, and retention of pharmacy personnel.[6] Another useful resource is *Hard-wiring Excellence*, a book written by Quint Studer that has several chapters related to employee satisfac-tion, development, and recognition.[7] Each of these resources provides numerous suggestions on specific ways to recognize and reward staff.

Above all, employees need to feel valued and appreciated. Many managers often forget to take time to directly acknowledge and thank staff for their efforts. More importantly, a sincere, verbal expression of gratitude is generally valued highest by employees and costs the department nothing. Another simple, highly effective, and inexpensive way to recognize staff is through the use of thank-you notes. Handwritten notes thanking employees for specific accomplishments are quite valuable because they express to employees that their manager cares enough to individually recognize the contributions they have made. Some even recommend sending a thank-you note to the employee's home address for an added personal touch. For significant accomplishments, it can also be effective for managers to ask their supervisors or even the hospital president to write a note to an employee detailing their appreciation. A related method that recognizes each employee on an annual basis is sending birthday or employment anniversary cards with a handwritten note thanking staff members for successes they have achieved throughout the year.

Another useful tool is "rounding" on direct reports. Studer considers this one of the "must-haves" for employee satisfaction.[7] The concept is relatively simple and involves informal but structured visits with individual staff members to develop professional relationships with them, identify potential improvements that can be made, and seek out specific people for recognition. Simple questions like, "What is going well today?" or "What can we do better?" are a great way to get staff talking about important aspects of the work environment or ideas for improvement. Asking staff members about co-workers who deserve acknowledgment is another way to identify strong performers. (Managers can then follow-through with a thank-you note to those employees who were recommended by a co-worker.) Effective rounding also improves the perceived availability of the manager, which is a characteristic that employees value highly.

As a final point, addressing issues associated with high, middle, and low performers is an additional management strategy that is essential to a positive, productive work environment.[7] High performers are those pharmacists and technicians who consistently go above and beyond their daily job requirements. These are the staff members that a manager hates to lose under any circumstances. Middle performers represent the majority of the pharmacy team, and they often meet and occasionally exceed expectations. They are also essential to department operations and services. Low performers represent the small percentage of staff members who consistently miss the mark with respect to productivity and quality of work. This group presents a significant liability to the department because their low output (and typically poor attitude) negatively affects other staff members and can also be a poor reflection on the department as a whole. One of the most frustrating job aspects for any good employee is having to work alongside a consistently low performer who always seems to exert the minimal amount of effort to get the job

done. Tolerance for employees who exhibit poor job performance saps departmental morale. One effective way to improve overall performance and to eliminate these low performers is consciously addressing each of these 3 types of staff members.

Many managers will simply deal with low performers through the performance-management process and hope that over time the employee will improve or leave. Although documentation of poor performance is important, there is a better way of tackling low performers. Once or twice per year, a manager should meet formally with each of his or her direct reports after categorizing them into a high-, medium-, or low-performing rank. These meetings should be brief and focused. For high and medium performers, the meeting is very positive and complimentary in tone, with a manager specifically recognizing the employee's contributions to the department and adding emphasis for high performers. Meetings with low-performing staff are different. In a direct and specific way, a manager must meet with each low performer and straightforwardly tell these employees that their behavior and performance are not adequate. Examples of poor behavior should be cited whenever possible, along with unambiguous improvement expectations. Then a follow-up meeting should be scheduled, preferably in 2 to 3 weeks, and the employee made aware that progress must be demonstrated. Low performers will (and should) feel uncomfortable after the initial meeting, but more importantly, they will clearly understand that their work habits need to immediately improve. This discomfort may make low-performing staff realize that their work ethic and attitude might not be a good match for the department and a better fit could be found elsewhere.

DEPARTMENT-LEVEL STRATEGIES

The ideal pharmacy department is one that is efficient and productive, allowing each employee to practice at their full potential. Pharmacy leaders must constantly strive to improve pharmacy operations and, ultimately, the work environment. Just as with individual managers, it is important to select and develop a strong leadership team that understands the collective effect they can have on employee retention. The following strategies are important baseline elements for any pharmacy department, regardless of size or management structure.

Employees should always be guaranteed the opportunity to start off right. Special attention and planning for the new employee's first day, week, month, and year are the initial steps toward helping each staff member achieve their full potential. Make sure existing staff members are appropriately introduced to new team members, and it is often effective to assign the new person a "mentor" or trainer to assist them with the learning process. New staff should receive regular communication and feedback—both formally and informally—throughout the training period. It is important to "re-recruit" new staff members and ask them for their input on department operations. New employees see the department from a different perspective and can be an invaluable resource for improvement opportunities.

Effective communication is essential for positive morale. Regular staff meetings, a newsletter, weekly e-mail communications, and semiannual department reports are a few ways to keep employees informed. These venues are ideal for communicating hospital news and department-specific initiatives and reinforcing the vision and goals of the department. Effective communication should be a planned function, and the method of communication should be selectively and strategically employed to deliver the appropriate message. For example, it is wise to present a formal department report or "state of the union" to the staff at least once a year. Use presentation software to review the significant accomplishments of the department, review key metrics such as staffing levels and financial performance, and discuss hospital goals with aligned department tactics created to achieve those goals.

As discussed, employee recognition is an important factor for staff retention. Staff meetings and other department events are excellent venues to recognize individuals or pharmacy teams who have been successful. National Pharmacy Week is another time when hospital-wide recognition of the department can be valuable. Plaques, gift cards, and other small but meaningful awards are low cost but will be appreciated by staff. Many departments also use giveaways like t-shirts, sweatshirts, or other items with the hospital logo or a department-specific design to recognize staff members.

Creating an ongoing staff development program is a functional way to engage employees and demonstrate the department's commitment to their success. Developmental goals for every staff member should be individualized and integrated into the performance-management process.

Arranging journal clubs, using invited speakers, and providing staff with opportunities to cross-train in new areas are all ways to foster an atmosphere in which employees feel as though they have opportunities to grow professionally. Creating meaningful staff competencies on renal dosing, pharmacokinetics, anticoagulation, or other clinical subjects is an excellent way to standardize performance and encourage employee growth. As an added incentive, these programs can be approved as pharmacist or technician continuing education (CE). This can be accomplished at a relatively low cost, and staff are provided the added CE benefit for completing department-sponsored competencies or other training programs. Most state health system pharmacist associations can assist with CE approval needs.

There are many other methods that foster staff development. Encourage employees to develop a poster or platform presentation that can be delivered at a local, state, or national meeting. If a presentation is not possible, sponsor the employees' attendance at the meeting and ask them to provide a summary of what they learned from the meeting at a subsequent staff luncheon. Recognizing staff members for noteworthy interventions and reviewing unique or significant interventions at staff meetings are additional tactics that increase staff awareness and knowledge related to patient care and drug therapy.

Scheduling is another important employee satisfaction element. Offering unique, flexible scheduling options such as job sharing, part-time options, compressed work weeks, and self-scheduling are generally highly valued by today's workforce and may help retain employees who might otherwise resign. Progressive departments are open to staff suggestions regarding scheduling ideas and coverage options. Although no particular set of solutions can meet every employee's needs, department schedules and shifts should always be fair and equitable.

The impact of daily work responsibilities on job satisfaction is significant. Pharmacists and technicians want to feel productive and be able to contribute to patient care without having to develop work-arounds to get their tasks done. Staff must have the tools and resources they need. Thus, it is imperative that all pharmacy automation is fully optimized to prevent unnecessary daily frustration. Technician responsibilities should be maximized, allowing pharmacists to increase their direct patient-care capabilities. Talented department leaders are constantly focused on ways to improve the delivery of pharmacy services throughout the health system and to challenge staff professionally. For example, decentralizing pharmacy operations and allowing pharmacists to work more directly with the health care team will not only improve pharmacist job satisfaction but can also improve the department's recruiting capabilities.[8]

Great departments also offer opportunities for advancement and promotion. These can be formal or informal, depending on department size and organizational structure. Even when a formal promotion is not possible, allowing a pharmacist to lead a protocol development team or a performance improvement project is an excellent way to "promote" staff. Encourage, recognize, and pay for Board certification. Groom a pharmacist to become the residency program coordinator or director. In every department, formal succession planning, as well as leadership mentoring, should be implemented.

HEALTH SYSTEM RETENTION FACTORS

Ideally, the pharmacy department is seated within a health system that is also focused on employee recognition and retention. Hospital-wide efforts will only augment those offered by the department and can be leveraged for added effect.

The hospital's benefits package is important for recruitment and retention. Aggressive vesting schedules for retirement programs, parking perks, incentives for carpooling or using mass transit, cafeteria discounts, and retention bonuses for hard-to-fill positions are ways to improve employee loyalty. Unique offerings such as child care services can be invaluable to staff members who have to balance work and family.

None of the retention tactics discussed thus far have addressed salary issues. Many department heads view salary as the most important aspect of retention, but data suggest otherwise.[5] Employees rarely leave because of salary issues when they perceive their salaries as competitive. There are numerous examples of pharmacy departments across the United States in which salaries are barely competitive, yet turnover is minimal. The leaders in these departments realize that all the other elements discussed in this article are generally more important than salary alone. Even when a staff member resigns, citing salary as the key reason, it is important to delve further into the decision to leave during an exit interview. Oftentimes, there are several other work environment–related reasons for the resignation that the employee feels will be different at their new position.

On the other hand, it is incumbent upon pharmacy leadership to ensure competitive pharmacist and technician salaries. Tracking pharmacist and technician salaries is imperative. Working with the human resources (HR) department is the best way to accomplish this. Most HR departments have access to local or regional salary surveys that can be used to benchmark pharmacy department pay. It is also helpful to seek out and document local, pay-related incentives (eg, PRN rates, shift differentials, holiday pay, and other additions to base pay) at other facilities and share these with HR as appropriate. Remember that any pay raise will directly cost the hospital but may indirectly improve other parameters such as overtime, contract labor costs, or the inherent cost of turnover. If pharmacy salaries are truly causing turnover, then it may be necessary to create a written proposal justifying an increase. This proposal will have a much greater likelihood of success if measurable reductions in other expenses are projected and later documented.

Lastly, the pharmacy's status within the health system can have a significant impact on job satisfaction and morale. A pharmacy's reputation and relationship with physicians, nurses, administration, and other health professionals is important and can be improved by consistently creating opportunities for pharmacy staff to impact patient care and outcomes. Developing and expanding progressive, patient-focused programs and collaborative services that allow pharmacists to regularly participate in health care decisions and improve medication therapy are essential.

SUMMARY

Caring for patients is important work, and pharmacists and technicians should feel appreciated for the contributions that they make each day. Recognizing turnover as a controllable metric for overall satisfaction and department efficiency is essential. An effective director understands that focused, individualized strategies implemented by pharmacy management, the department, and the hospital all have a considerable influence on staff motivation, retention, and turnover.

REFERENCES

1. Weber RJ. Human resources management for the pharmacy director. *Hosp Pharm.* 2006;41(12):1206-1214.

2. White SJ. Effective pharmacy department leadership. *Hosp Pharm.* 2007;42(1):77-79.

3. Pedersen CA, Schneider PJ, Scheckelhoff DJ. ASHP national survey of pharmacy practice in hospital settings: prescribing and transcribing—2007. *Am J Health Syst Pharm.* 2008;65(9):827-843.

4. American Society of Health-System Pharmacists. 2006 ASHP Pharmacy Staffing Survey Results. http://www .ashp.org/s_ashp/docs/files/ PPM_2006StaffSurvey.pdf. Accessed June 1, 2008.

5. Buckingham M, Coffman C. *First Break All the Rules: What the World's Greatest Managers Do Differently.* New York, NY: Simon & Schuster, Inc.; 1999.

6. Hawkins B. *Best Practices for Hospital and Health-System Pharmacy.* Bethesda, MD: American Society of Health-System Pharmacists; 2007.

7. Studer Q. *Hardwiring Excellence: Purpose, Worthwhile Work, Making a Difference.* Gulf Breeze, FL: Fire Starter Publishing; 2004.

8. Sanborn M. Strategies for developing clinical services—implementing a decentralized pharmacy program. *Hosp Pharm.* 2006;41(9):895-898. ∎

Management and Leadership

Developing a Meaningful Strategic Plan

Michael Sanborn, MS, FASHP *

The *Director's Forum* series is written and edited by Michael Sanborn and Robert Weber and is designed for guiding pharmacy leaders in establishing patient-centered services in hospitals and health systems. Another specific goal of this column is addressing many of the key challenges that pharmacy directors currently face, while also providing information that will foster growth in pharmacy leadership and patient safety. Previous articles in this series have discussed the many different aspects of pharmacy management and leadership challenges. This feature addresses the importance of developing and effectively executing a pharmacy strategic plan.

The famous oil tycoon T. Boone Pickens once said that "an idiot with a plan is far better off than a genius without one." Perceived intelligence aside, utilization of an active planning process for patient-focused pharmacy services is typically the hallmark of exceptional pharmacy programs. The planning process takes time, but progressive pharmacy directors know that the rewards associated with strategic planning are required to move the department forward in an effective and deliberate way. Active pursuit of a strategic plan is often the difference between a pharmacy department that reaches new levels of performance every year and one that merely struggles to maintain the status quo.

Strategic planning is the formal process of developing a department's direction, future allocation of resources, and priorities. This process aligns department efforts toward a set of common goals, accelerating cultural change and reducing the time spent on lower-priority work. There are many methods and techniques for developing a plan, which is usually designed to answer a variety of functional questions, including the following:

- What is the department currently doing?
- What should we be doing?
- Who are our customers and how can we serve them better?
- Are there risks and opportunities that we must address?
- How can the pharmacy align its goals with those of the organization?

Answering these questions can help set the department's future course and, more importantly, can do so in a way that allows the pharmacy to control much of its own destiny and potential.

BACKGROUND

The *American Journal of Health-System Pharmacy* ran a series of monthly articles from 1986 to 1989 that described strategic planning for clinical pharmacy services in a variety of pharmacy settings and situations.[1-5] Since that time there have been only a few publications that described effective utilization of this important function. Previous *Director's Forum* articles have discussed more focused department planning efforts, such as the development of a patient safety program, expanding clinical services, and automation and technology planning, but none have focused on

---

*Corporate Vice President, Baylor Health Care System, Dallas, Texas.

the specifics of developing and implementing a comprehensive strategic plan.

In 2001 Shane described the use of a strategic planning process for addressing financial challenges associated with the rapid release of new drugs, expanded indications for existing therapies, and increased annual expenditures for pharmaceutical products.[6] Also described in this article were prospective strategics, educational efforts, environmental analysis, and the effective use of task forces and other management strategies for providing better control and predictability of the pharmacy budget.

In 2008 Glazier discussed positioning the pharmacy as a clinical department, as well as the importance of developing a clear vision of departmental services and anticipated outcomes.[7] The article suggested that although many pharmacy directors have made efforts in describing a desired practice model, others have not taken the next step of developing a formal plan for achieving the desired level of practice. Specific elements were outlined in the proposed annual planning document, including defining the benefits of the department's objectives, developing metrics for measuring performance, creating strategies to achieve the overall goals, and assessing the skill mix and pharmacy interaction with other disciplines. The conclusion was that "a pharmacy patient care practice model and an annually updated pharmacy strategic operating plan are critical foundations needed to define [a pharmacy department's] commitment to the delivery of the value of which [they] know [they] are capable."

Another helpful document details a framework for high-performance pharmacy practice, which serves as a roadmap for the strategic approach to improving the medication-use process.[8] Seven dimensions of pharmacy practice are outlined, and an expert panel was used to develop 69 weighted performance elements that can be employed in the justification of existing services and identification of opportunities for improvement. Another useful tool includes a rating scale that assesses feasibility and financial, quality, and safety return metrics associated with each performance goal. The authors also describe how the framework can be used in a self-assessment and the development of a strategic plan.

There are several examples of strategic plans specific to health care and pharmacy, which illustrate the leverage that can be achieved through utilization of this process. A case in point is the American Society of Health-System Pharmacists' (ASHP's) Health-System Pharmacy 2015 initiative.[9] The overall goal of this initiative is to "significantly improve the practice of pharmacy in health systems" through the implementation of 6 large goals and 31 supporting objectives in health systems across the country. Details of each goal, as well as progress made toward accomplishing those goals, are available on the ASHP Web site.

Generally, a strategic plan has a timeline of 3 to 5 years, with forward-looking intentions. Any plan should be updated on at least an annual basis. However, for situations in which there is significant change and uncertainty, developing a plan that addresses the coming 18 months to 2 years may be worthwhile. For example, for a department that has stable leadership and fairly extensive patient care services, a long-term plan is appropriate. In contrast, a new leader in a department with limited services and significant operational challenges may initially want to develop a plan that is of shorter duration but more aggressive in its implementation timeline.

DESIGNING A STRATEGIC PLAN

A good strategic plan is fact based, goal oriented, and rooted in broad thinking. As mentioned, the pharmacy strategies also should complement and align with the overall goals of the health system and, ultimately, should be focused on improving medication use and patient care. In light of the multiple pressures that affect the health care system and pharmacy specifically, an executable strategic plan sets the tone and direction of the department and can be used as an effective staff communication tool.

The first step in developing a plan is creating or refining the mission and vision statements of the department. The mission is 1 or 2 sentences that summarize why the department exists; the vision outlines the desired future state of pharmacy services. It is important that each of these describes the real future of the department, and they may also be accompanied by broad, realistic goals and objectives. The strategic plan then provides the specifics regarding how the mission and vision will be realized.

The next step is identifying and analyzing the significant elements that affect the department. An excellent method for accomplishing this part of the planning process is the Strengths, Weaknesses, Opportunities, and Threats (SWOT) Analysis. In general, strengths and weaknesses are typically internal issues, whereas opportunities and threats often have a more outward focus. **Figure 1** lists questions that can help further quanti-

fy each of these areas. As the strategic plan is developed, the ultimate objective is to build on strengths, overcome weaknesses, explore new opportunities, and minimize threats.

After the SWOT Analysis is complete, construction of the strategic plan can begin. Most strategic plans consist of broad goals that are further defined by specific objectives. The plan subsequently can be developed so that it includes specific tactics for achieving those goals. For example, a broad goal for the department could be expanding pharmacy services throughout the organization to improve patient care. A specific objective related to that goal could be establishing an emergency department (ED) pharmacy program in the following 18 months. Tactics that support this objective might include developing a pro forma to justify the services, gaining medical staff support of the program, outlining specific ED pharmacist responsibilities, and designing metrics of program success. Sample elements that can be considered and included in a strategic plan are listed in **Table 1**.

Many organizations use "pillars" as categories for aligning particular objectives. Structuring a department's strategic plan in a similar way can ensure congruence with health system priorities. For several years, the Baylor Health Care System has tied both goals and performance to 4 pillars: Service, Quality, People, and Finance. Every year the organization sets specific goals around each of these pillars and then "cascades" the goals to individual departments for integration into specific department goals. The department goals are then cascaded to management and staff as annual performance goals. To assist in prioritization, each goal is weighted based

STRENGTHS	OPPORTUNITIES
What do we do well?	What services should we be providing?
What advantages and resources do we possess?	What prospects are we aware of that we have not yet addressed?
What do other departments and customers consider our strengths?	Are there emerging trends on which we can capitalize?
	Are there external forces (publications, regulations, etc) that we can leverage?
WEAKNESSES	THREATS
What could we do better?	What is the current financial climate?
For what are we often criticized?	Is significant change coming?
What are our vulnerabilities?	Do any of our weaknesses pose significant risk?
What specific services could be improved?	What roadblocks to progress exist?

Figure 1. Strengths, Weaknesses, Opportunities, and Threats Analysis questions for pharmacy strategic planning.

on the level of importance. Of course, departments and individuals can have goals and objectives that are not entirely related to the health system goals, but usually, fitting a goal into 1 of the 4 pillars is relatively easy.

Once a complete set of goals and objectives is developed, it should be incorporated into a document that effectively summarizes the entire plan. This includes the mission and vision statements, as well as the goals, objectives, and tactics. These can be listed in order of priority or weighted and incorporated into the pillar structure, as previously discussed. Some plans also may include a summary of the SWOT Analysis, but this is not essential.

THE IMPORTANCE OF STAFF INVOLVEMENT

Involving staff throughout the strategic planning process is essential to the department's overall success and always results in a more accurate and executable strategic plan. In addition, staff involvement immediately begins building ownership with regard to the department mission and vision. Brainstorming exercises with staff for each of the 4 sections of the SWOT Analysis can identify areas that may not have been readily apparent to department leadership. Techniques such as multivoting—in which staff members are asked to assign a limited number of votes to identified issues and goals—also can be worthwhile

Table 1. Elements for Potential Inclusion in a Pharmacy Strategic Plan

Issue	Sample Considerations
Personnel management	Staffing and labor allocations
	Recruitment and retention
	Use of technicians
	Residencies and teaching
Automation and technology	Optimization of existing technology
	Long-term automation planning
	Technology assessment
	Decision-support tools
Clinical services	Improvement of existing services
	Expansion into new areas
	Pharmacist education and development
	Antibiotic stewardship programs
Quality initiatives	Pharmacist's role
	Evidence-based care
	Tracking and monitoring improvement
Finance	Department budget
	Drug expense reduction
	Reimbursement maximization
	Facility improvement
Drug-use policy	Pharmacy and Therapeutics effectiveness
	Regulatory compliance
	Therapeutic initiatives
	Disaster and pandemic response
Patient safety	Pharmacy role in hospital efforts
	Medication-use safety
	Technology for improving safety
Pharmacy image	Service improvement
	Turnaround time
	Department marketing
	Publications and research

when prioritizing elements that will be included in the plan.

For example, Guerrero et al used a staff survey and small group meetings to develop a prioritized list of goals that could be incorporated into a strategic plan.[10] The department also conducted a work sampling study to identify relative amounts of time that staff spent on certain tasks (eg, dispensing, clinical services). They found that 19.7% of pharmacist time was spent on clinical services. Although this function was a priority for staff, it was perceived that management did not prioritize clinical functions effectively and that staff development opportunities were necessary. Using this information, the department developed a strategic plan that included goals such as a career ladder system, enhanced staff development opportunities, and improved clinical documentation systems.

Using a slightly different approach with staff, Chrymko recently described a virtual method for garnering staff involvement in strategic planning.[11] Each of the 4 elements of the SWOT Analysis were posted in the department conference room for several weeks, and staff could anonymously add items to each section. Staff meetings were used to discuss the elements that were identified. Staff then assisted in goal development and prioritization in a similar fashion. This virtual process allowed most staff to participate in the strategic planning process regardless of their shift, days off, and other scheduling challenges.

Oftentimes, assigning specific objectives of the plan to staff or managers is helpful and encouraging. For instance, if developing a technician-based patient interview process to improve medication reconciliation is a goal, a group of technicians and pharmacists can assist in the development of an action plan. The group should identify helpful reference articles, design the list of patient interview questions, and develop some sample work schedules that will accommodate the new service.

TRACKING PROGRESS AND SUCCESS

Strategic planning should not be a 1-time event, and a good plan consists of a working, operational document. Reviewing the strategic plan on a regular basis and measuring movement toward each goal is essential for achieving the desired out comes. This can be accomplished through the use of dashboards or scorecards that document progress. In some cases, measuring progress against defined benchmarks can be helpful. Results

and progress should be shared at staff meetings to reinforce the utility benefit of the plan.

Most strategic plans contain short-, medium-, and long-term goals and objectives. Ideally, each should have metrics that are bound by time. For instance, a goal under the finance pillar may be reduction of the pharmaceutical budget by 3% during the fiscal year. An objective of this goal may be establishing a formal renal dosing program, which would not only reduce drug utilization, but also would improve patient care (quality pillar). Measuring the number of renal dosing consults each month and posting a run chart to show progress keeps staff engaged and motivated. Celebrating successes as each of these smaller milestones is completed can build additional momentum toward further achievement.

Ongoing planning is necessary for any strategic plan. Circumstances change, and as progress is achieved, updates to the plan are necessary. The addition of new hospital services may require significant pharmacy support that must be incorporated into the plan. As objectives are completed, new ones can be developed that further expand pharmacy department services. At a minimum, the plan should be reviewed and updated annually, and a complete redraft should be considered every 2 to 3 years.

SUMMARY

A working strategic plan is a fundamental tool for departments that want to improve their overall performance. A good plan provides a detailed assessment of the current practice environment, as well as future opportunities for growth and expansion. Developing a plan with staff involvement, implementing the plan, and continuously tracking progress are essential elements needed for advancing patient-centered pharmacy services.

REFERENCES

1. Hutchinson RA, Witte KW, Vogel DP. Development and implementation of a strategic-planning process at a university hospital. *Am J Health Syst Pharm.* 1989;46(5):952-957.

2. Linggi A, Pelham LD. Strategic planning for clinical services: St. Joseph Hospital and Health Care Center. *Am J Hosp Pharm.* 1986;43(9):2164-2168.

3. Kelly WN. Strategic planning for clinical services: Hamot Medical Center. *Am J Hosp Pharm.* 1986;43(9):2159-2163.

4. Anderson RW. Strategic planning for clinical services: the University of Texas M.D. Anderson Hospital and Tumor Institute. *Am J Hosp Pharm.* 1986; 43(9):2169-2173.

5. Pierpaoli PG, Anderson RW, Kelly WN, Linggi A, Pelham LD. Strategic planning for clinical services: panel discussion. *Am J Hosp Pharm.* 1986; 43(9):2174-2177.

6. Shane R. Strategic management of pharmaceutical expenses. *Am J Health Syst Pharm.* 2001;58(5):406-409.

7. Glazier HS. Creating a plan—delivering on pharmacy value. *Am J Health Syst Pharm.* 2008:65(4):340-342.

8. Vermulen LC, Rough SS, Thielke TS, et al. Strategic approach for improving the medication-use process in health systems: the high-performance pharmacy practice framework. *Am J Health Syst Pharm.* 2007;64(16):1699-1710.

9. Health-system pharmacy 2015. American Society of Health-System Pharmacists Web site. http://www.ashp.org/2015. Accessed May 3, 2009.

10. Guerrero RM, Nickman NA, Bair JN. Using pharmacists' perceptions in planning changes in pharmacy practice. *Am J Hosp Pharm.* 1990;47(9):2026-2030.

11. Chrymko MM. Virtual strategic planning. *Am J Health Syst Pharm.* 2007;64(2):136. ∎

Effective Pharmacy Department Leadership

Sara J. White, MS, FASHP*

The *Director's Forum* series is written and edited by Robert Weber and Michael Sanborn and is designed to guide pharmacy leaders in establishing patient-centered services in hospitals and health systems. Another specific goal of this column is to address many of the key challenges that pharmacy directors face today, while providing information to foster growth in pharmacy leadership. This month's *Forum* was written by guest author Sara J. White and focuses directly on some of the critical elements that exemplify strong pharmacy leadership, as well as the director's role in staff development.

Effective pharmacy department leadership has never been more critical than it is today. Leadership focuses not only on a single patient's drug therapy but on processes to maximize positive patient outcomes for all patients. Strong leadership allows the pharmacy staff to use their drug expertise to prevent harm to patients and maximize therapeutic success. It is what has been responsible for pharmacists going on patient care rounds; compounding intravenous admixtures; ensuring rational, cost-effective therapeutics through formulary systems; and promoting patient safety through the use of computers and automation. Without leadership, pharmacists would be practicing in the basement pharmacy, having nurses prepare medications from stock bottles, with physicians prescribing medications at will without any review, and pharmacists merely processing all orders manually. Effective departmental leadership is required for the continued evolution of pharmacy services.

It is important to distinguish between leadership and management. They are dramatically different; however, both must be performed. Management is ensuring things are done right, and leadership is doing the right things. Management's emphasis is on tasks and safely executing them consistently. Management is a job description, while leadership is beyond that; it is a life decision. Leadership includes justifying and planning for medication use automation, physician order entry, and bedside bar coding. Leadership requires the courage to embark into the unknown and the ability to instill that courage in others. Leaders are people, regardless of their job title, or their situation in life, who see the opportunities to make positive changes and then take action to bring about those changes. Obviously, every Director of Pharmacy needs to be both a manager and a leader; they must prioritize, so they have time to spend on both.

Specifically, what is effective pharmacy departmental leadership? Leadership is more of an art than a specific science, so in every department of pharmacy someone has to be willing to stand up and put it on the line as the leader, because playing it safe from the sidelines is not always in the best interest of patients and pharmacy staff. While many books, articles, and college courses are devoted to leadership, in a pragmatic way it

*Pharmacy Leadership Coach, 550 Ortega Ave., B123, Mountain View, CA 94040, E-mail RxSJW@Yahoo.com.

can be divided into two areas; 1. Being responsible and accountable; and 2. Growing and developing people. While this article focuses specifically on the Director of Pharmacy, in larger departments, some of these activities may be delegated to middle managers within the pharmacy. However, the Director is still ultimately accountable. Many health system pharmacies do not have middle managers, and the Director must take on many roles, which can seem daunting. The upside is that in these departments, it is often easier to really know the staff and what is actually going on than in bigger departments. Regardless of the department's size, each Director owes it to their patients and staff to do their best, given their circumstances. It is amazing what can be achieved when the Director commits to providing true leadership.

TIPS ON BEING RESPONSIBLE AND ACCOUNTABLE

Effective departmental leadership means being in charge and holding oneself accountable for all aspects of the pharmacy services even when delegated to other middle managers. Embracing responsibility is an attitude and approach. This accountability entails ensuring that operations are running smoothly, departmental reporting relationships are clear for all staff, regulatory standards are being met, and there are enough trained and competent staff to provide the patients with safe and quality pharmacy services. The leader must serve as a continuous role model for pharmacists by being responsible and accountable.

The leader consciously establishes the departmental culture and tone by their philosophy, actions, and character. Being true to one's values results in the consistency and dependability that the staff need to feel comfortable in their daily decisions. This culture ensures that everyone is treated fairly and consistently. An effective leader leads from the front, but not by doing other's jobs.

Leaders ensure that decisions are made; actual results are achieved; and that all issues are quickly resolved. They also ensure that changes are well-planned, implemented, and fine tuned (including good cooperation by all involved).

Effective leadership ensures there is a current, written department vision in which all staff have had input and participate in its periodic updating; people commit to causes not just plans. Frequently, staff should discuss their specific contributions towards achieving the vision to keep the focus on the big picture—in addition to the day to day problems.

The leader continually thinks strategically,[1] thus anticipating changes versus reacting to them. An effective strategist looks at what is happening now in the context of where they want to go. Thinking strategically means planning long-term or declaring your intent at the same time as maintaining the short-term results; mapping out the route to future success; ensuring day to day decisions lead to the desired future vision; focusing the available resources appropriately; and identifying, prioritizing, and implementing needed change. It also means tapping the creative energy and knowledge of the pharmacy staff; assessing the pharmacy "customer's needs" (administration, nurses, physicians, patients, and pharmacy staff); making, assessing, and seizing opportunities; looking for future threats; aligning the pharmacy strategic plan with the organization's strategic direction; developing and communicating action plans that contain milestones; and documenting and sharing progress with staff and others.

Effective leaders strive to achieve excellence[2] and do not stop at good enough. Achieving excellence means working to fulfill their potential; identifying their personal career vision; having significant but attainable personal goals; having targets for both achievements and career moves; learning from mistakes; and having confidence in themselves. It also means giving themselves credit for what they do well; improving with training; knowledge and skill areas where they feel inadequate; mastering risk taking to make significant gains by looking in all directions before they leap; developing drive by determination and persistently channeling their energy toward a chosen purpose; seeing the strategic plan through to completion; getting people to work with them; giving the staff permission to challenge the status quo; insisting on high standards for themselves and others; accepting challenges; fostering and trusting their intuition in addition to their logical thinking; improving verbal communication skills; being innovative with other ways to organize and process pharmacy work; and using or being a mentor to continually improve their leadership effectiveness. Excellence also means being proactive and constantly marketing the value of the pharmacy services and pharmacy staff throughout the organization— especially to senior administration.

TIPS ON GROWING AND DEVELOPING PEOPLE

People are a leader's main asset and must be a top priority especially given the pharmacist shortage. An effective leader should get to know the staff as individuals. A way to build this staff relationship is to regularly spend time out in the work areas to assess things first hand and to be available to the staff. An effective leader establishes an atmosphere of trust,[3] as it is the foundation of good working relationships (both in the department and throughout the organization). The leader's character, especially integrity, and competence are vital to establishing this trust.

The leader must be open to alternate, flexible schedules, such as job sharing, less than full time, 10-hour shifts, and telecommuting to assist the staff in balancing their personal life and career. Offering schedule options can be a significant recruiting and retention strategy. The leader should have a candid discussion (on all topics) with the staff, so they understand what is important from the staffs' viewpoint.

Developing a practice model that will attract and retain a full staff including departmental middle managers, as appropriate, is a key leadership function as is continually assessing current staff capabilities and hiring and developing for the future needs.

The time investment up front to ensure a complete orientation, training, competency assessment, on-going staff development, and meaningful performance evaluation program is an important investment. Providing performance feedback on a regular basis and not just at the annual review meeting is a good use of the time it takes in helping people grow and develop.

Effective leadership inspires, mobilizes, and unlocks staffs' potential to achieve the established departmental vision versus just commanding. Eliciting cooperation and teamwork comes from finding out what the staff want and why. People are willing to follow a leader who is attuned to their aspirations, fears, and ideals. Leadership improves the level of human dignity in the group being lead. The staff are inspired when they are engaged in meaningful work and frequently receive encouragement, credit, appreciation, and recognition. No one likes being taken for granted; the leader should employ all the available organizational programs for staff recognition and develop pharmacy specific ones as appropriate. One way to provide this inspiration is to periodically ask the staff, "What have been our successes?" Another approach is to keep track of pharmacy successes and list them all for the staff at the end of the year. While the individual accomplishments are important, the cumulative results can be quite impressive.

The effective leader role models, by their own actions; integrating personal life and career, working efficiently (handling E-mail, voice mail, pagers, and paper), and being emotional intelligent, so people want to be around them. They also exhibit integrity and honesty in everything they do, listening sincerely to people and frequently communicating information regarding the organization and its challenges and directions.

The effective leader should not only have their own succession plan, but also one for each middle manager and pharmacist. A good succession plan invests in mentoring and coaching programs, so the person can reach their full potential. Everyone wants to create a lasting legacy[4] or impact by having their work make a difference and leaving the world a better place.

This quest to leave a lasting legacy is the journey from success to significance. Leaders who see their role as serving others leave the most lasting legacy. By asking how a person wants to be remembered, or what they want their legacy to be, we plant the seeds for them living their lives as if they matter and assisting them in achieving that legacy.

An effective leader builds new leaders, which means instilling the attitude that every pharmacist can be a leader on their shift or in their practice. An effective leader explains to the staff what they do on a daily basis, why they do it, and the impact pharmacy has throughout the whole organization. To build every pharmacist as a leader, the department provides leadership experiences, training, and coaching to set the pharmacists up for success.

Leadership is ensuring the quality of the next generation of pharmacy staff by offering clerkships (clinical and leadership), residencies, pharmacy technician externships, and lecturing at schools of pharmacy—no matter where the school is located.

CONCLUSION

There are two kinds of people; those who make things happen, and those who wonder what happened. Which kind of a leader does every pharmacy department deserve? What a leader does with the future means the difference between leaving a track record or a legacy. If a leader is doing what they love, it is an important part of achieving their personal satisfaction and success. The effective leader must discover their own approach and core values. They need to rally the staff through their example, values, and success stories, while also mobilizing strength, courage, and willingness to do what is necessary to fulfill the pharmacy vision by combining their mind, heart, skill, and appropriate tools.

REFERENCES

1. Bruce A, Langdon K. *Strategic Thinking.* New York, New York: Dorling Kindersley Publishing, Inc.; 2000.

2. Heller R. *Achieving Excellence.* New York, New York: Dorling Kindersley Publishing, Inc.; 1999.

3. Covey SMR, Merrill R. *The Speed of Trust, the One Thing that Changes Everything.* New York, New York: Simon & Schuster, Inc.; 2006.

4. Kouzes JM, Posner BZ. *A Leader's Legacy, How Would You like to be Remembered?* New York, New York: John Wiley & Son's, Inc.; 2006. ■

Succession Planning: The Forgotten Art

Scott M. Mark, PharmD, MS, MEd, FASHP, FACHE, FABC*

The *Director's Forum* series is edited by Michael Sanborn and Robert Weber and is designed to guide pharmacy leaders in establishing patient-centered services in hospitals and health systems. Another specific goal of this column is to address many of the key challenges that pharmacy directors face today while providing information that will foster growth in pharmacy leadership and patient safety. This month's *Forum* focuses on succession planning. As part of a long-term strategy, succession planning can provide a pipeline of leadership talent that will support the future of a department, organization, and, ultimately, the profession of pharmacy.

THE QUIET CRISIS

The recent report on the pharmacy leadership crisis has once again generated concerns about the future of pharmacy leadership in health systems.[1] There may not be enough young people entering the workforce to compensate for the exodus. The data indicate that the shortage of pharmacy managers has increased from 27% in 2003 to 36% in 2004. Additionally, an estimated 70% to 80% of directors are expected to turnover within 10 years.

Pharmacy leaders occupy a unique position in health systems because they manage a department that is a key clinical contributor and an operating budget that represents a significant portion of the overall health system budget.[2] Developing the many skill sets required to fulfill this role requires time and careful planning. After months of unsuccessful recruiting, many health systems are finding it very difficult to recruit a qualified director of pharmacy from outside of the organization. Some have come to the conclusion that pharmacy leadership will have to be developed internally. This development will not happen by chance. It requires deliberate mentorship and opportunity.[3] In the past, even small health systems maintained a middle management layer of assistant directors, operations managers, and clinical coordinators. Years of cost cutting has eliminated these positions, which historically served as a training ground for future directors.

If the profession of pharmacy is going to survive this leadership gap, there will need to be a renewed emphasis on succession planning. Research indicates that 50% of pharmacy directors report that they have not identified a successor.[1] The lack of leadership development and the oversight of succession plans have become the quiet crisis in pharmacy.

ROLE OF SUCCESSION PLANNING

Succession planning is perhaps best understood as any effort designed to ensure the continued effective performance within a department of pharmacy by making provisions for the development, replacement, and strategic application of key people over time. It can be defined as a deliberate and

*Director of Pharmacy and Director of the Pharmacy Practice Management Residency at the University of Pittsburgh Medical Center; Assistant Professor and Vice Chair of Pharmacy Systems at the University of Pittsburgh School of Pharmacy.

systematic effort to project leadership requirements: identify a pool of high-potential candidates, develop leadership competencies in those candidates through intentional learning experiences, and then select leaders from among the pool of potential leaders.

Many pharmacy departments confuse workforce planning with succession planning. Workforce planning is anticipating human capital needs and assuring that you have the human resources to operate effectively. Generally speaking, workforce planning is more focused on quantitative measures. For example, a director might ask "How many management positions do I need to hire for this year?"

Succession planning however focuses more on selectively identifying individuals with certain attributes, qualities, and abilities who are capable of taking over specific role responsibilities as they become available. It addresses both quantitative and qualitative measures. For example, a director might ask "What skills do I need on my management team this year, and who has the aptitude to develop them?"

It is also critical to ensure that succession planning is integrated with strategic planning. When evaluating the potential loss of skills from the team, it not sufficient to replace the skills that will be lost. Rather, it is necessary to anticipate skills that may be needed as a result of implementing the strategic plan. As a result, effective strategic succession planning must focus not on the skills that are needed on the team today but on those that will be needed at the time of anticipated leadership change.

It is also important to point out that strategic succession planning is not an episodic activity that has to be done to assure some level of compliance. Strategic succession planning is an integral part of how one must do business to survive. It also is not an option. It is a management practice and an imperative. It is how human capital resources are anticipated and proactively managed. According to the late Peter Drucker, "Effective management of our human resources is the last source of increasing our competitive advantage as too few organizations are very good at it!"[4]

NONTRADITIONAL LEADERSHIP ROLES

In addition to growing high-talent workers, succession planning also improves employee retention, and employee satisfaction. As discussed, succession planning also focuses on matching key skill sets needed to advance the organizational strategic plan. This is particularly pertinent in pharmacy, a field in which as few as 30% of current clinical pharmacy practitioners are willing to consider pharmacy management as a career option.[1] Many cite a key reason as their reluctance to give up their clinical practice. To address this concern, it may be strategically necessary to retool succession plans to develop nontraditional leadership roles in which practitioners can continue to practice while providing much needed leadership. By evaluating individual required skills, the responsibilities required of the leadership role can potentially be filled with 2 or more practicing clinicians.

Considerations would include anything that may need evaluation in addition to the needed skill sets. This may include the diversity of the team, cultural fit of the new employee, or the existing leadership model itself. The desired outcomes represent not only the skill set development but also the continual replenishment of talent, the sequential progression of personnel at the right time, and the tangential development across service lines to ensure a breadth of skills.

ELEMENTS OF SUCCESSION PLANNING

There are 6 key elements to succession planning:

1. Assessment of key positions
2. Identification and assessment of key talent
3. Identification of future skill requirements and strategic plans
4. Assessment of developmental gaps
5. Generation of development plans
6. Development of monitoring and review

ELEMENTS DEFINED
1. Assessment of Key Positions

Within any pharmacy department, there are key positions that are critical to the core mission. These are positions that, if they suddenly became vacant, would present a challenge in terms of maintaining seamless pharmacy operations. It is essential that these positions be identified and the critical competencies and experiences needed for the position cataloged. The department should never be "one deep" at any critical position. Sports enthusiasts refer to this as bench strength. If a starting player gets injured, is there anyone on the bench that can play the role? Stated another way, there should never be only one person who knows how to do a job. Proper cross-training will ensure that there is always someone on the bench who can step in if needed.

Historically in pharmacy, individu-al skill sets were thought of as they relate to clinical skills but not management. For example, when evaluating a clinical team, one may recognize that many of the clinical specialists on the team are knowledgeable about infectious diseases and that there is a limited amount of expertise in oncology. One would then recruit accordingly to fill that gap. Similarly, if the pharmacy management team has a relative void in key knowledge areas such as reimbursement, benchmarking, and project or inventory management, it would seem intuitive that the recruiting would follow a similar targeted approach. Often, however, the recruiting is generic and not designed to add specific skills to the pharmacy management team.

2. Identification of Key Talent

Knowing what personnel are available for advancement is essential to developing a comprehensive succession plan.[5] It is not enough however to have a personnel directory handy, but rather, it is important to know where each employee is in their development and their career aspirations and what potential they have to progress. For example, a team may consist of several strong clinicians but none of them currently possesses the skills necessary to become a clinical coordinator should the need arise. To understand which skills may need to be developed, it will be necessary to critically evaluate the skills needed for a successful clinical coordinator and compare this list with the inventory of skills present in existing staff. It is imperative to understand that the skills needed to be a successful clinician are not the same as the skills needed to be a successful clinical coordinator.

3. Identification of Future Skill Requirements and Strategic Plans

It is important to consider both the departmental and organizational strategic plans when evaluating succession planning. Omitting this step is a key mistake that many organizations make. Effective succession planning is not simply ensuring that the existing skill sets on the management team are replicated but rather that the skill sets needed in the future are available. To achieve this, it is necessary to know the direction that the organization is heading. For example, the organization may be expanding its ambulatory programs with plans to open ambulatory surgical centers and human immunodeficiency virus, diabetes, and anticoagulation clinics. In light of these growth plans, it may be apparent that in addition to needing to hire an effective pharmacy leader for these areas, a team must develop the necessary expertise related to 340b programs, medication therapy management, and outpatient reimbursement.

4. Assessment of Developmental Gaps

Once the future direction of the department is known and the future skill sets are identified, this can be contrasted to existing personnel to establish which skill areas are under represented. These skill sets can then be prioritized to form the road map for training, development, and advancement. Individual personnel can be moved through a tailored program, which will ensure that the needed skill sets are acquired. Each person identified for succession planning should have an Individual Development Plan (IDP) developed for them that codifies the intended experiences and timelines. It is important that each employee understand the path,[6] which

will engender additional commitment and buy-in. It is also important that each position have a primary person identified, as well as a secondary person. Given the level of turnover in pharmacy today, it is not uncommon for more than one person to be subsequently recruited away from a health system simultaneously.

5. Individual Development Plans

Essentially, IDPs are documents that outline specific activities that will be part of the employee's professional development program over a specified timeline. These are mutually agreed upon by employer and employee and are intended to define a career path for advancement. These help the employee achieve the necessary experiences. They also serve as formal commitments on the part of the organization to the employee. Sometimes employees invest their time in activities and fail to see a return on their investment in the form of a promotion. In addition, employees may not know what they need to work on to improve their candidacy for advancement. As a result, they select skills to improve upon that are not considered essential at the next level. An IDP satisfies both of these oversights by identifying which skills will need to be developed and formally acknowledging the organization's investment in the employee's advancement.

One final point of caution: it is important that the employee have a substantial say in which opportunities are being selected for them in a development plan. A common organizational mistake is "tapping" a staff member for a particular promotion pathway that is undesirable to the employee. If the employee does not have a say and their desire is to grow in another direction, then they will ultimately be unhappy. Ironically, the organization's efforts to create promotion opportunities for the employee may actually force the person to leave the company in search of the opportunity that will better satisfy their passion.

6. Development of Monitoring and Review

It will be necessary to ensure that the development program is advancing as designed. Individual personnel who were felt to have aptitude may falter, and staff who had been initially overlooked may emerge. Because the strategic plan is a living document, it will be necessary to continually evaluate the changing departmental or corporate landscape to ensure that the training remains aligned with the direction.

Additionally, although experience demonstrates that certain initiatives, such as stretch assignments, provide a greater probability of skill development, the outcome is not guaranteed. It is also true that some individuals learn better in certain environments. As such, although a particular assignment may have worked in the past, it may not work for every employee.

WHERE TO START?

One of the simplest succession planning starting points involves a thorough evaluation of the department's organizational chart. For each position, identify the skill sets that are currently needed for success and the necessary skill sets that are anticipated over the next 5 years. This exercise involves much more than simply evaluating how many people directly report to a given manager. For example, a pharmacy information technology manager may have several direct reports, all of whom are excellent in their roles. None, however, may have the necessary political savvy, systems-thinking skills, or negotiation finesse to move into the manager role if it were to become vacant. In contrast, another person on the organizational chart may have no direct reports; however, their skill set may be more easily replicated and therefore more readily found in other personnel.

The next step is to rearrange the organizational chart so that each key position has a list of names below it that represent potential successors. For each employee identified for succession planning, a skill development assessment and associated timeline should be estimated to better represent how much investment is needed.

During this phase, it is often helpful to use predication methods to evaluate candidates who may best suit a particular position. This involves various behavioral trait assessments and emotional suitability analysis for a given role. Peer assessments, self assessments, and managerial sponsorship may also influence decisions. Substantive assessment methods may include job knowledge tests, performance appraisals, promotability ratings, interview simulations, and review boards. A 360-degree assessment, which evaluates feedback from a variety of coworkers, has also been used.[7] It is important to stress that job knowledge tests and performance appraisals are tools to evaluate an employee's performance in their current job and not necessarily the future position. Similarly, seniority is also a poor predictor of advancement success.

It is important to note that as a leader moves up the organizational chart, their primary skill set needed for success will likely change.[8] This often includes a stepwise transition from managing self to managing others; managing others to leading managers, leading managers to leading pharmacy function (such as operations); leading function to leading a business unit (such as the inpatient pharmacy); and finally leading business to leading business group (the entire pharmacy enterprise).

A mistake that is commonly made is overlooking this simple reality. It is frequently assumed that if an employee is highly successful in their current role, a promotion to the next level will correspond with equivalent or greater success. As an example, most people can appreciate that just because Michael Jordan was a successful basketball player, it was not guaranteed that he would be a successful baseball player. Clearly, different skills are required for each sport. Similarly, just because Magic Johnson was as successful basketball player did not guarantee that he would be a successful coach. In pharmacy, however, it is common for outstanding clinicians to be promoted to the position of clinical coordinator, overlooking the fact that these roles require much different skills.

Because the skill sets required at each level are completely different, many highly successful people are promoted only to fail miserably later. This concept is known as the *Peter Principle*, named after Laurence Peter who first described it.[9] Essentially, employees will continue to excel in their jobs until someone promotes them into a job that they are not able to perform well due to mismatched skills. As a result, they are never promoted again. To avoid this, it is imperative that the focus, mentoring, and development efforts be on the skill set re-quired in the new job and not those that made the person successful in their prior position.

SUCCESSION PLANNING TIPS

1. *It is important to involve top management, employees, and other stakeholders in development, communication, and implementation of the strategic workforce plan.* Because top management sets the overall direction and goals of workplace planning, it is critical that a departmental initiative be appropriately aligned. This congruence is also important because it will often be necessary to give developing leaders stretch assignments and experiences in which they may frequently interact with those at higher levels within the organization. It will be necessary to have hospital leadership support to ensure that the mentee has the appropriate access to meetings and information. Because the stakeholders should also have a vested interest in the success of a program, it will be necessary to develop a communication strategy. For example, it may be necessary to provide an aspiring clinician with some experience in presenting and leading higher-level meetings. This could include leading a Pharmacy and Therapeutics meeting, co-chairing a performance improvement team, or presenting at the Medical Executive Committee meeting. Without the proper prior communication and coaching, this may seem threatening. Additionally, assigning a key initiative to a clinician may not be interpreted by senior administration as a developmental opportunity but rather a sign that the initiative was not

given top priority. Effective communication will clarify this distinction.

2. *Determine the critical skills and competencies that will be needed to achieve the future programmatic results.* Pharmacy departments can use various approaches for making a fact-based determination of the critical human capital skills and competencies needed for the future. Partnering with the senior leadership team and the corporate HR department can help manage risks. For example, it is not uncommon for hospitals to commit to a given technology vendor and then subsequently change course as a result of unsatisfactory contracting or performance. This information would therefore be critical to a pharmacy director who is building an informatics team. The value and selection of future candidates would obviously differ greatly if the department suddenly needed expertise in the architecture of a completely different operating system.

3. *Develop strategies tailored to address gaps and human capital conditions for critical skills and competencies that need attention.* This is more than simply developing a comprehensive training and development program. This involves aligning the department's hiring, training, strategic planning, and other human capital planning strategies. For instance, a given department may know that they are expecting the existing clinical coordinator to retire within the next year. The leading clinician, who is best prepared to succeed the clinical coordinator, is a cardiology practitioner who is intimately involved in the launch of a new clinical service line in a recently built patient tower. This initiative is important and highly visible. In this situation, the clinician, although interested in the promotion, may not be available to learn the new skill sets or responsibilities. It might be possible to solve this dilemma with proper foresight and the support of administration to allow a new cardiology clinician to be hired now. This will allow the new clinician to grow into the role and be able to support the new patient tower expansion, thus allowing the existing clinician to prepare for the new coordinator role.

4. *Build the capability needed to address administrative, educational, and other requirements important to supporting workforce strategies.* It would be a mistake to assume that because the department has excellent leaders at key positions, it will automatically be possible to train future leaders. Not everyone is a good teacher, nor do they want to be. The system itself may not have the capacity to take on a formal mentoring responsibility and the culture within the department may not be ready. Seasoned leaders can become territorial and, as such, may not be willing to mentor a fledgling leader. For a mentee to gain practical experience in a specific task, it may be appropriate for someone else to give up that responsibility for a specified period of time. If not presented properly, this change in roles can be viewed as a threat to the seasoned manager's self esteem or prestige. Therefore, it is important to build and foster a culture of

sharing and encouragement where succession planning is readily accepted and appreciated.

5. *Monitor and evaluate the department's progress towards its succession planning efforts and the contribution that human capital results have made toward achieving programmatic goals.* This is a step that is often overlooked. Successful leadership planning requires the development of meaningful outcome-oriented performance goals and then collecting performance data to measure levels of goal achievement. Many organizations fail to make these goals specific. As a result, they provide leadership experiences intended to build skill sets but never really know if the skills were developed. It is only after the employee is promoted that the skill deficit is identified.

   For example, one important skill set needed for the role of clinical coordinator may be to develop a clinical vision for the department and to establish and nurture political relationships needed to realize the plan. Although it is fairly easy to evaluate whether an individual has thought through a plan, it is much more difficult to evaluate their political savvy and their ability to leverage relationships. Careful attention must be paid to the mastery of these "softer" skills to ensure the employee's success in their new role.

6. *Engage others in the development and support structure.* Many factors contribute to the success of a formal employee development program. As previously mentioned, visible support from the top is important. However, it is also important to have support from line management and sometimes staff. These people may be asked to participate in the developmental training or to collaborate with the candidates. If not addressed proactively, resentment, frustration, or general lack of cooperation can result. Incorporating employee and line management input will help mitigate such challenges. Similarly, it is also critical to prepare mentees emotionally. For example, it may not be apparent that their relationships with their peers will change dramatically as they transition into new roles. Unprepared successors can find this unsettling as preexisting friendships may change.

7. *Succession planning programs should also be based on the objective assessment of candidates.* A high level of honest evaluation and transparency will help clarify how candidates are selected and the overall progress that they achieve. Accountability, follow-up, and integration with other human resource systems is also important.

OUTCOME MEASURES

Outcome measures can essentially be divided into 2 major categories, competencies, and results. Competencies are generally further divided into hard and soft skills. Hard skills represent technical skills like financial acumen, computer skills, ability to write a business plan, and more. Soft skills are just as important but are more often undervalued in the decision process and also harder to assess. They include abilities such as interpersonal skills, strategic thinking, judgment, emotional intelligence, and more. When newly promoted managers fail, it is generally a result of insufficient soft skills rather than hard skills.

The second major outcome measure is results. These too can be further divided into 2 primary categories, objective and subjective measures. Objective measures include work group results, production, customer satisfaction, and others. Subjective measures involve the importance of the work product to achieving the organization's goals, organizational effectiveness, or improved team capacity.

MANAGEMENT AND LEADERSHIP DEVELOPMENT ACTIVITIES

Employees selected for advancement are generally sent through a series of structured activities. These are intended to close any remaining developmental gaps and prepare employees for job levels as opposed to specific positions. Activities may involve skill-building classes, coaching, mentoring, formal education, developmental experiences, short-term assignments, and action learning. Organizations spend millions of dollars on developmental programs with a wide range of success.

According to the War for Talent Survey, job experience is the single most effective method of developing leaders.[10] This is further supported by employee responses in which 65% cited on-the-job experiences and challenging job assignments as the single greatest contributor to their development. While coaching and mentoring were felt to be important, providing employees with new, challenging assignments is essential. It is also important to point out that formal classroom training was felt to be one of the least effective forms of development. It is also interesting to note that when pharmacy practitioners were recently surveyed, 70% indicated that they did not have a mentor. Similarly, 63% of middle managers also did not have a mentor. This is in stark contrast to the 55% of pharmacy students who did.[1]

OBSTACLES TO PLANNED SUCCESSION

Certainly with all the positive benefit to succession planning, it seems logical that everyone would be actively engaged in it. Unfortunately, as noted, most are not. Primary reasons include:

- Managers do not want to think about getting older or retiring.
- It is perceived that the department could not possibly survive without the incumbent in that role.
- Many feel that they are too busy doing their job to mentor anyone.
- Fear of obsolescence.
- Reluctance to release power and control.
- Threat to personal identity.
- Bias against the program.
- Inability to choose among successors.
- Fear of retirement.
- Jealousy and rivalry.
- Fear of downstream consequences to the department.

Successors, of course, have their own set of worries:

- Will I live up to expectations?
- Will I be able to establish my independence?
- Will I be able to establish good working relationships with my new colleagues?
- Will my former colleagues respect me?
- What if I fail?

For any program to succeed, organizations need to emphasize teamwork, mentoring, and honesty. People often struggle with candor but it is at the heart of success.[11]

It is also important to note that a common concern of many of the involved leaders in succession planning is a fear of long-term consequences to the department. Many leaders spend years building and perfecting a department. As the incumbent leader's departure approaches, they certainly want to know that they will be missed when they are gone; they also want to ensure that what they have built will withstand the transition. However, studies show that how a leader departs an organization can have a critical impact on operational success metrics in the years that immediately follow.[12–16]

Exiting leaders essentially fall into 1 of 4 main categories.[17] *Monarchs* are leaders that leave their post under some exigent circumstances. They are fired or otherwise pushed out. As a result, their relationship with the organization is usually severed.

Generals are leaders that leave but retain some position of interference. They may be in a vice presidential capacity, be active in the Foundation, take an emeritus position with the school of pharmacy, or be in some other role that allows them to remain and continue to gain glory, as well as meddle in department affairs. They periodically feel the need to rescue the department from the real or imaginary inadequacy of the successor. In a sense, this validates their leadership skill by showing that the department cannot function without them. However, the reality is that a leader's true lasting value is best measured by the effectiveness of their succession planning within an organization.[18] True leaders leave a department that can function seamlessly without them, rather than implode in their absence.

The third type of exiting leader is the *Ambassador*. Ambassadors leave their post quietly and gracefully and serve as postretirement mentors. They may maintain a minimal presence but do not try to sabotage their successor. They take great effort to detach from any decision-making responsibility.

The fourth and final category is the *Governor*. Governors complete their rule in office and then disappear. They maintain very little ongoing contact with the department once they have left and allow it to function independently.

Data collected on leadership exit strategies indicate that organizations perform better in major categories such as asset management, sales, income, and employee turnover when the exiting leader assumes the role of the Ambassador and provides continued mentorship without meddling.[17] Although the data are less clear, Generals who linger and meddle create environments in which it is hard for the successor to independently lead, and as such, the department flounders. These observations can provide valuable insight for pharmacy directors who are promoted into hospital administrative roles but retain responsibility for pharmacy services.

CONCLUSION

Pharmacy is on the brink of an impending leadership crisis and the lack of young leaders entering formal leadership training programs will not compensate for the expected exodus. For many health systems, it will simply not be possible to externally recruit qualified people to replace key staff lost to other organizations or to retirement. An effective solution to this challenge is to develop these replacements internally. If the profession of pharmacy is going to survive this leadership gap, a renewed emphasis on succession planning is essential.

REFERENCES

1. White SJ. Will there be a pharmacy leadership crisis? An ASHP foundation scholar-in-residence report. *Am J Health Syst Pharm.* 2005;62(8):845–855.

2. Zilz DA, Woodward BW, Thielke TS, Shane RR, Scott B. Leadership skills for high-performance pharmacy practice. *Am J Health Syst Pharm.* 2006; 61(23):2562-2574.

3. Young D. Effective leadership is vital to pharmacy's future. *Am J Health Syst Pharm.* 2004;61(12):1212-1214.

4. Drucker PF. *The Essential Drucker: The Best of Sixty Years of Peter Drucker's Essential Writings on Management.* New York, NY: Harper Collins; 2003.

5. Smith JE. Integrating human resources and program-planning strategies. *Am J Health Syst Pharm.* 1989;46(6):1153-1161.

6. Chase PA. Human resources management for a hospital pharmacy department. *Am J Health Syst Pharm.* 1989;46(6):1162-1169.

7. ASHP: CareerPharm. Identifying top performers for succession and workforce planning. 2005. http://www.careerpharm.com/employer/resources/top-performers.cfm. Accessed May 12, 2008.

8. American Journal of Health-System Pharmacy. ASHP Report: Proceedings of the 2005 Conference for Leaders in Health-System Pharmacy. http://pt.wkhealth.com/pt/re/ajhp/fulltext.00043627-200608150-00015.htm;jsessionid=LyHX1Zbw8Ly2GMr1ThPxZ2rGyPXGzYLppvvXy1Q5VTdTwS0khJBL!298990308!181195629!8091!-1. Accessed May 12, 2008.

9. Peter LJ, Hull R. *The Peter Principle.* New York, NY: Bantam; 1970.

10. Fast Company. War for talent II: seven ways to win. *Fast Co.* 2000;42(12):98.

11. Welch J, Welch S. *Winning.* New York, NY: Harper Collins; 2005.

12. Conger JA, Fulmer RM. *Growing Your Company's Leaders: How Great Organizations Use Succession Management to Sustain Competitive Advantage.* New York, NY: AMACOM; 2004.

13. Corporate University Xchange. *Sixth Annual Benchmarking Report.* New York, NY: Corporate University Xchange; 2004.

14. Hiltz T. Use of a balanced scorecard at the U.S. Army Corps of Engineers. http://unpan1.un.org/intradoc/groups/public/documents/aspa/unpan015901.pdf. Accessed May 12, 2008.

15. Donald Chrusciel D, Field DW. Critical success factors into criteria for performance excellence—an organizational change strategy. *J Indust Tech.* 2003; 19(4):1-11.

16. Weiss DS, Finn R. HR metrics that count: aligning human capital management to business results. *Human Res Plan.* 2005;28(1):33-38.

17. Sonnefeld J. *The Hero's Farewell—What Happens When CEOs Retire.* New York, NY: Oxford University Press; 1988.

18. Thielke TS. Searching for excellence in leadership transformation. *Am J Health Syst Pharm.* 2005;62(16):1657-1662. ∎

Working Effectively With Consultants

Michael Sanborn, MS, FASHP*

The *Director's Forum* series is written and edited by Michael Sanborn and Robert Weber and is designed to guide pharmacy leaders in establishing patient-centered services in hospitals and health systems. Another specific goal of this column is to address many of the key challenges that pharmacy directors currently face, while providing information to foster growth in pharmacy leadership and patient safety. This *Director's Forum* article focuses on the use of consultants in pharmacies and in health care. This is a unique topic that most directors will address at one time or another during their careers.

It has been said that a consultant is someone who looks at your watch and tells you the time. In fact, consultants are typically hired to serve as an outside, objective resource that can provide expert advice on a given area without bias or emotion. As with any type of service, different consultants and consulting companies offer varying levels of expertise, experience, types of consulting, and results. When effectively utilized, consultants can serve as a very valuable resource and change agent to improve department and hospital performance. This article will address ways in which to leverage improvement efforts with consultants and maximize the impact of their recommendations.

BACKGROUND

Health care consulting is big business because health care is such a significant contributor to our overall economy. Nationally, health care consulting revenues continue to grow at nearly double-digit rates and these revenues are estimated to approach nearly $25 billion in 2008 and over $30 billion by 2010.[1,2] Health care

consultants may be engaged in an organization for a multitude of reasons, a few of which include: human resource management, facilities planning, patient satisfaction improvement, efficiency analysis, risk reduction, revenue enhancement, and information technology expansion. Oftentimes, consultants are hired to improve specific aspects of an organization's financial position and such engagements can range from billing to marketing analysis, to a focus on operational costs (usually including supply and/or labor costs). There are 2 salient situations in which hospital consultants are engaged—at the request of the pharmacy or of someone outside of pharmacy.

Typically, consultants are engaged at a high level within the organization as part of a specific improvement effort and are not employed as the result of the management of any individual department. In circumstances where cost reduction or operational improvement is the explicit focus, it is not unusual for an individual department head to initially feel threatened. Anger or frustration is not uncommon, due to the implication that an outsider, oftentimes a non-pharmacist, is needed to advise how to run the department. In these situations, it is important for the manager to quickly move past the initial anxiety and to focus on clearly understanding why the consulting group was engaged and the specific outcomes expected by the hospital. Be objective and open-mind-

*Corporate Vice President, Baylor Health Care System, Dallas, Texas ed as to how these expectations relate directly to your department. This can help the overall experience flow much more smoothly and will increase the likelihood that the end result is something that all parties can accept.

It is also important to realize that financial and operational consultants will often encourage senior leadership to include the pharmacy as part of the engagement regardless of the department's perceived level of performance, since it is an area with significant labor costs (due to the relatively high expense of pharmacist and technician salaries versus other health care workers) and very high supply costs. There are also a number of companies and individuals that specialize in pharmacy consulting and these groups may be selected by the pharmacy department, or the hospital, to assist with a particular problem or opportunity.

Pharmacy directors may choose to employ consultants within the department for a variety of reasons. Providing evaluation or justification for new clinical programs, facilities planning for USP <797> compliance, developing strategies for medication error reduction, and management of new technology or information system implementation are all examples of situations in which consultants can be helpful. In general, a partnership with a consultant company might be considered in situations where there is a lack of time, personnel, financial support, information, expertise, or visibility that is necessary to move a project or service forward.[3]

If your facility has elected to work with a particular consulting group, or if your department is considering the use of a pharmacy consultant, there are a variety of steps that can be taken to make sure you get the most out of the consulting experience. These steps include consultant selection, understanding the consultant's methodology, preparation and data collection, active participation in the consulting process, and assisting with the development of specific recommendations.

CONSULTANT SELECTION

There are many ways to select a health care consultant. Obviously, if a consultant group is selected by the hospital's senior leadership, then there is typically little opportunity for the pharmacy department to influence that decision. If, however, the pharmacy is employing the consultant, or if pharmacy has some influence in the hospital's consultant selection, it is best to treat the process similar to that of selecting an employee for a key position. When carefully selected, the consultant will be able to serve as an expert advisor and can offer recommendations that will meet or exceed the desired result.

The selection process should start with a thorough review of the consultant's credentials and past experience. There are organizations that accredit and credential both consulting companies and consultants and these include the American Association of Health-care Consultants and the National Society of Certified Healthcare Business Consultants. While such credentials may assist in winnowing down a large list of potential companies, not all firms or individuals seek certification by these organizations. This is especially true of smaller, more specialized consultant groups, so it is worthwhile to determine upfront if a specific set of credentials is required.

References are probably one of the most important consultant selection tools and some specific questions regarding previous clients should be considered. Has the company worked with facilities or departments like yours before (eg, academic teaching hospital, long-term care facility, widespread ambulatory services, extensive pharmacy consult services)? What specific references do they have? What were the consulting outcomes at each of those reference sites and how did they compare with the organization's initial expectations? Was the quality of their recommendations such that they could all be implemented and the projected benefits realized? Were the recommendations durable and practical enough that they are still in use today? Have there been sites where the company did not meet a facility's expectations, and if so, why? Once a list of references has been provided, it is very important to follow through and contact the facilities with a set of predetermined questions that will allow you to compare the potential success of your experience with theirs.

When working with large consulting firms, it is also imperative to understand the backgrounds and expertise of the specific individuals that will be executing the consulting effort. Many companies will sell their consulting process, but will then use relative apprentices at the site that have been trained to use that particular process. While this strategy can be effective, it is not the same as working with someone that has a high level of expertise in the desired area. It is important to decide whether this level of expertise is necessary before agreeing to work with an individual company. At a minimum, it is worthwhile to ask for resumes of those individuals that will be onsite.

Another requirement for selecting a consultant involves an analysis of each company's consulting methodology. This is typically discussed at a general level during the initial deliberation process. However, it is important to clearly understand how the work will be performed and how long it may take to reach the expected results. There are many different consulting methods and varying techniques are employed depending on the type of processes or areas being analyzed. Best practice implementation, time and motion studies, skills training, process mapping, and comparisons to known benchmarks are some examples of techniques that can be used as part of a larger consulting process. There are also more formal consulting philosophies that were developed in the manufacturing industry and are now being applied to health care. For example, the Six Sigma methodology is becoming more popular in hospitals and uses data and statistical analysis to measure and improve operational performance. The "lean" methodology has also been applied to health care and focuses on the elimination of waste and the improvement of quality. There is no single best method for health care consulting but it is important to critically evaluate the proposed process to be sure it will deliver the desired results.

Finally, it is important to understand how the consultant is typically paid for their services. Consultants may work strictly on an hourly rate or may quote a cost for the entire product. Others may suggest minimal upfront funding but are later compensated based on a percentage of total (or projected) savings generated. Premiums and incentives based on predetermined performance goals are also common, depending on the type of expected outcomes. A comprehensive contract with the detailed expectations of both sides, as well a specific end points to measure performance, is an essential part of any consulting engagement.

PREPARATION AND DATA COLLECTION

Once a consulting group has been selected, the next step is to prepare for the consulting effort. Oftentimes the consultant will have detailed recommendations regarding resources needed as well as a draft timeline for project execution. For example, they may recommend that one or more staff members are available full-time during onsite visits or that certain staff are available for individual interviews. Prior to the consultant's arrival, it is also important to effectively communicate the purpose, timeline, expectations, and other pertinent information with the pharmacy staff.

Data are often requested by the consultant in advance to allow for pre-visit analysis and potential comparisons to a database of previous clients. The types of data requested will always depend on the type of consulting planned. A comprehensive department analysis will often require the production of extensive department data; however, an engagement that is more narrowly focused, such as supply chain management, may require more specific data that includes line-item drug expenses, purchase velocity reports, formulary activity, and department policies surrounding inventory control and purchasing.

During the preparation process, it is often helpful to make a formal inventory of various programs and best practices that are currently in place as well as services and practice changes that are planned or needed in the future. This type of information is help-ful in setting the pre-consulting baseline and can also allow the consultant to focus efforts on specific department goals or other areas that have not yet been improved. Likewise, if additional justification is needed for a planned service or for department expansion, be prepared to share this information with the consultants to see if it can be addressed during the visit and then included as part of the final recommendations.

The goal of advanced preparation is to be completely organized and ready to work with the consultants immediately upon their arrival. Any data provided to the consultants should also be internally scrutinized in advance of the initial meeting so that specific questions and comments can be readily addressed. If other members of the staff are required as part of the project, make sure they clearly understand their role and expectations as well as have the necessary time to participate.

During any onsite data collection sessions, make sure that data being collected adequately reflects your typical operation. For example, if chemotherapy volume data are collected during a week when one of the hospital's primary oncologists is on vacation, then it will likely be necessary to make adjustments or to postpone data collection. Be aware of data fluctuations that may occur by time of day, day of week, type of drug, or by individual personnel productivity variations and make appropriate adjustments in the data sample size to accommodate this variability. Additionally, be conscious of costs that are fixed versus variable. Certain labor and supply costs are necessary regardless of the volumes produced and these should be identified in advance as fixed costs. Any data-collection tools used during the process should be discussed in advance to ensure their applicability to your operation. Finally, make sure all staff involved in data collection fully understand his or her responsibility and the importance of comprehensive, accurate measurements.

ACTIVE PARTICIPATION IN THE PROCESS

As mentioned, consulting services are typically employed for a variety of reasons. Active participation is an important part of any consulting project so complete knowledge transfer takes place. If the project is related to facility improvements, work directly with the consultants to understand all of the pertinent regulations and requirements and how each will be addressed. When working with technology consultants, make sure they understand all hospital processes and procedures associated with acquisition and implementation as well as strengths or limitations of the information-systems infrastructure.

In situations where consulting services are forced upon the department (oftentimes for focused cost reductions), a common reflex is to resist all requests and efforts made by the consultant. This type of behavior is not productive and can often lead to a strained and potentially negative relationship with the consultants, hospital administration, or both. It can also lead to long-term detrimental results for the department. In 1995, McAllister published an instructive article on working with consultants that were focused only on labor reduction.[4] Even when faced with potential budget cuts, as a department leader it is important to engage the consultants honestly, understand their purpose, and work directly with them to assure

a satisfactory outcome for all parties. An advanced understanding of potential benchmark statistics used by many consulting companies is helpful.

For example, labor consultants will often focus efforts towards tying pharmacy labor expenses to a hospital or department statistic such as patient days or doses billed. Supply chain consultants will frequently compare overall hospital supply costs as well as pharmacy supply costs versus a national average and will also commonly associate department data with a hospital statistic such as drug cost per discharge. In both cases, such statistics have shown to have only a limited value for interfacility comparison, primarily because they do not account for the level of clinical pharmacy services (and other non-distributive tasks and services) and because many of the statistic definitions are subject to some degree of variation.[5-8] While it is not possible to discuss all caveats associated with certain parameters, **Table 1** summarizes many of the common statistical benchmark denominators that are used and some of the advantages and disadvantages of each that should be considered. Prior to using any of these denominators, it is helpful to meet with hospital finance staff to fully understand how each value is determined. There is no ideal pharmacy benchmark statistic, so when possible, ascertain in advance which benchmarks will be used as well as specific high and low targets that are typical for a comparable facility.

DEVELOPMENT OF RECOMMENDATIONS

The goal of any consulting engagement is to develop meaningful and actionable recommendations that will have long-lasting benefit to the

Table 1. Considerations with Common Pharmacy Productivity Ratios

Ratio Denominator	Advantages and Disadvantages
Licensed Beds	A published, recognized number; however, there can be significant differences between this number and the number of beds that are actually staffed and used by the facility. This does not include outpatient volumes unless adjusted.
Occupied Bed	A measure of beds that are actually used. Typically more reliable than licensed beds but does not account for variations in length of stay by patient type or from one facility to another. May or may not include short-stay patients. Does not include outpatient volumes unless adjusted.
Admissions	Number is a standardized hospital statistic. It may or may not include various patient types that require pharmacy services (eg, newborns, short stay) Can also be adjusted to include outpatients.
Discharges	Similar to admissions but may exclude expired patients or certain types of transfers. May or may not include short-stay patients.
Patient Days	Typically better than admissions because length of stay is incorporated into the statistic. Can be skewed by inordinate numbers of low-or high-acuity patients if not case-mix adjusted.
Adjusted Patient Days	Same as patient days but adjusts for contributions by outpatient volumes. Should be calculated using pharmacy revenue rather than hospital revenue.
Doses Dispensed	Relatively easy to obtain from most pharmacy information systems. Gives equal importance to an oral-unit-dose tablet and a complex-chemotherapy preparation or TPN. Does not account for non-dispensing workload (clinical services). May include non-drug or other atypical pharmacy items that can vary dramatically from one facility to another. Billing units may also vary.
Doses Billed	Same considerations as doses dispensed but does not contain medications that are returned after dispensing nor the workload associated with the return process.
Case-Mix Index	An adjustment factor that can be incorporated into most statistics that takes patient acuity into account. Calculated using diagnosis related group (DRG) weights for the hospital's DRG-based claims. Improves the reliability of most ratios but may not be directly related to pharmacy workload and may not include all patient types.

organization. Once data collection and the onsite analysis are complete, a listing of recommendations is typically produced. Some of these recommendations may have been discussed during the onsite activities, whereas others may be completely new and unexpected. Each recommendation should be carefully and objectively reviewed. Some recommendations may initially appear impossible or impractical but it is important to not reject these recommendations out of hand. There may be ways to modify the recommendation such that it can be effectively implemented. For those recommendations that seem questionable or unachievable, ask for reference facilities that may have successfully implemented the program or service.

It is also worthwhile to point out that consultants hired to analyze a specific area do not always consider the impact of their recommendations to other areas. For instance, a supply chain consultant may recommend the implementation of a syringe-based admixture delivery system without taking into account changes in staffing or technology that would be needed to compound enough syringes for all patients. In this scenario, will the existing pumps be compatible with a syringe system? Will there be any positive or negative effects on nursing labor? What are the implementation costs of such a change? While the initial recommendation may look good on paper, it is the responsibility of the director to make sure that each recommendation is fully scrutinized for all costs.

Once a set of recommendations has been agreed upon, a detailed plan and timeline should be established for implementation. Oftentimes, it is necessary to present the findings to hospital administration, particularly when resources are needed or significant change is planned. In addition, a communication plan for the staff should be developed with a focus on those staff members that will be directly affected, as well as feedback to the staff who participated in the process.

Remember that improvement does not stop once the recommendations are implemented. Good consultants will leave behind tools and techniques that can be used long-term for future projects. When possible, data collected prior to implementation should be compared with post-implementation data to measure the impact of the consulting effort and to plan for future incremental improvements.

SUMMARY

There are a number of situations where health care consultants might be employed and they can serve as a valuable pharmacy resource when selected and effectively used. When initiating any consulting arrangement, it is important that both the methodology and the goals are clearly understood. Pharmacy directors should focus on effective project planning, active participation in the consulting process, and the development of clear, achievable recommendations to ensure a positive outcome that delivers long-lasting department improvements.

REFERENCES

1. Kennedy Information, Inc. The Healthcare Consulting Marketplace 2007. http://www.consultingcentral.com/research/industry-practices/health care-consulting-marketplace-report. Accessed January 13, 2008.

2. Newsblaze.com, LLC. Healthcare Consulting Leads Industry Recovery Vital Signs Approach Double-Digit Growth; $25B by 2008. http://newsblaze.com/story/2005071208302200001.mwir/topstory.html. Accessed January 13, 2008.

3. O'Connor PJ, DiBona JR. Balancing costs and outcomes through partnerships with consultants. *Am J Health Syst Pharm.* 2005;62(2):139-141.

4. McAllister JC 3rd. Collaborating with re-engineering consultants: maintaining resources for the future. *Am J Health Syst Pharm.* 1995;52(23):2676-2680.

5. Gupta SR, Wojtynek JE, Walton SM, et al. Association between hospital size and pharmacy department productivity. *Am J Health Syst Pharm.* 2007;64(9):937-944.

6. Glazier HS, Malen J. Pharmacy staffing and productivity. *Am J Health Syst Pharm.* 2007;64(22):2320, 2322-2323.

7. Felkey BG, Liang H, Krueger KP. Data mining for the health system pharmacist. *Hosp Pharm.* 2003;38(9):845-850.

8. Knoer SJ, Couldry RJ, Folker T. Evaluating a benchmarking database and identifying cost reduction opportunities by diagnosis-related group. *Am J Health Syst Pharm.* 1999;56(11):1102-1107. ∎

Building Your Financial IQ

Matthew W. Eberts, PharmD, MBA*; Scott M. Mark, PharmD, MS, MEd, FASHP FACHE, FABC†; and Robert J. Weber, PharmD, MS, BCPS, FASHP‡

The *Director's Forum* series has been written and edited by Robert Weber and Michael Sanborn and is designed to guide pharmacy leaders in establishing patient-centered services in hospitals and health systems. Effective this issue, Scott M. Mark, PharmD, MS, MEd, FASHP, FACHE, FABC, will assume the responsibilities of editing the column along with Robert Weber, PharmD, MS, BCPS, FASHP. Michael Sanborn, MS, FASHP, will step down as coeditor of this column with this issue. We would like to acknowledge the excellent work done by Mr. Sanborn in originating and editing this column for the last 4 years. His contributions significantly influenced the leadership direction of hospital and health-system pharmacists. Dr. Mark is currently the Director of Pharmacy at the University of Pittsburgh Medical Center and Associate Professor and Vice Chair of Pharmacy at the University of Pittsburgh School of Pharmacy. His practice and teaching are in the area of pharmacy leadership and practice management. We welcome Dr. Mark as a co-editor of the *Director's Forum*. This month's article focuses on assessing the ability of the pharmacy director in managing the pharmacy's financial operations—a key skill set necessary in developing patient-centered pharmacy services.

A successful pharmacy leader is able to establish a vision for the department and transform that vision into reality. This individual possesses the ability to connect with people, operational expertise, and a mastery of the medication delivery process. However, if the vision requires investments such as additional staffing, new automation, or information technology expenditure, capital and full-time equivalents (FTEs) must be provided by the "C-suite" (the senior executives such as the chief executive officer [CEO], chief financial officer [CFO],

and chief nursing officer [CNO]). The pharmacy director knows investments in pharmacy services will produce desirable outcomes, including decreased drug expenses and medication errors, quicker turn around time, and better regulatory compliance.[1-3] This understanding is not intrinsic to the hospital's executive leadership.

Imagine spending the past year as the hospital's CFO. It has been a struggle to generate any profit or at least to minimize losses. Perhaps layoffs, budget cuts, frozen salaries, cut benefits, and delays for important projects were some of the difficult decisions that needed to be made over the past year.[4,5] Ahead lies uncertainty regarding health care reform, economic conditions, pay for performance, and declining reimbursement rates. The challenge that faces the CFO is ensuring the long-term success of the organization.

With this in mind, imagine receiving a request from the pharmacy for five new pharmacist FTEs to roll out a unit-based pharmacy model. The request from pharmacy came in the same week as a request from imaging to purchase a computed tomography machine that performs a specialized test offered by the hospital across town, a request from nursing to purchase infusion pumps compli-

*Pharmacy Manager, University of Pittsburgh Medical Center, Adjunct Instructor, Department of Pharmacy & Therapeutics, University of Pittsburgh School of Pharmacy, Pittsburgh, Pennsylvania; †Director of Pharmacy, University of Pittsburgh Medical Center, Associate Professor and Vice Chair, Department of Pharmacy & Therapeutics, University of Pittsburgh School of Pharmacy, Pittsburgh, Pennsylvania; ‡Executive Director of Pharmacy, University of Pittsburgh Medical Center, Associate Professor and Chair, Department of Pharmacy & Therapeutics, University of Pittsburgh School of Pharmacy, Pittsburgh, Pennsylvania.

ant with new safety guidelines, and a request from maintenance to replace the boiler that keeps failing. The CFO believes the hospital is only able to support one of these requests. If the CFO chooses a priority other than pharmacy, the pharmacy director's vision may need to be put on hold or watered down.

The goal of this article is to provide the pharmacy director with knowledge and strategies for utilizing financial tools to justify investments in pharmacy services. The aims of this article are to (1) review key financial terms relevant to the pharmacy director, (2) demonstrate financial tools that can be used to show the value of investing in pharmacy, (3) discuss strategies the pharmacy director can utilize to negotiate resources, and (4) present case studies to better demonstrate these skills.

FINANCIAL TERMS

The pharmacy director should be familiar with the following financial terms[6,7]:

- **Revenue:** Income that an organization receives for its normal business activities (eg, money collected from payers for the provision of care).
- **Expenses:** Outflow of cash from the organization to individuals or other organizations (ie, employee wages).
- **Operating income:** Profit from the organization's operations (revenue minus expenses).
- **EBITDA (Earnings Before Interest, Taxes, Depreciation, and Amortization):** The earnings before interest, taxes, depreciation, or amortization are subtracted. This metric reveals the earnings of an organization without the effects of variables not related directly to operations.

- **Cash flow:** Time-specific movement of cash in and out of the business. The organization needs to know when money will be flowing so they can be sure to have adequate amounts at all times.
- **Net present value:** The difference between the present day value of expenses and revenues for a particular project. Over time money loses value because of inflation; net present value (NPV) allows the entire lifespan of a project to be evaluated in today's dollars.
- **Internal rate of return:** The rate of growth a project is expected to generate. This can be used to compare and rank projects based upon the growth an organization is expected to realize.
- **Time to payback:** The amount of time it will take an investment to pay for itself.
- **Run rate:** How an organization or service line's financial results would look if a small sample was extrapolated over a longer period of time, for example, using one quarter's performance to predict an entire year. See **Table 1** as an example of a one quarter profit and loss statement used to predict 1 year of results.
- **Return on investment:** The amount of return an organization realizes from an investment (income divided by cost). Return on investment is also included in **Table 1**.
- **Cost of capital:** The expected return on money/investments held by the company (needed for calculated NPV).
- **Inventory turns:** Number of times the inventory is sold or turned over during a specified time period.

Table 1. One-year run rate for investigational drug service based upon one quarter's profit and loss statement

Revenue (top line)

Description	First quarter	1 year projected	How calculated
Setup/dispensing	$45,000	$180,000	Q1 result × 4
Audits	$2,500	$10,000	Q1 result × 4
HIV grant	$10,000	$40,000	Q1 result × 4
Total revenue	$57,500	$230,000	Sum of above
Expenses			
Salary	($42,000)	($168,000)	Q1 result × 4
Rent	($3,000)	($12,000)	Q1 result × 4
Telephone/pager	($60)	($240)	Q1 result × 4
Supplies	($905)	($3,620)	Q1 result × 4
Total expenses	($45,965)	($183,860)	Sum of above
Net income (bottom line)			
Excess revenue over expenses	$11,535	$46,140	Total revenue – Total expense
Return on investment	25.1%	25.1%	Excess revenue/Absolute value of total expense

FINANCIAL TOOLS

The following are financial tools the pharmacy director should have at his or her disposal when requesting resources from the organization.[6,7]

- **Pro forma:** Models the financial effect that a transaction such as leasing a new piece of equipment will have on cash flow. A pro forma is an estimated financial statement illustrating the effect an investment will have on an organization. **Table 2** is an example. Note that the values in this example are from a case found later in this article.
- **Profit and loss statement (income statement):** A statement that illustrates how the revenues (top line) are transformed into the net income (bottom line) over a specific period of time. The statement includes detailed revenue numbers and subtracts detailed expense numbers to result in the net income. **Table 1** is a profit and loss statement for an investigational drug pharmacy.

- **Business plan:** A tool that allows an organization to look ahead, allocate resources, and prepare for problems and opportunities. Business plans can be utilized for new service lines, significant capital investments, or expanding current operations. The plan should follow the accepted format as outlined in the box titled "Business Plan Format." The length and amount of detail included in the plan is dictated by the organization's culture and the scope of the project.

STRATEGY

The ability to demonstrate the value of pharmacy services and equipment utilizing the previously described financial tools is a vital skill set.

- **Align project with priorities:** At any given time, the hospital executives have a list of priority issues to address. The hospital executives are under significant pressure to accomplish these goals. In addition to

Table 2. Pro forma for 5-year lease of two carousel units

Time period (year)[a]	0	1	2	3	4	5	Total
Expenses related to the project							
Lease price	($75,000)	($75,000)	($75,000)	($75,000)	($75,000)	–	($375,000)
Service charge	($10,000)	($10,000)	($10,000)	($10,000)	($10,000)	–	($50,000)
Shipping/installation	($20,000)	–	–	–	–	–	($20,000)
Interface build	($5,000)	–	–	–	–	–	($5,000)
Cost savings (revenue) realized by the project							
Increase in inventory turns	–	$410,000	$0	$0	$0	$0	$410,000
Decrease in medication errors[b]	–	$93,420	$93,420	$93,420	$93,420	$93,420	$467,100
Cash flow							
Total investment/Return	($110,000)	$418,420	$8,420	$8,420	$8,420	$93,420	$427,100
(Cost savings – Expenses)							
Return on investment							
Cumulative net cash flow	($110,000)	$308,420	$316,840	$325,260	$333,680	$427,100	$427,100
(Cumulative cost savings – Expenses)							
Metrics for valuing project							
Time to payback, years							0.26
Internal rate of return							283%
Net present value							$364,669
Cost of capital (enter as %)						7.5%	

[a]Time period 0 represents day 1 of the project; time periods 1–5 represent the end of that particular year. [b]Decrease in medication errors calculated as ($2,595/adverse drug events) × 36 errors per year. [c]Can be calculated by *Microsoft Office Excel* utilizing formulas.

hospital-wide goals, executives have specific goals they are challenged to meet. Frequently these goals are linked to their bonus pay. For a pharmacy director, it is important to find out what these priorities are and link the department's projects to them. This "help me, help you" approach can be a smart strategy for moving projects forward.

- **Stepwise approach:** In many cases, a proposal that moves a project directly to the finish line is too aggressive to earn executive support. As such, it makes sense to develop a step-by-step plan that incrementally moves toward the goal. The initial steps should be focused on low investment/big win items. This will allow the pharmacy director to build momentum and gain support for future investments. As the project is successful, it is critical that the pharmacy department markets this message to the C-suite so they understand the investment in pharmacy has been a wise one.
- **Establish a relationship with the C-suite:** A mentoring relationship with a hospital executive team member, for instance the CFO or the chief information officer (CIO), can be a useful relationship for the pharmacy director. The obvious benefit to establishing a mentoring relationship with the CFO is a conduit to an individual who is an expert in the area of finance. The pharmacy leader can learn to see through the eyes of the executive, as well as educating the leader as to the importance of pharmacy services in patient care. Another benefit is a personal relationship with an individual who controls how the hospital will allocate its resources. This relationship with the C-suite

will give the pharmacy leader a level of credibility that will aid in earning resources from the organization.

CASE STUDIES
Case Study 1
Background

The pharmacy director at a 290-bed suburban hospital would like to implement a decentralized pharmacist model. The plan is to continue dispensing medications from the central pharmacy while positioning the pharmacists on the units. The hospital currently has one satellite pharmacy covering the critical care areas (intensive care unit and critical care unit) from 7 AM to 11 PM 7 days a week.

Description of the problem

The pharmacy director believes that the value pharmacists bring is their ability to serve on the care team as medication experts. Moving the pharmacists to the units will increase their capacity to fill this role. The ultimate goal would be decentralized coverage on all care units from 7 AM to 11 PM every day. To achieve this goal, the pharmacy director needs to hire five pharmacist FTEs.

Strategy

The pharmacy director realizes that a request for five additional pharmacist FTEs will be dead on arrival; therefore the director will utilize a stepwise approach. Thanks to a relationship the pharmacy leader has built with the hospital's CFO, he knows one of the biggest priorities for the hospital is decreasing malpractice lawsuits related to anticoagulation therapy against the hospital. The director can propose adding two pharmacist FTEs to cover the areas most likely to see anticoagulation therapy as a method to decrease malpractice lawsuits. This will align the pharmacy's vision with the hospital's priority. The success of this initial phase can be used to support future growth.

Financial tools

A business plan would be a prudent tool to use in this situation. The plan can include benchmarking data from other institutions with unit-based models and financial information directly linking the investment in pharmacy to the decrease in malpractice lawsuits.

Case Study 2
Background

The pharmacy director at a 120-bed rural hospital would like to implement carousel technology for storing and dispensing medications. The hospital currently performs a manual daily cart fill and has automated dispensing cabinets on the units for storing emergent medications, controlled substances, and as-needed medications.

Description of the problem

The pharmacy director wants to add automation to the medication delivery process to improve safety, efficiency, and inventory management. The pharmacy has seen a steady increase in medication errors, and the director feels that carousel technology is the best solution to the problem. The director postulates that carousel technology will eliminate 36 medication errors annually. Additionally, the pharmacy is currently turning their inventory seven times annually. The hospital CFO has read that a small hospital pharmacy should turn their inventory 10 times per year.[8] The director has been challenged with increasing the yearly inventory turns to

10. An analysis of the current condition reveals that two carousel units are required. The pharmacy director needs to get support from their vice president for the project. Terms of the lease are included in **Table 3**.

Strategy

The pharmacy director has been challenged with increasing inventory turns. The director could link the investment in carousel technology to meeting that goal. As an example of how to quantify this project, **Table 4** shows the cash freed up by increasing the turns.

An increase in medication errors is alarming news throughout the organization. The pharmacy director can focus attention on carousel technology and how it will decrease medication errors; this strategy can work to gain support from nursing and medical staff for the investment.

Business Plan Format

I. **Executive Summary:** High level overview (write this last).

II. **Company Description:** Background information, legal establishment, etc.

III. **Product or Service:** Describe the service or technology. Focus on customer benefits.

IV. **Analysis:** Benchmark data, current condition, etc.

V. **Strategy and Implementation Plan:** Be specific. Include management responsibilities with dates and budgets. Make sure you can track results.

VI. **Management Team:** Describe the organization and the key management team members.

VII. **Financial Analysis:** Demonstrate the financial impact of the project utilizing financial tools such as pro forma and profit and loss statements.

The director may argue that this technology will increase efficiencies in the pharmacy. However it is impor-

Table 3. Lease terms for two carousel units

Lease cost per year	$75,000
Yearly service charge	$10,000
Shipping/installation fee (one time)	$20,000
Interface build (one time)	$5,000

tant to note that increased efficiency justification can be a double-edged sword when trying to gain executive support for a project. Unless the director is clear on how the resources will be reallocated, the executive leader may remove staffing resources from the pharmacy's budget.

Financial tools

A pro forma is included for a 5-year lease (see **Table 2**). The pro forma shows that the carousel investment has a positive return of $427,100 for the hospital. In today's dollars that represents $364,669 (as demonstrated by the net present value). This document includes cost savings realized from error avoidance. This number can be obtained through literature research or an internal number can be utilized.[9] Cost avoidance can be seen as "soft dollars" by executive leaders, therefore it is important for the director to use errors specific to the

hospital to help tell the story of how medication errors negatively affect the organization.

CONCLUSION

Every director has a vision for the pharmacy department. The ability to transform the vision into reality is linked to the leader's "financial IQ" in terms of gaining support from the executive leadership team. This is achieved by linking pharmacy investments directly to the hospital's overall performance.

Imagine the CFO mulling through a stack of requests from different departments knowing there are limited resources to share. The prioritization of those requests will be based upon the return the organization realizes from its investment. The hospital has had three major lawsuits over the past 5 years related to anti-coagulation medications. The board of directors has communicated to the executive team that eliminating these lawsuits is high priority. As the CFO reviews the pharmacy director's request to develop a unit-based model, it is clear how the program will decrease the lawsuits. Now the pharmacy department has the upper edge in gaining support for their project.

Table 4. Effect on inventory realized by increasing turns to 10

CURRENT CONDITION		
2009 purchases	Actual inventory (performed 12/1/2009)	Inventory turns
$9,500,000	$1,360,000	7[a]
PROJECTION WITH 10 INVENTORY TURNS		
2009 purchases	New on-hand inventory	Inventory turns
$9,500,000	$950,000[b]	10
PROJECTED FREED CASH	$410,000[c]	

[a]Calculated by dividing total purchases by actual inventory. [b]Calculated by dividing total purchases by desired number of inventory turns. [c]Calculated by subtracting new inventory on hand from actual inventory.

The emphasis in this *Director's Forum* has been to assist pharmacy leaders in developing patient-centered pharmacy services. Having a good handle on financial terms, applications, and strategies enhances the director's financial IQ and helps to justify new services. A pharmacy leader who is regarded as a competent health care provider who takes their fiduciary responsibility seriously will be successful in any organization.

REFERENCES

1. De Rijdt T, Willems L, Simoens S. Economic effects of clinical pharmacy interventions: a literature review. *Am J Health Syst Pharm.* 2008;65(12):1161-1172.

2. Maviglia SM, Yoo JY, Franz C, et al. Cost-benefit analysis of a hospital pharmacy bar code solution. *Arch Intern Med.* 2007;167(8):788-794.

3. Van den Bemt PM, Postma MJ, van Roon EN, et al. Cost-benefit analysis of the detection of prescribing errors by hospital pharmacy staff. *Drug Saf.* 2002;25(2):135-143.

4. Evans M. A little off the top. While overall healthcare hiring is up, some health systems are being forced to cut jobs, workers and find other savings. *Mod Healthc.* 2008;38(22):6-7, 14, 1.

5. Levin SA, Dickey K. Financial strategies for weathering the economic downturn. Leaders will need to focus on operations, financing options and long-term plans. *Health Prog.* 2009; 90(2):61-64.

6. Wilson AL. *Financial Management for Health-System Pharmacists.* Bethesda, MD: American Society of Health-System Pharmacists; 2009.

7. Investorwords Web site. http://www. investorwords.com. Accessed January 2010

8. Hawkins B, ed. *Best Practices for Hospital & Health-System Pharmacy 2008-2009: Positions & Guidance Documents of ASHP.* Bethesda, MD: American Society of Health-System Pharmacists; 2008.

9. Bates DW, Spell N, Cullen DJ, et al; Adverse Drug Events Prevention Study Group. The costs of adverse drug events in hospitalized patients. *JAMA.* 1997;277(4):307-311. ∎

A Pharmacy Director's Primer on the American Recovery and Reinvestment Act of 2009

Lindsey R. Kelley, PharmD, MS*; Shelby L. Corman, PharmD, BCPS†; and Robert J. Weber, MS, FASHP‡

The *Director's Forum* series is written and edited by Michael Sanborn and Robert Weber and is designed for guiding pharmacy leaders in establishing patient-centered services in hospitals and health systems. Another specific goal of this column is addressing many of the key challenges that pharmacy directors currently face, while also providing information that will foster growth in pharmacy leadership and patient safety. Previous articles in this series have discussed the many different aspects of pharmacy management and leadership challenges. This feature addresses the impact of the American Recovery and Reinvestment Act (the Stimulus Program) on hospital pharmacy practices.

INTRODUCTION

The United States is a leader in the world economy, with an estimated annual gross domestic product (GDP) of approximately $14 trillion.[1] In March 2008 financial backing of housing mortgages failed, leading to a recession that was temporarily slowed by the government's $700 billion Troubled Asset Relief Program (TARP). Even though top banks who received TARP funding have been granted approval to pay back $68 billion of the funds received, the struggle for economic stability is ongoing as indicated by the May 2009 bankruptcy filing by General Motors.[2] To further manage and assist the struggling US economy, President Barack Obama signed into law the American Recovery and Reinvestment Act (ARRA; also known as the Stimulus Program) in February 2009.[3] This act provides money for maintaining and building important society infrastructure to drive economic stability.[4]

The US economic struggles have had global impact. Fallout from US economic instability has seriously impaired liquidity in interbank markets. The standards that govern bank lending operations are tightening in US and Western European markets. This effect has been most profound for banks in Western Europe and other countries where financial institutions are strongly tied to US subprime securities. Even US bonds and equities, once noted for their resilience, have lost favor with investors because of a lack of confidence in their liquidity and ability to produce the returns they once created. Low-income countries and other countries relying on short-term, cross-border trading also have been affected, and those that are integrated into the world economy have experienced a decrease in demand for exports.[5]

Because of its size and complexity, the US health care system is especially vulnerable to the current economic downturn. In 2005 the United States spent 6.9% of its GDP on health care

*Pharmacy Manager, UPMC Shadyside, University of Pittsburgh Medical Center; †Assistant Professor of Pharmacy & Therapeutics, University of Pittsburgh School of Pharmacy; Clinical Specialist, Drug Information, University of Pittsburgh Medical Center; ‡Chief Pharmacy Officer, University of Pittsburgh Medical Center; Associate Professor and Chair, Department of Pharmacy & Therapeutics, University of Pittsburgh School of Pharmacy, Pittsburgh, Pennsylvania.

when the average for high-income countries was 6.7%. Furthermore, compared with other countries, the United States spent the largest additional amount on health care from private expenditures.[6]

US hospitals and health systems already have felt the effects of the current economic deficits. According to the American Hospital Association, 9 of 10 hospitals have made cutbacks to address economic concerns. These cutbacks include reductions in staffing, cuts to administrative expenses, and reductions in services that require subsidies, such as behavioral health. In addition, indicators of hospitals' abilities to meet their financial obligations (such as total and operating margins, cash on hand, and debt service coverage ratio) are slipping, and nearly all hospital respondents reported their capital situation as unimproved or having continually deteriorated since December 2008.[7]

Not surprisingly, pharmacy directors are being asked to respond to their organizations' requirements for reduction in the cost of operations. A survey published by the American Society of Health-System Pharmacists (ASHP) in April 2009 found that, of 541 hospital pharmacy respondents, 37% had staffing budgets reduced, 10% laid off personnel, and 22% had vacant positions frozen.[8] Other possible actions include cutting clinical services, reducing drug budgets, and implementing drug cost initiatives that target less-costly therapeutic equivalents. Directors of pharmacy who understand the ARRA are in a unique position for developing strategies that effectively capitalize on the resources provided by initiatives of the act.

The objective of this article is to provide pharmacy directors with practical knowledge of the 2009 ARRA and its potential applications to hospital pharmacy. Specifically, the article provides a brief overview of the ARRA, describes the key health care provisions within the act, predicts possible barriers to the implementation of its initiatives, lists provided incentives, and discusses resulting opportunities for hospital pharmacies.

OVERVIEW OF THE AMERICAN RECOVERY AND REINVESTMENT ACT

The ARRA was signed by President Obama on February 17, 2009. The ARRA appropriated $787 billion for the recovery of the economy, which will be allocated among various areas of infrastructure within the United States. The oversight of distribution of funds was assigned to a 12-person group called the Recovery Accountability and Transparency Board. More specifically, this group is charged with coordinating and conducting the management of funds distributed under this law to prevent fraud, waste, and abuse.[3] The board members (listed in **Table 1**) are US inspectors general from the US Government Accountability Office; the board is led by Chairman Earl E. Devaney. Devaney is a former police officer and retired member of the US Secret Service. There are no health care professionals on the board.

The $787 billion act is an attempt at fiscal stabilization through the creation and preservation of jobs, reinforcement of infrastructure, investment in energy research, and assistance to unemployed Americans who have been most affected by the recession. The ARRA covers 8 primary areas, including tax relief (for individuals and companies), state and local fiscal relief, infrastructure and science,

Table 1. Members of the Recovery Accountability and Transparency Board

Member	Title
The Honorable Earl E. Devaney	Chairman
The Honorable Richard L. Skinner	Vice Chairman, Inspector General of Homeland Security
The Honorable Phyllis K. Fong	Inspector General Department of Agriculture
The Honorable Todd. J. Zinser	Inspector General Department of Commerce
The Honorable Gordon S. Heddell	Acting Inspector General Department of Defense
The Honorable Gregory H. Friedman	Inspector General Department of Energy
The Honorable Daniel Levinson	Inspector General Department of Health and Human Services
The Honorable Glenn A. Fine	Inspector General Department of Justice
The Honorable Calvin L. Scovel III	Inspector General Department of Transportation
The Honorable Eric M. Thorson	Inspector General Department of Treasury
The Honorable J. Russell George	Treasury Inspector General for Tax Administration
Mary Mitchelson	Acting Inspector General Department of Education
Mary L. Kendall	Acting Inspector General Department of the Interior

protection of the vulnerable, health care, education and training, energy, and other areas. Notably, a small portion ($148.2 billion) of the ARRA is devoted to health care. **Table 2** shows how the money from the ARRA for health care has been appropriated.

Table 2. American Recovery and Reinvestment Act Appropriations for Health Care

Category	Amount ($ billions)
Medicaid	87
Health insurance 65% subsidy	24.7
National Institutes of Health	10
Health Resources and Services Administration	2.5
Veterans health affairs	1.4
Comparative effectiveness research	1.1
Health prevention and wellness	1
Training of health care professionals	0.5
Health services on Native American reservations	0.5
Medicare	0.3
Total	148.2

KEY HEALTH CARE PROVISIONS IN THE AMERICAN RECOVERY AND REINVESTMENT ACT
Comparative Effectiveness Research

Comparative effectiveness research (CER) is an attempt to evaluate the place in therapy of various treatment options for conditions in which similar treatments exist without a clear indication for a best practice. Though it has been subject to various interpretations, the latest draft definition from the CER Council states the following[9]:

Comparative effectiveness research is the conduct and synthesis of systematic research comparing different interventions and strategies to prevent, diagnose, treat and monitor health conditions. The purpose of this research is to inform patients, providers, and decision-makers, responding to their expressed needs, about which interventions are most effective for which patients under specific circumstances. To provide this information, comparative effectiveness research must assess a comprehensive array of health-related outcomes for diverse patient populations. This research necessitates the development, expansion, and use of a variety of data sources and methods to assess comparative effectiveness.

The goal of CER is to provide evidence for situations in which prior head-to-head comparisons do not exist. This is accomplished in 2 ways: comparing agents or interventions that are therapeutic alternatives and evaluating outcomes in clinical practice.[10] Funding applications may include medications, procedures, medical and assistive devices and technologies, behavioral change strategies, and delivery system interventions. Furthermore, these funds fill gaps where the industry may have been reluctant to contribute research dollars in the past, as well as opening the door to studies evaluating therapies, such as medication versus surgery, for which obtaining support may have been difficult previously. Funding this type of research is consistent with the aim of the ARRA to support methods of clinical decision support and, according to the American Medical Association, "provide a meaningful, initial down payment on CER that will strengthen the delivery of evidence-based medicine while preserving physician decision-making autonomy."[11]

Funding for research comparing therapeutically equivalent treatment modalities has been set aside in the amount of $1.1 billion. The funds will be administered by the Agency for Healthcare Research and Quality, the National Institutes of Health, and the Office of the Secretary of the US Department of Health and Human Services (DHHS) through a competitive grant process managed by the Federal Coordinating Council for Comparative Effectiveness Research (FCC-CER). The FCC-CER is a 15-member group representing various federal agencies in which at least half of the members are clinical experts or physicians. The funding is intended to hasten development and dissemination of research comparing treatments; more importantly, it is also an effort to reduce redundancy and encourage collaboration. Because it is likely that many of the studies will focus on pharmaceutical treatment options, the outcomes are of great importance to pharmaceutical manufacturers, insurers, pharmacists, and policy-makers. Notably, any and all outcomes, reports, and/or recommendations found through this newly funded research or made by the FCC-CER must not be taken as mandates or used as guidelines for coverage or reimbursement.[12]

Rural Health Initiatives

Several initiatives contained within the ARRA focus on improving health services in rural areas of the United States. Among them are increased funding for community health infrastructure and service, support of prevention and wellness programs, and training of health care professionals. Rural community health centers have been allotted $2 billion for use in infrastructure and service expansion, with monies being obtained through a competitive grant process. Infrastructure funds make up three-fourths ($1.5 billion) of the total funding and must be used for renovations and improvements to health information technology (HIT). Renovations include construction and equipment upgrades, as well as acquisition of new technology systems. It is required that the remaining $500 million be used to increase services at existing sites and to create new sites, including supplemental pay to community health centers that experience spikes in uninsured populations.

Prevention and wellness programs will receive $1 billion to support efforts by states and localities in fighting preventable chronic diseases and infectious diseases. The appropriations are available through competitive grants and include immunization programs, as well as any state efforts, for reducing health care–related infections.

Significant funds ($300 million) have been allotted to the National Health Service Corps (NHSC). The NHSC provides incentives (in the form of loan repayment, salary support, and scholarships) to health care professionals so that they can practice in underserved areas. Despite lobbying efforts by organizations such as ASHP, pharmacists are not eligible for NHSC assistance. However, additional appropriations that have been made for health care workforce training are eligible to pharmacists. This additional $200 million has been set aside for the training of health professionals and includes all professionals recognized under Titles VII and VIII of the Public Health Service Act. Another $250 million has been directed toward the training of health care workers via the US Department of Labor. Priority for these funds has been set for projects that prepare workers for careers in the health care sector.

Health Information Technology

Following increases to Medicare and Medicaid funding, the most significant contribution to the $150 billion appropriated for health care is $19.2 billion for the development of HIT for Medicare and Medicaid. This funding includes the previously mentioned rural HIT initiatives.

In addition to mapping out a wish list for better quality of health care, the Health Information Technology for Economic and Clinical Health Act (HITECH) provisions of the 2009 ARRA create new offices and new committees to assist in the fair and transparent distribution of funds. Though created by the Bush administration in 2004, the Office of the National Coordinator for Health Information Technology (ONCHIT) within the DHHS is officially established by HITECH. Appointed by the secretary of the DHHS, the national coordinator for HIT will lead efforts and the HIT Policy and Standards Committees will provide recommendations for actual policy frameworks, standards, implementation specifics, and certification criteria.

Although primarily charged with developing nationwide HIT infrastructure that allows for the electronic use and exchange of information, ONCHIT has been tasked with several other responsibilities. Included in these is working with the National Institute of Standards and Technology and other agencies to update and execute the initial Federal HIT Strategic Plan (developed June 3, 2009) and publishing a report evaluating estimated resources required for meeting the strategic outcomes described. The following are other areas for consideration by ONCHIT: post-marketing surveillance, telemedicine technologies to assist in reducing requirements for travel in remote areas, technologies that assist in home health care and at-home patient monitoring, technologies that work to reduce medication errors, and a general focus toward continuity of care and better communication between all health care practitioners caring for patients, including any family or guardians acting on the patient's behalf.

BARRIERS TO IMPLEMENTING INITIATIVES OF THE AMERICAN RECOVERY AND REINVESTMENT ACT IN HEALTH CARE

The major barriers to implementing the ARRA initiatives include fears about the final use of CER and skepticism of long-term goals for HIT initiatives.

Implementation of CER will be challenging for a number of reasons. There are concerns from physician groups that guidelines and decisions made based on CER will dictate how treatment of patients will proceed. Some speculate that the government and private insurers will use the results of CER to dictate payment strata and/or coverage. Additional concerns exist because even properly conducted scientific research does not translate into changes in clinical outcomes.

From a health information standpoint, ONCHIT acknowledges that the goals outlined within the HITECH portion of the act represent a "far-sighted commitment" to health care, and the appropriation of funding for these endeavors "will require careful thought and planning" to ensure their success.[13]

Anecdotally, technology in health care has been met with mixed reviews. Though nearly all health care providers agree that technology represents safer methods of practicing medicine, it also has been acknowledged that the systems currently available lack key aspects that would make any of them ideal. Current systems are proprietary, and switching vendors or creating interfaces between parts of a system can be difficult if not impossible. Further technology concerns that must be addressed include bandwidth availability, regulations for governing data sharing and ownership, protective measures for safeguarding patient health information, and a lack of protocols to which all parties agree.

Outside of technological challenges, attempts at implementing health care technology (eg, electronic medical records, bedside bar-code administration) in the past have not been properly incentivized nor have they had the full support of the entire health care team. Collaboration is crucial in health care. Not gaining the buy-in of all involved can sabotage a plan for implementation. Indeed, ONCHIT acknowledges that, in addition to staffing concerns, buy-in from stakeholders in the private and public sectors is the second of 2 key steps for successful and effective implementation of HIT initiatives.

INCENTIVES IN THE AMERICAN RECOVERY AND REINVESTMENT ACT INITIATIVES

Given the robust HITECH goals, offering incentives to providers and health systems is vital to success. Financial incentives are available through Medicare to encourage physicians and hospitals to adopt and use a certified electronic health record in a meaningful way, and according to projections from the Congressional Budget Office, these incentives will increase adoption of comprehensive electronic health records by 25% compared with adoption without incentives. ONCHIT can provide competitive grants to states for loans to reimburse early promoters with more money. The payment structure is such that if adopted in 2011 or 2012, provider payment eligibility is up to $18,000; in 2014 the limit is $12,000; and if not adopted until 2015, then no incentive is available. If adopted in a rural area, there is an additional 10% increase in incentive. If adopted late, there will be penalties: in 2015 there is a –1% penalty to payment; in 2016, a –2% penalty; in 2017, a –3% penalty; and in 2019 there is potential for further penalties. Furthermore, Medicare and Medicaid provide these payment incentives, but physicians cannot receive funding from both agencies.[14]

OPPORTUNITIES FOR PHARMACY

Much effort has been put into the identification of pharmacists as the medication experts for patients and colleagues. The greatest opportunities for pharmacy center on 3 basic concepts: input, planning, and monitoring. Organizations representing physicians, physician assistants, and pharmacists already have submitted support and recommendations to ONCHIT. Among the comments was language for the inclusion of pharmacists in NHSC loan forgiveness programs.[15] Included in strategic planning for ONCHIT are 3 ways that stakeholders may become involved: listening to and participating during the public comment periods at meetings of the Health IT Policy Committee and the Health IT Standards Committee, commenting on draft program descriptions, and providing expert input and information. Areas of pharmacy expertise and input at the hospital or health system level include quality and safety of medication use, patient access to medications, and integration of pharmacy needs into current and future HIT plans.

CER has the potential for assisting in the resolution of a long-standing frustration of pharmacists and physicians involved in formulary management and therapeutic guideline development: a paucity of primarily placebo-controlled trials for evaluation of the efficacy of medications. With access to the results of comparative trials, Pharmacy and Therapeutics committees would be able to make better-informed decisions about the relative efficacy of medications and provide valuable information that can be applied to pharmacoeconomic decision making, potentially leading to drug budget reductions. This is an opportunity for pharmacists to not only use better information to select from a number of therapeutic options but to obtain funding to conduct these studies if they have the necessary skills and training. Although some may argue that the availability of CER will reduce the need for clinicians with specialty training in drug information and literature evaluation, this is unlikely because there will still be a need for critical evaluation of CER and comparison of the populations studied with each institution's patient population and case mix. Therefore, it is important that pharmacy directors continually allocate resources to personnel involved in interpreting and performing CER.

Pharmacy automation requires interfaces with HIT and electronic health record systems; automated dispensing machines must be able to pull needed medication information, barcode point-of-care systems must be user-friendly and reliable. There are also opportunities upfront to request builds for reports and research tools used to perform medication utilization evaluations and adverse drug event reporting. Also, pharmacy involvement upfront allows for projection of and planning for future staffing needs.

The last area of opportunity is arguably the most important; all pharmacists and directors should stay ahead of changes pertaining to the ARRA. This will allow for anticipation by the health care profession of further opportunities in an environment in which the overall effects of the ARRA on health care are yet unknown. Several professional pharmacy organizations, such as ASHP, the National Community Pharmacists Association, and the American Pharmacists Association, provide resources via their Web sites to facilitate engagement from pharmacy professionals. These organizations also represent avenues for further advocacy of pharmacists and directors.

CONCLUSION

John P. Kotter, widely regarded as the world's foremost authority on leadership and change, claims that the first error in failed transformation efforts is the failure to create a sense of urgency.[16] The Obama administration has certainly created a sense of urgency around the implementation of the ARRA and the utilization of the appropriated funds. Of the many initiatives in the 407-page document, those that most likely will affect health care and pharmacy remain CER, expansion and increases in rural health services, and HIT initiatives. Though barriers have existed in the past and will continue moving forward, staffing issues can be overcome and buy-in gained to attain successful implementation. The pharmacy director plays an important role in ensuring that pharmacy is involved when discussions of implementation of new initiatives are taking place; this is accomplished by taking advantage of extra funding to secure pharmacy resources, remaining informed, and providing input and expertise to national organizations and senior administrators within hospitals and health systems.

REFERENCES

1. National income and product accounts. Gross domestic product: second quarter 2009 (advance estimate). Comprehensive revision: 1929 through first quarter 2009 [news release]. Washington, DC: Bureau of Economic Analysis; July 31, 2009. http://www.bea.gov/newsreleases/national/gdp/gdpnewsrelease.htm. Accessed June 30, 2009.

2. US Government Accountability Office. Troubled Asset Relief Program: June 2009 status of efforts to address transparency and accountability issues. http://www.gao.gov/new.items/d09658.pdf. Published June 2009. Accessed July 9, 2009.

3. US Government. Recovery timeline. http://www.recovery.gov/?q=content/timeline. Accessed June 30, 2009.

4. US Department of the Treasury. Financial stability impact: additional transactions. http://www.financialstability.gov/impact/DataTables/additionaltransactions.html. Updated July 28, 2009. Accessed June 30, 2009.

5. International Monetary Fund. World economic outlook April 2009: crisis and recovery. http://www.imf.org/external/pubs/ft/weo/2009/01/pdf/text.pdf. Published April 2009. Accessed July 1, 2009.

6. World Health Organization. The world health report 2008: primary health care now more than ever. Geneva, Switzerland: World Health Organization; 2008. http://www.who.int/whr/2008/whr08_en.pdf. Accessed July 9, 2009.

7. American Hospital Association. The economic crisis: the toll on the patients and communities hospitals serve. http://www.aha.org/aha/content/2009/pdf/090427econcrisisreport.pdf. Published April 27, 2009. Accessed July 9, 2009.

8. Impact of the current economy on pharmacy services in hospitals and health systems. Bethesda, MD: American Society of Health-System Pharmacists; March 26, 2009. http://www.ashp.org/economy-survey. Accessed July 9, 2009.

9. US Department of Health and Human Services. Draft definition, prioritization criteria, and strategic framework for public comment. http://www.hhs.gov/recovery/programs/cer/draftdefinition.html. Accessed July 7, 2009.

10. Schumock GT, Pickard AS. Comparative effectiveness research: relevance and applications to pharmacy. *Am J Health Syst Pharm.* 2009;66(14):1278-1286.

11. American Medical Association. H.R. 1, the "American Recovery and Reinvestment Act of 2009" explanation of comparative effectiveness research (CER) pro visions. http://www.ama-assn.org/ama1/pub/upload/mm/399/arra-cer-provisions.pdf. Accessed July 9, 2009.

12. US Department of Health and Human Services. Federal Coordinating Council for Comparative Effectiveness Research: report to the President and Congress. http://www.hhs.gov/recovery/programs/cer/cerannualrpt.pdf. Published June 30, 2009. Accessed July 10, 2009.

13. Office of the National Coordinator for Health Information Technology. Health information technology: American Recovery and Reinvestment Act (Recovery Act) implementation plan. http://www.hhs.gov/recovery/reports/plans/onc_hit.pdf. Accessed June 10, 2009.

14. American Medical Association. H.R. 1, the "American Recovery and Reinvestment Act of 2009" explanation of health information technology (HIT) provisions. http://www.ama-assn.org/ama1/pub/upload/mm/399/arra-hit-provisions.pdf. Accessed July 10, 2009.

15. American Society of Health-System Pharmacists. Senate Finance Committee: description of policy options. Transforming the health care delivery system: proposals to improve patient care and reduce health care costs: ASHP comments. http://www.ashp.org/DocLibrary/News/news_cap_Comments_Finance05202009.pdf. Published May 13, 2009. Accessed June 10, 2009.

16. Kotter JP. Leading change: why transformation efforts fail. In: Kotter JP, ed. *Harvard Business Review on Change.* Boston, MA: Harvard Business School Publishing; 1991:3-6. ■

Industry Relationships and the Pharmacy Director: Striking the Right Balance

Meredith Mulvanity, PharmD, * *and Robert J. Weber, MS, FASHP*[†]

The *Director's Forum* series is written and edited by Michael Sanborn and Robert Weber and is designed for guiding pharmacy leaders in establishing patient-centered services in hospitals and health systems. Another specific goal of this column is addressing many of the key challenges that pharmacy directors currently face, while also providing information that will foster growth in pharmacy leadership and patient safety. Recent public highlight of inappropriate relationships between health care professionals and the industry requires that the pharmacy director actively promote an environment of unbiased practice. The article features ways the pharmacy director can further recognize and react to potential workplace conflicts of interest.

INTRODUCTION

In the past decade, significantly more attention and scrutiny have been paid to the marketing practices of the pharmaceutical industry, biotechnology companies, and medical device industry. Much of this attention is due to the substantial and growing body of evidence demonstrating the adverse consequences of interactions between health care providers and industry.[1] While health care professionals may not believe that they are personally biased by the industry's marketing (eg, gifts, meals), these practices are designed to sell products and advance the interests of the company's shareholders.[2,3]

In general, pharmacists' perceptions of the pharmaceutical industry have been quite skeptical. A study of physicians and pharmacists serving on Pharmacy and Therapeutics (P&T) committees in Pennsylvania showed that 75% of pharmacists reported being skeptical and unsatisfied with industry drug information and marketing. The pharmacists also were concerned that industry bias and conflicts of interest could affect formulary decisions.[4] In an editorial, authors describe the exposure of most pharmacists to industry as only "raindrops of influence." However, some pharmacists, such as clinical specialists, drug information pharmacists, P&T committee members, clinical coordinators, and directors, are in positions of value to industry. These individuals are often involved in conducting clinical research, developing drug use policy, and speaking at professional meetings; money and attention could be spent "courting" these "thought leaders." From an industry perspective, a hierarchical approach to marketing is more efficient since the opinions of these individuals carry considerable weight.[5]

While keeping the concerns of industry influence in the health care setting in mind, it is just as important to understand that pharmaceutical and medical device manufacturers promote the welfare of patients through their commitment to research and

*Pharmacy Practice Management Resident University of Pittsburgh Medical Center; [†]Executive Director of Pharmacy University of Pittsburgh Medical Center Associate Professor and Chair Department of Pharmacy & Therapeutics University of Pittsburgh School of Pharmacy.

product development. Their research and investments in discovery, development, and distribution of new pharmaceutical agents and medical devices continue to benefit countless patients. Their support for continuing medical education (CME), clinical guideline development, and sponsorship of professional medical societies are additional societal and health care industry benefits.[1] The recent rapid response of the pharmaceutical industry in testing and distributing the vaccine for H1N1 influenza is a very tangible example of the valuable role that the pharmaceutical industry plays in improving the health of the public.

The objective of this article is to provide the pharmacy director with information and strategies for managing relationships with industry. These relationships are not limited to the individual or personal connections a pharmacy director may have, but rather extend to include the relationships of their staff, department, hospital or health-system, and academic affiliation with industry. For the purposes of this article "the industry" discussed includes The Pharmaceutical Research and Manufacturers of America (PhRMA) as well as technology and device, and distribution vendors (eg, McKesson Automation Solutions, Cardinal Health Distribution). The specific aims of this article focus on helping the pharmacy director to manage relationships with industry by providing a background on the evolution of issues associated with industry relationships, describing the guiding principles for evaluating appropriateness of such relationships, and providing tools that can be implemented in practice to prevent conflicts of interest and ensure both professionalism and responsibility to patient care.

EVOLUTION OF INDUSTRY RELATIONSHIP ISSUES

Historically, lavish dining, ski trips, hunting and fishing excursions, and various other "big ticket" items were not uncommon as part of the marketing and "gifting" practices of the pharmaceutical companies, medical device manufacturers, and hospital supplier groups. In 2000, the industry sponsored 314,000 events specifically for physicians, and reports suggest that in 2004 PhRMA spent $23 billion dollars in marketing to physicians.[6,7] Recent lawsuits, congressional investigations, and even federal prosecution have made documents public demonstrating how company practices often "cross the line." Concerned consumers, health care professionals, and the government are wary that such practices geared towards profit-seeking may actually jeopardize patient welfare.[1]

Although highly regulated by the Food and Drug Administration (FDA) and Federal Trade Commission, such transgressions have prompted the industry to stricter self-regulation. In 2008, PhRMA adopted a newly revised "Code on Interactions with Healthcare Professionals." The strengthened code is aimed at helping the industry in "maintaining the highest ethical standards and in all marketing practices and to promote the best patient care possible."[8] According to industry data in 2006, total promotional spending was $12 billion compared to $58.8 billion spent in research and development in 2007. Direct to consumer advertising made up $4.8 billion with office promotion, hospital promotion, and journal advertising comprising $7.2 billion.[9]

Various organizations, medical societies, and even state legislatures have also put regulations in place that limit the value of gifts and food industry provides to the health care community. Minnesota, Maine, Vermont, and West Virginia were the first among many to require drug manufacturers to report all consulting payments made to doctors, and Congress was quick to follow suit.[10] Many would agree that although physician groups, the manufacturers, and federal government have instituted self-regulation of marketing, other research related to the psychology of gifting and the receipt of even the smallest of gifts, such as pens and free lunch, suggest even more stringency is required. Authors of a 2006 article in the *Journal of the American Medical Association* called for action and regulation that includes elimination or modification of common practices related to small gifts, pharmaceutical samples, continuing medical education, funds for travel, speakers bureaus, ghostwriting, and consulting and re search contracts. They also proposed a policy under which academic medical centers would take the lead in eliminating conflicts of interests that remain a part of the relationships between health care providers and industry.[1] Therefore, in light of this changing climate and whether your practice site is an academic medical center or a small community hospital, chances are your interactions and the interactions of your pharmacy department with industry will be in question.

GUIDING PRINCIPLES FOR EVALUATING INDUSTRY RELATIONSHIPS

Developing and maintaining relationships with industry is an important role of the pharmacy director. The responsibility of ensuring the appropriateness of interactions between the department, the health system, and the individual with industry falls primarily on the shoulders of the pharmacy director because much of their day-to-day decision making regarding formulary management, purchasing, and contracting hinges on critically evaluating available information from various vendors. In the process of evaluating such relationships, the following guiding principles of autonomy, disclosure, and professionalism are undeniably important and essential to consider in order to strike the right balance within your practice with regard to industry relations.

Autonomy

Maintaining autonomy in all aspects of practice is critical. This entails making independent decisions that are free of bias and ensure all possible alternative options have been explored. An autonomous decision does not have to be the sole responsibility of a single individual; rather, it should include an independent and thorough investigation, evaluation, and analysis of all available data and allow for ample time to weigh all possible options.

Disclosure

Relationships with industry are inherent to the practice of pharmacy and it is virtually impossible to identify an individual that is truly free of potential conflicts of interest. Many practitioners are actively involved in activities such as consulting, writing, and others that encompass various aspects of industry relations. Some individuals may be shareholders or even board members of particular companies. While considering these inevitable challenges and in order to avoid elimination or prohibition of such activities, ensuring appropriate disclosure of these relationships and financial ties is of utmost importance.

Professionalism

Although professionalism may be perceived as a thoughtless principle and guiding doctrine, there are many instances in which it could be called into question. Maintaining your ability to use professional judgment and make ethically sound decisions regardless of incentive, allegiance and even something as simple as comfort level or personal preference with a particular product or vendor representative can be more difficult than others may have alluded to.

Case Study 1
Background

A well-known and well-regarded pharmacy director has just undergone a successful implementation of a new-to-market intravenous (IV) dispensing robotic system in her department. Based on her knowledge and experience in the area of various automation technology implementations, she has also been asked to speak at her state pharmacy association's annual meeting on this particular topic.

Description of the Problem

When the robotics company representative hears of the speaking engagement, he decides to make a special visit to the director's institution and offers to help provide information and slides for the presentation that highlight his particular product. He also offers NFL football tickets for an upcoming game that he knows is bringing the director's husband's favorite team into town as a kind gesture for her continued support of their new product launch. The director is taken by surprise and, although she knows the tickets would be a welcome surprise for her husband, she feels conflicted about what to do and if the information the representative is suggesting she include in her presentation is appropriate and unbiased.

Recommendation

The first sign that this interaction may not be appropriate is that the director is questioning the motive for offering the tickets and the willingness of the representative to provide proprietary information for her upcoming presentation. In this case the most professional approach is for the director to decline the offer for the football tickets and create her own slide deck highlighting nonproprietary information about the various types of dispensing automation technology available on the market. She should submit her slides for peer review prior to the presentation and disclose any financial or consulting relationship she may have with particular vendors. At the conclusion of her presentation it would, however, be considered entirely appropriate for the director to answer any questions that arise regarding her experience in the implementation of certain commercially available products.

TOOLS AND STRATEGIES TO PREVENT CONFLICT OF INTEREST
Structure and Content of a Conflict of Interest Policy

Depending on an institution's size, practice model, and academic affiliation, there may or may not exist a policy that specifically deals with conflict of interest and industry relations. In case your institution may be in the process of developing such a policy or in the periodic review of an existing policy, the following recommendations for the structure and content of the policy and supporting documents may be useful. It is also important to consider the necessary involvement of the pharmacy department in development of this type of policy when the interactions between staff and industry are both frequent and warranted. **Figure 1** outlines recommended components to include in the general obligations of a conflict of interest policy. **Figure 2** includes additional components relating to personnel, faculty, staff, and students in the clinical setting. These activities are common in academic medical centers and may pertain to certain research activities as well.

In addition to the policy, an institution-specific statement of purpose is an essential accompaniment that highlights the mission of the organization

I. **Policy Statement**
II. **Scope**
III. **Specific Activities**
  a. Gifts and provision of meals
  b. Consulting relationships
  c. Drug or device samples
  d. Site access
  e. Support of continuing education
  f. Industry sponsored meetings
  g. Industry support for scholarships or fellowships and other support of students, residents or trainees
  h. Frequent speaker arrangements (speakers bureaus) and ghost-writing
  i. Other industry support for research
IV. **Reporting and Enforcement**

Figure 2. Conflict of interest policy—interaction between representatives of certain industries and faculty, staff, and students of the schools of health sciences and hospital-employed personnel.

and commitment to patient care. It should also outline the reasons behind the policy development, which is designed to eliminate potential conflicts of interest and ensure that practitioners remain free from influence created by financial relationships with, or gifts from, industry. If at all possible, posting the policies in a central repository, preferably electronically, such as an intranet site, along with frequently asked questions and links to other pertinent resources (eg, disclosure forms, contact information for a site-specific compliance officer) may provide added benefits. Incorporating the review of such policies at new hire and resident orientations and distributing a related mandatory competency to staff and faculty is also essential.

Contracting and Competitive Bidding

In the arena of contracting, related activities and interactions with industry are often in question and come under great scrutiny when discussing

I. **Policy Statement**
II. **Scope**
  a. Entities covered by the policy
  b. Individuals covered by the policy
III. **Definition of a Conflict of Interest**
IV. **Disclosure and Identification of Interests**
  a. Disclosure of individual interests
    i. Required periodic disclosure (annual basis)
  b. Identification and querying of interests
V. **Review and Evaluation Process**
VI. **Violations of the Policy**
VII. **Examples of Decisions and Transactions Requiring Review**
  a. Decisions made by the institution's board of directors
  b. Corporate fundamental change transactions
  c. Supply chain
  d. Commercial services and strategic business initiatives
  e. Medical and health sciences foundation
  f. Clinical trials office
  g. Grants and contracting
  h. Investments through treasury

Figure 1. Conflict of interest policy—general obligations.

conflicts of interest. In general, using the principles of autonomy, disclosure, and professionalism as guidance for important and strategic decisions such as selection of a pharmacy information system or automated dispensing cabinet vendor, and contracts with wholesalers and distributors, will help to minimize any potential conflicts of interest. Insisting on an independent review of all available information and proposals, and requiring whenever possible that the department submit requests for competitive bidding is necessary.

One particular area of concern and potential oversight for the pharmacy department when accepting anything of value from a pharmaceutical company is ensuring they are in compliance with federal anti-kickback laws. According to the Office of the Inspector General, pharmacists and other health care providers who knowingly and willfully solicit or receive remuneration from a drug company in exchange for federal health care program businesses are in violation of the law. Potential unlawful situations include accepting a pharmaceutical company's off-contract or hidden price reductions in the form of educational and research grants, free drug product, or payments for consulting and speaking services in an attempt to avoid meeting Medicaid's best price requirements.[11]

Pharmacy and Therapeutics Committee

The pharmacy director is often in the position of chair or other voting member of their institution's P&T committee. The director's responsibilities, along with those of supporting medical staff and other voting members, are critical in the management of the drug formulary. In its yearly published "Projecting Future Drug Expenditures" analysis, the American Society of Health-System Pharmacists (ASHP) predicted an increase of 1% to 3% in 2009 for the drug budget of hospital pharmacies. They also reported that 14 new drugs were expected to be approved by the FDA and released for use in 2009 alone.[12] Taking these predictions into account represents the daunting tasks and responsibilities of the P&T committee at various institutions.

The pharmacy director should ensure the appropriate membership of the committee, including representation from the various specialties and departments. Re quests for additions to the formulary should be managed by this committee and require independent review of all available clinical data before being eligible for a vote. Whenever possible the independent review should be completed by an individual or group of individuals not directly involved in the request for the addition to the formulary and would include pertinent comparative effectiveness research, grading of all available clinical data, as well as safety concerns for the agent in question.

Case Study 2
Background

A certain institution is known for excellence in clinical research, attracting world renowned physicians, and having a very active P&T committee.

Description of the Problem

The P&T committee and pharmacy director who serves as cochair receive a request for the addition of a new fast-acting IV antihypertensive agent to the institution's formulary. The request is made by a physician who is a voting member of the committee. It is also known that this physician served as a coinvestigator of a trial evaluating this agent for use in the intensive care unit (ICU) setting. The pharmacy director is not surprised by the request to add this new drug to the formulary, but he is conflicted on how to proceed and whether include this physician in the P&T voting process.

Recommendation

This particular request is somewhat challenging. In order to minimize potential bias of the committee, it is important that the review of the drug is completed by an independent third party. In this case an appropriate approach would be for the pharmacy director to assign the completion of a formulary review document for this drug to someone such as a pharmacy resident or clinical pharmacist. He should ensure that all available published data and the results from comparative research trials of the different studies evaluated by the FDA upon approval of this drug are included in the review. Asking the physician to provide his rationale for addition of this drug to the formulary and disclosure of his relationship with the manufacturer, as well as his role in the clinical research is appropriate. During the voting process, it is also recommended that the physician in question be exempt from the decision regarding this particular agent.

Management of Drug Samples

Discussion surrounding both the influence and usefulness of prescription drug samples is quite controversial. It has been reported that in 2004 PhRMA provided an estimated $15.9 billion in free drug samples as part of the marketing practices and physician detailing.[7] Many institutions

have banned the distribution of drug samples all together. Others, such as the University of California, Los Angeles' (UCLA) Medical School, have adopted guidelines that prohibit shipping drug samples to individual doctors and allow their use only in cases in which a patient is indigent or there is another significant barrier to care.[13]

In April 2009, the University of Pittsburgh Medical Center (UPMC) enacted a ban that does not prohibit distributing samples and vouchers to patients but ends regular sales and delivery visits by pharmaceutical representatives to physician offices. Their unique approach is aimed at eliminating perceived conflicts of interest between UPMC providers and drug companies and is in addition to policies banning industry provided gifts and meals to hospital personnel. UPMC is using a Web-based platform operated by a private firm, which allows physician offices to order samples from a Web-based central distribution center, in hopes of re placing sales representatives' visits.[14]

The decision whether or not to allow a prescription drug samples varies from institution to institution, but in the role of director of pharmacy it is likely that you and your department will be engaged in the discussion. You may even be asked to actively manage the issue, as well as the available inventory of samples in your everyday practice.

CONCLUSION

Pharmacy directors hold an important leadership role and position of authority, and they must accept responsibility for ensuring appropriate interactions and relationships with the pharmaceutical industry, technology and device, and distribution vendors.

True freedom from influence is very difficult to achieve and almost impossible for practical purposes. A reasonable and manageable goal is to try to strike a balance with regard to industry relations in order to minimize potential bias in both financial and therapeutic decisions. This approach will ensure the continued development of a patient-centered pharmacy service.

REFERENCES

1. Brennan TA, Rothman DS, Blank L, et al. Health industry practices that create conflicts of interest: a policy proposal for academic medical centers. *JAMA*. 2006;295(4):429-433.

2. Dana J, Loewenstein G. A social science perspective on gifts to physicians from industry. *JAMA*. 2003;290(2):252-255.

3. Wanzana A. Physicians and the pharmaceutical industry: is a gift ever just a gift? *JAMA*. 2000;283(3):373-380.

4. Poirier TI, Giannetti V, Giudici RA. Pharmacists' and physicians' attitudes toward pharmaceutical marketing practices. *Am J Hosp Pharm*. 1994;51(3):378-381.

5. Haines ST, Dumo P. Relationship between the pharmaceutical industry and pharmacy practitioners: undue influence? *Am J Health Syst Pharm*. 2002;59(19):1871-1874.

6. The National Institute for Health Care Management Research and Educational Foundation. Prescription drugs and mass media advertising. 2000. http://www.nihcm.org/finalweb/DTCbrief2001.pdf. Accessed October 4, 2009.

7. Underwood A. Thanks, but no thanks–why more doctors, medical schools and hospitals are just saying no to drug-company promotions. October 29, 2007. *Newsweek*. http://www.newsweek.com/id/57342. Accessed September 25, 2009.

8. Pharmaceutical Research and Manufacturers of America. Code on Interactions with Health Care Professionals. http://www.phrma.org/code_on_interactions_with_healthcare_professionals. Accessed September 25, 2009.

9. Pharmaceutical Research and Manufacturers of America. The facts about pharmaceutical promotion and marketing. July 2008. http://www.phrma.org/files/Marketing%20and%20Promotion%20Facts_071108_FINAL.pdf. Accessed October 4, 2009.

10. Harris G. Minnesota limits on gifts to doctors may catch on. *New York Times*. October 12, 2007. http://www.nytimes.com/2007/10/12/us/12gift.html. Accessed September 25, 2009.

11. Young D. Pharmacists should heed anti-kickback law, experts advise. *Am J Health Syst Pharm*. 2004;61(9):878, 880.

12. Hoffman JM, Shah ND, Vermeulen LC, et al. Projecting future drug expenditures—2009. *Am J Health Syst Pharm*. 2009;66(3):237-257.

13. Aleccia J. Free drug samples cost more in the long run. MSNBC. March 25, 2008. http://www.msnbc.msn.com/id/23783105. Accessed September 25, 2009.

14. Roche WF. UPMC to stop reps' delivery of drug samples. *Pittsburgh Tribune Review*. March 20, 2009. http://pittsburghlive.com/x/pittsburghtrib/news/cityregion/s_616956.html#. Accessed September 25, 2009. ∎

Medication Safety

Developing a Medication Patient Safety Program, Part 1: Infrastructure and Strategy

Scott M. Mark, PharmD, MS, MEd, FASHP, FACHE* and
Robert J. Weber, MS, FASHP†

The *Director's Forum* series is written and edited by Robert Weber and Michael Sanborn and is designed to guide pharmacy leaders in establishing patient-centered services in hospitals and health systems. Another specific goal of this column is to address many of the key challenges that pharmacy directors face today, while providing information to foster growth in pharmacy leadership and patient safety. This month's *Forum* is co-authored by Scott Mark and focuses directly on the importance of a patient safety infrastructure.

INTRODUCTION

Growing evidence of the number of medical errors that occur throughout the US health care system has prompted stakeholders' interest in hospitals' approach to improve safety. A significant concern of patients, health care organizations, and clinicians is medication errors that occur at an average of 19% to 36% in hospitals; in fact, every patient will experience at least one medication error during their hospital stay.[1] In the United States Pharmacopeial Convention's 2004 published report, almost 2% of all reported medication errors (approximately 4,000 yearly) resulted in significant harm to patients.[2]

The Institute of Medicine (IOM) recently released a report commissioned by the Center for Medicare and Medicaid Services titled *Preventing Medication Errors*. This report suggests a national agenda for preventing medication errors including improving pa-

tients' understanding of medications using technology to improve information related to medication use, improving drug packaging and labeling, employing human factors engineering concepts to drug-related technologies, funding medication safety research, and providing monetary incentives for quality and safety in health care.[3] Patient safety experts Drs. Lucian Leape and Donald Berwick, in a commentary published a year before the IOM report was released, noted progress in the health care environment of patient safety that focused on a systems-based approach. However, they warned that significant improvement in patient safety would only be recognized by an ambitious national agenda.[4]

As a result of the call to action by the IOM and others, hospitals and health care organizations must establish their own agenda to prevent medication errors based on collaboration among caregivers through an effective organizational culture of patient safety. Building a culture of safety remains a somewhat elusive construct, and health care organizations often struggle with how to develop a safety culture infrastructure that will result in continuous improvements in quality of care.[5] Additionally, most hospitals

*Assistant Professor of Pharmacy and Therapeutics, University of Pittsburgh School of Pharmacy, Director of Pharmacy, University of Pittsburgh Medical Center; †Associate Professor and Chair, University of Pittsburgh School of Pharmacy, Executive Director of Pharmacy, University of Pittsburgh Medical Center.

do not have sufficient infrastructure and a clear strategy for preventing medication errors.

When considering patient safety in hospitals, the goal is to create a strong safety culture throughout the organization, with everyone developing a sense of responsibility for patient safety rather than considering safety the primary responsibility of a separate committee like the Quality Assurance Department. Related to this concept, many health care workers may view patient safety efforts as "extra" work and not an integral part of their job function. Building a safety culture is not a sudden transformation; a culture emerges as a collective learning process from working together over a long period of time.[6] Finally, an organization's safety culture is often the product of individual and group values, attitudes, perceptions, competencies, and the hospital staff and leadership's patterns of behavior.[7]

Many organizations do not have a clear and focused strategic plan for patient safety, including the area of medication patient safety. In reviewing the literature, only one peer-reviewed publication was found that described the importance and process for developing an organizational strategic plan around medication safety.

This article begins a series in the *Director's Forum* describing the pharmacy director's role in implementing a patient medication safety program. Previous articles in the *Director's Forum* stressed the importance of the pharmacy director's thorough knowledge in core competencies of hospital pharmacy practice in order to promote a patient-centered pharmacy service. An example that relates to patient safety involves the pharmacy director having knowledge of essential department and hospital data, which are related to the types and causes of serious medication errors and adverse drug events. Firsthand knowledge of this information will establish the initial steps in creating a strategy to improve medication safety. Regional and national data on medication errors may provide the pharmacy director with important strategies to establish a patient safety program. For example, the Pittsburgh Regional Health Care Initiative has identified important data related to medication errors and found four drugs that contribute to nearly 45% of all serious medication errors.

This first article will focus on practical considerations in developing a culture, strategy, and infrastructure for a medication patient safety program. A second article will focus on the examples of patient safety programs that can be implemented in a pharmacy department and have an organizational impact on patient safety.

Building a medication patient safety program requires a patient-centered approach to develop a collaborative and comprehensive program. The goal of this article is to help hospital pharmacy directors understand their organization's patient safety culture and develop a strategic medication safety plan. The specific aims of this article are to (1) describe how to promote a blame-free medication error reporting system; (2) describe how to review essential department and hospital data to determine priorities for patient safety; (3) show how establishing a pharmacy medication safety officer will help establish an infrastructure for patient safety; and (4) outline the steps to establish a medication safety strategic plan. Given the critical nature of medication error prevention in hospitals, it is imperative that the pharmacy director be a leader in implementing and assessing the hospital's medication safety program.

MEDICATION ERROR REPORTING SYSTEMS AND "BLAME FREE" CULTURE

In order to design safer medication delivery systems, information on medication errors must be collected and analyzed. While it is essential that data be collected and trended for analysis, the difficulty in detecting errors has long been recognized as a barrier to studying the problem effectively. Medication errors should be identified and documented, and their causes must be studied in order to develop systems that minimize recurrence. Most hospitals and health systems use a variety of methods to gather information on medication safety, including computerized surveillance, voluntary reporting, and observing medication processes.

These systems identify errors and track a variety of information on the errors, including the person who committed the error. Despite much rhetoric on the systems-approach to improving patient safety, the actions of individuals involved in an error are routinely reviewed. The perception and action taken regarding an individual's involvement in an error establishes the patient safety culture for that organization. The pharmacy director plays a key role in promoting blame-free analysis of medication errors within the organization by establishing a pharmacy department culture of open communication around medication errors.

One key cultural paradigm centers on blame-free reporting of errors. When people feel they can openly communicate about medication errors without fear of punishment or disciplinary action, then it is likely that they will share information about the actual contributing factors. To some, investigating an event implies a punitive direction as opposed to studying an event which implies learning. As a result, some hospitals have adopted standardized words for use when discussing medication-related events in an attempt to minimize any negative connotations. Importantly, conversations and information related to medication errors need to stay de-personalized and non-judgmental.

Hospital executives and physicians need to be personally involved if a culture of safety is going to be established.[8] This means educating the board of trustees and medical staff on the importance of patient safety while making a significant place for patient safety initiatives in the budget. For example, creating an economic analysis of the cost of an error can help to justify expense allocation. Importantly, involving physicians and leadership in root-cause analyses provides them with an insight that medication errors are multifactorial in nature.

It is also essential that it be culturally acceptable to question other health care professionals, orders, or situations. Too often, a root cause analysis conducted after a major error reveals that one or more health care professionals thought there was a problem, but they did not feel comfortable questioning it, or they were "scolded" for questioning and therefore did not escalate their concern. A well-established process for questioning a medication order needs to be outlined.

The pharmacy director plays an important role in establishing a "blame-free" and open environment in dealing with errors. First, the pharmacy director should remove any reference to punitive consequences of medication errors in performance evaluations and job descriptions. Second, the pharmacy director should establish a regular forum to discuss medication errors with department staff. Third, the pharmacy director should educate the medical staff, through the hospital's Medical Executive Committee, on the medication order review process while gaining their support on pharmacists' questioning orders that may be unsafe. Finally, the pharmacy director should routinely publicize successes in medication patient safety to provide staff with tangible outcomes for their error-prevention efforts. **Table 1** summarizes how the pharmacy director can promote a "blame free" process for reporting and discussing medication errors.

ESSENTIAL DEPARTMENT DATA AND MEDICATION SAFETY

Understanding the nature of medication errors and adverse drug events for a given hospital is critical to implement interventions that improve safety. Determining causes of medication errors should be coupled with assessment of the severity of the error. While quality management processes should include programs to prevent all medication errors, effort should be concentrated on eliminating the causes of errors associated with greater levels of severity. There should be established mechanisms for tracking drugs or drug classes that are involved in medication errors. Correlations between errors and the method of drug distribution and dispensing should also be reviewed (eg, unit dose, floor stock, injectable medication, etc). A previous article of the *Director's Forum* stressed the importance of the director of pharmacy's knowledge and understanding of essential department data including medication error information.

Table 1. Strategies for Promoting a "Blame-Free" Organizational Culture for Reporting and Discussing Medication Errors

Remove references to punitive consequences for committing medication errors from all performance appraisals; consider adding a performance standard to promote the reporting of medication errors

In collaboration with the medical staff, nursing staff, and hospital leadership, develop a statement promoting the open and honest discussion of medication errors

Educate hospital governance on the concept of establishing a "no blame" patient safety culture

Approve a policy by the hospital and medical leadership that empowers pharmacists to refuse to dispense unsafe orders until an appropriate review process is employed (eg, review by Chief of Medical Staff and Director of Pharmacy)

Review all medication sentinel events in the appropriate forum (eg, Medical Executive Committee) stressing the systems-based factors that contributed to the error

Publish a quarterly review of medication errors focusing on the types, severity, and causes of medication errors; distribute this report to all hospital and medical staff

Participate in a national medication error reporting system that provides additional information on errors across a broad scope of hospitals and patients to best establish safety priorities for the organization

From this information, the hospital can establish some targeted drugs or drug classes for safety efforts. If institution-specific data are not available, then national and regional data on problem medications are available through the United States Pharmacopeia (USP) and the Institute for Safe Medication Practices (ISMP). **Table 2** lists the drugs most commonly associated with serious medication errors.

A similar list should be developed for each health system and a concentrated effort made across all disciplines to eliminate the more common root causes, which attribute to each error involving a medication on this list. For example, as a result of an analysis of their internal data, it may be determined that insulin is the most common medication associated with a severe medication error.

HOSPITAL AND DEPARTMENT INFRASTRUCTURE FOR MEDICATION PATIENT SAFETY

A unified hospital vision for medication safety is critical to the institution's success. To drive change, hospital leaders must create organizational infrastructure to provide patient safety. Importantly, hospitals must also establish an infrastructure for communicating medication safety concerns.

Table 2. Medications Commonly Associated with Serious Medication Errors[11]

Insulin
Albuterol
Morphine sulfate
Heparin, warfarin
Potassium chloride
Cefazolin
Furosemide
Levofloxacin, vancomycin

Quality Councils or Patient Safety Steering Committees are examples of the type of governing body created to evaluate medication safety concerns. Often such entities report directly to the hospital board to ensure that they can function autonomously and avoid conflicts of interest.

Many organizations have formed multidisciplinary groups designed to talk about frontline medication safety concerns. These Unit-Based Medication Safety Teams or Safety Action Teams then hold patient safety dialogues, which serve to define issues. Approaching the issues from the bottom up generally promotes an increased level of support. For example, this serves to engage the expertise of the people doing the work. It is important that these groups develop a common goal, such as the reduction of medication errors involving insulin within a given unit or patient population. Finally, the pharmacy department needs to establish a structure that allows them to participate in various medication safety programs throughout an organization.

The University of Pittsburgh Medical Center (UPMC) established a medication safety pharmacist position in 2001 to address the organization's need for direct pharmacist involvement in patient safety. The job functions of this position are listed in **Table 3**. This position has become an integral part of the hospital's medication patient safety program and has positively impacted medication error reporting rates and implementation of medication safety initiatives.[9]

DEVELOPING A MEDICATION SAFETY STRATEGIC PLAN

The medication safety strategic plan is a collaboration of various depart-

Table 3. Job Functions of a Medication Safety Pharmacist

Identify and implement best practices for medication safety
Analyze current practices that may contribute to medication error occurrence and take proactive steps to prevent errors before they occur
Facilitate process and system changes and prevention activities to reduce the likelihood of occurrence/recurrence of error
Manage medication error reporting and investigation
Review reports and collect additional information to determine root cause
Manage medication error data entry into internal and external databases to provide reports to clinical staff and committees as appropriate
Educate pharmacy staff and other health care professionals to promote safe medication practices
Participate in departmental and interdisciplinary hospital, health system, and regional committees related to emergency medications, adverse events, medication errors, policy review, safe medication use, and patient safety
Assist in the development and review of medication use policies and adapt to current practice
Address issues of non-compliance and recommend corrective actions
Monitor compliance with medication control and security standards in the pharmacy and hospital patient cares areas

ments and is primarily the champion efforts of the director of pharmacy and the chair of the Pharmacy & Therapeutics Committee. Although the strategy to prevent medication errors may be different for each initiative, a standard approach is suggested by the ISMP to address all patient safety initiatives (see **Table 4**).[10]

Whether the institution uses benchmark data received from other hospitals, comparative data from surveys such as the ISMP survey, internal data from variance reports, or information gathered from the flow diagrams, it should be possible to get a sense of the safety needs and the prioritization of the risk associated with each. Using a multidisciplinary team, solutions should be identified to reduce or minimize the identified risks. These proposals are then consolidated and mapped along a timeline to create a Medication Safety Strategic Plan. This Safety Plan then serves as the guide for decisions and sets the vision for upcoming years. Importantly, the plan integrates the many ways to improve medication safety, including incorporation of automation and technology, expansion of clinical pharmacy services, policy development, and forma-

Table 4. Medication Error Prevention Methods and Their Effectivenesss

Method	Effectiveness
Forcing functions and constraints	Most effective
Automation and computerization	Most effective
Standardization and protocols	Effective
Checklists and double-check systems	Effective
Rules and policies	Least effective
Education and information	Least effective
Be more careful; be vigilant	Not effective

*Adapted from recommendations by the Institute for Safe Medication Practices

tion of unit-based teams. **Appendix A** provides an example of a medication safety strategic plan for preventing insulin medication errors.

SUMMARY AND CONCLUSION

Developing a systematic and strategic approach to preventing medication errors must be a 2007 organizational imperative for hospital pharmacy directors. A successful medication safety strategic plan must incorporate an effective use of hospital and departmental data, be supported by an adequate infrastructure, and embrace a culture of "no blame" in reporting and analyzing medication errors. The pharmacy director plays a key role in this plan by providing expert advice on medication errors and supporting an open environment within the pharmacy department. Finally, a pharmacist position dedicated to medication patient safety activities may provide the necessary focus and resource to make significant improvements in an organization's patient safety outcomes.

REFERENCES

1. Barker KN, Flynn EA, Pepper GA, Bates DW, Mikeal RL. Medication errors observed in 36 health care facilities. *Arch Intern Med.* 2002;162:1897-1903.

2. Hicks RW, Santell JP, Cousins DD, Williams RL. *MEDMARX™ 5th Anniversary Data Report: A Chartbook of 2003 Findings and Trends, 1999-2003.* Rockville, MD: USP Center for the Advancement of Patient Safety; 2004.

3. Aspden P, Wolcott J, Bootman JL, In: *Preventing Medication Errors: Quality Chasm Series.* Washington, DC: Institute of Medicine of National Academies, the National Academies Press; Anticipat-Checklists and double-check systems Effective ed 2007 publication. Available at: http://www.nap.edu/catalog/11623.html. Accessed January 8, 2007.

4. Leape LL, Berwick DM. Five years after to err is human: what have we learned? *JAMA.* 2005;293:2384-2390.

5. Manasse HR Jr, Eturnbull J, Diamond LH. Patient safety: a review of the contemporary American experience. *Singapore Med J.* 2002;43:254-262.

6. National Quality Forum. *Safe Practices for Better Health care: A Consensus Report.* Washington, DC: National Quality Forum; 2003.

7. Schein E. *Organizational Culture and Leadership.* 2nd ed. San Francisco, CA: Jossey–Bass; 1992.

8. Mark SM, Mercado MC. Medication Safety. In: TR Brown, Ed. *Handbook of Institutional Pharmacy Practice.* Bethesda, MD: ASHP; 2006:229-249.

9. Kowiatek JG, Weber RJ, Skledar SJ, Sirio CA. Medication safety manager in an academic medical center. *Am J Health Syst Pharm.* 2004;61:58-64.

10. Cohen MR, Levine SR, Mandrack MM. *Confronting the Challenges of Neonatal and Pediatric Medication Safety.* Huntingdon Valley, PA: ISMP; 2003.

11. American Society of Health-System Pharmacists. *Incorporating Safe Medication Principles into Daily Practice: Teaching Tool for Health Care Practitioners.* Bethesda, MD: ASHP Research and Education Foundation; 2004. ∎

Appendix A: Sample Medication Safety Strategic Plan for Preventing Insulin Medication Errors

GOAL: PREVENT MEDICATION ERRORS FROM INSULIN PRESCRIBING AND ADMINISTRATION

Intervention: Design and Implement Insulin Ordering Form
Cost: Low—mostly staff time for form development, education
Champion: Dr. Blue
Measurement of success: All insulin orders received after June 30, 2007 must be written on an insulin order form. Those not received on this form will not be processed.
Evaluation: All insulin orders will be tracked for 1 fiscal year, and reports will be provided to each department head monthly. Data will also be reviewed at the P&T committee monthly.

Intervention: Modify Insulin Warnings in Hospital Computer Systems
Cost: Minimal internal programming costs
Champion: Dr. White
Measurement of success: Programming completed by June 30, 2007. All insulin errors will be compared to computer reports of warning acknowledgements
Evaluation: Incidence of insulin errors will be tracked.

Intervention: Assess All Insulin-Related Procedures
Cost: Low—possible costs might include education, forms development, buying alternative products, etc
Champion: Dr. Green
Measurement of success: Review of steps and processes, changes where needed, presentation and approval of Med Error Performance Improvement Team.
Evaluation: This task has been completed and for the most part felt to be in compliance.

Intervention: Eliminate Abbreviations "U" and "IU"
Cost: None
Champion: Dr. Purple
Measurement of success: Monitoring of all insulin orders for compliance.
Evaluation: All orders must comply.

Intervention: Establish a Hospital-Wide Policy for Insulin
Cost: Low—mostly time of drafters of policy
Champion: Dr. Black
Measurement of success: Approval of policy.
Evaluation: This policy was approved and has since been revised in order to keep pace with the changing process of medication delivery at the hospital.

Intervention: Inservice all Staff on Insulin Handling and Prescribing
Champion: Dr. Red
Measurement of success: Successful inservice of affected groups (75% attendance)
Evaluation: Reduction in insulin errors by 10% in the first month.

Intervention: Implementation of Unit-Based Medication Error Reduction Performance Improvement Effort
Measurement of success: Completion of at least one error reduction project per year, which is focused on insulin
Evaluation: A reduction of insulin errors by unit by 10%.

Intervention: Reformat Medication Labels for Insulin
Measurement of success: Successful implementation of new label formats and fewer label-related errors with insulin reported
Evaluation: Specific focus in root cause analysis on label information and contribution to cause.

Developing a Medication Patient Safety Program, Part 2: Process and Implementation

Scott M. Mark, PharmD, MS, MEd, FASHP, FACHE* and
Robert J. Weber, MS, FASHP†

The *Director's Forum* series is written and edited by Robert Weber and Michael Sanborn and is designed to guide pharmacy leaders in establishing patient-centered services in hospitals and health systems. Another specific goal of this column is to address many of the key challenges that pharmacy directors face today, while providing information to foster growth in pharmacy leadership and patient safety. This month's *Forum* is co-authored by Scott Mark and focuses directly on processes for determining program priorities for patient safety and implementing a successful program.

This article continues a series in the *Director's Forum* describing the pharmacy director's role in implementing a medication patient safety program. The first article focused on practical considerations in developing a strategy and infrastructure for a medication patient safety program. This second article will focus on the process of targeting opportunities for error prevention and review the implementation strategies employed in a successful program at the University of Pittsburgh Medical Center (UPMC).

A key role of the Director of Pharmacy is to set the direction for medication safety improvement. The success of any medication safety program is aligning people and resources to focus on a specific patient safety goal. While the release of the Institute of Medicine report in July 2006 served as a wake-up call, 7 years later, many health systems have still failed to implement a comprehensive interdisciplinary system, which uses essential data to focus patient safety efforts. Most have implemented medication-error reporting systems, which evaluate and score medication errors but have not practically applied these data.

For a medication safety program to be effective, it must use medication-error reporting data effectively and be broad in its scope—since errors occur in all steps of the medication process. For example, a hospital may identify a "Top 10" list of drugs associated with serious errors as a way to target improvement. For any effort around the "Top 10" list to be effective, the entire organization must align to play a role in improving patient safety. Properly executed, this organizational coordination will involve changes to prescribing, storage, inventory selection, dispensing, administration, documentation, labeling, informatics, reporting, and education.

Everyone in the medication-use process plays a vital role in preventing errors, with each person depending on the other to promote safety. Even the most knowledgeable and diligent professional will, in all probability, make a number of medication errors over

---

*Assistant Professor of Pharmacy and Therapeutics, University of Pittsburgh School of Pharmacy, Director of Pharmacy, University of Pittsburgh Medical Center; †Associate Professor and Chair, University of Pittsburgh School of Pharmacy, Executive Director of Pharmacy, University of Pittsburgh Medical Center.

the course of a career. Most will be intercepted by another health care professional and most will not result in patient harm. However, serious errors occur when the checks at each point in the process fail. For this reason, it is essential to view medication safety improvements from the standpoint of system security, rather than individual departmental improvements. By taking a more comprehensive view, it will be easier to view the vulnerabilities of the entire system and subsequently make changes, which will result in true error reduction.

Implementing successful patient safety programs requires a patient-centered approach and is important in developing a collaborative and comprehensive program. The goal of this article is to provide hospital pharmacy directors with examples of successful medication patient safety programs. The specific aims of this article are to (1) present methods for identifying the targets of a patient safety program and (2) describe the steps in implementing a successful patient safety program in medication education at the UPMC, along with the impact of this program on organizational safety culture.

IDENTIFYING TARGETS FOR PATIENT SAFETY PROGRAMS

Once a culture of medication safety has been developed, the focus must be determined. This can be harder than it seems, as you will find many areas that you feel need improvement. Lack of focus, however, can lead to a lack of success. The key to implementing a medication safety program is in identifying the annual targets and ways in which everyone can participate. As with any other business plan, they must be developed through collabora-

tion around targets, which are agreed upon and meaningful to the organization. Medication safety strategic plans are rarely successful when developed in a vacuum; they should serve as the guide for decision making and change.

The ideas for selection of what items to include in a medication safety strategic plan can come from many areas. Departments that are new to this process may need to use population data for medication errors or published accounts of problem areas. Lists of medications commonly associated with errors, such as the one that was provided in part one of this series, is subsequently valuable. There are five key areas in which information is gathered to select the highest priority targets for medication safety improvements include (1) department and hospital data; (2) root cause analysis findings; (3) risk assessment in the medication use process; (4) internal survey results; and (5) staff surveys.

Departmental and Hospital Data

In departments that have been collecting data, one common source for target selection is inhouse medication error or incident reports. Trends may indicate that errors involving a specific or drug class have increased. The team may choose to target medications or classes that have increased all medication errors or identify a subset of these data such as "near-misses" (errors that were caught before they reached the patient) or serious medication errors (errors that required patient therapy intervention, caused permanent harm, or resulted in death). While quality management processes should include programs to decrease the incidence of all medication errors, often effort is concentrated on eliminating the causes of errors associated with greater levels of severity.

Alternatively, some targets are selected as a result of the method of drug distribution. For example, the goal may be to reduce medication errors associated with floor stock drugs, automated dispensing cabinets, or injectable products. It is also common for organizations to target specific elements of the medication use process. Medication errors are often categorized by the segment of the medication use process which has failed. Therefore, they can be categorized as prescribing, dispensing, administration, monitoring, and patient compliance errors. The Joint Commission on Accreditation of Health Care Organizations (JCAHO) has also adopted a similar approach in the revised 2004 medication management chapter standards. This format can provide focus if for example, the organization is experiencing a problem with medication administration errors. Studies indicate that 49% of medication errors occur during the ordering phase, 26% during the delivery (transcribing) phase, and 25% during the processing (preparing and dispensing) phase.[1]

Root Cause Analysis (RCA) Findings

Another common way to identify potential items for the medication safety strategic plan is from the results of recent RCA. RCA is a way to identify the cause that is most directly responsible for causing errors. The JCAHO now requires all institutions to perform an RCA on all sentinel events. RCAs are multidisciplinary reviews of serious errors, which help to identify all underlying causes or factors that may have contributed to the event. They are particularly use-

ful ways to determine both the causative factors but also the more subtle contributory elements that may not be immediately apparent. Trending the findings of RCA can also uncover patterns that thread through many errors.

RCA participants generally find the process particularly enlightening, as they learn to see the medication use process from the perspective of other professionals. The very nature of the discussion provides a point and counterpoint that reveal hidden defenses in the system and help to understand its complexity. Learning to evaluate the medication use process from systematic perspective helps to reduce overall risk and understand how the actions of one professional influence that of another. For this reason, many organizations conduct mock-RCA or focused-event studies on non-sentinel events. These less serious near misses can reveal a tremendous amount of information that can be used to prevent the next sentinel event. Often these studies are conducted with more than one facilitator to ensure that nonverbal behavior is observed. Even though there is a stated openness to the process, some may still be uncomfortable sharing and a perceptive facilitator can recognize nonverbal clues and ensure that points are fully explored. The fishbone diagram in **Figure 1** demonstrates information that can be learned from an RCA and how the contributing factors can be grouped into phases of the medication use process for improvement. According to the JCAHO, communication is now the leading root cause of all types of sentinel events.

A review of all organizational RCAs may also demonstrate that communication errors contribute to a significant number of sentinel errors. As a result, communication "hand-offs" may be selected as a point of focus in the medication-safety strategic plan.

Evaluating Risk in Medication Use Process

Another way to identify key areas of potential focus is to conduct an analysis of the medication use system. To fully understand the complexity of a given medication use system, it must be flowed out. This can be done for an individual medication or for a general process. Once completed, the multidisciplinary team will have a better understanding of the complexity of the problem and will understand the medication-use strengths and risk points. Flow diagrams are also useful for assessing changes that will occur with process redesigns. For example, the changes which may be proposed in the insulin ordering process can be assessed prior to implementation.

Health care has begun to utilize techniques adopted from other industries to proactively analyze systems and identify areas of weakness. Three such processes are Failure Mode and Effects Analysis (FMEA) commonly used in the aerospace and automotive industries.[2-4] FMEA is a systematic method of identifying and preventing product, equipment, and process problems before they occur. Interdisciplinary teams are assembled to evaluate complicated systems and identify areas of concern. Proactive changes are then taken to strengthen these areas. Applied to health care, FMEA provides a safety tool for risk managers to improve the patient care environment.

Probabilistic Risk Assessments are a similar process that utilize error prob-abilities. Systems are mapped and failure probability is assigned to each process point. Pathways deemed to have a high risk of failure then become a point of focus for process redesign.

Healthcare Failure Mode Effects Analysis uses a simplified tool, the Hazard Scoring Martix (Matrix) to assess risk. The Matrix applies hazard analysis principles that factor in the severity and probability of the potential failure mode occurring. The Matrix defines degrees of severity as: catastrophic, major, moderate, and minor. Degrees of probability are defined as frequent, occasional, uncommon, and remote.[5]

Some key areas that may be selected as a result of a medication use analysis would include high-risk practices with low frequency of use or areas in which new processes have been recently implemented into high risk areas. Examples might include the use of pediatric crash carts in an adult hospital or the introduction of new programmable pumps for infusing medications on the nursing units. The JCAHO requires all institutions to develop a process for managing high-risk medications. In a sense, this requires a proactive risk assessment.

Internal Baselines

Many organizations now use medication safety self-assessments as a means of measuring and tracking progress in key areas of the medication use process. In a sense, this becomes the backbone of the medication safety strategic plan. This will establish a baseline from which to evaluate the safety of the current system as well as the impact that changes or interventions may have. There are several ways to achieve this end. One commonly used method is to complete the com-

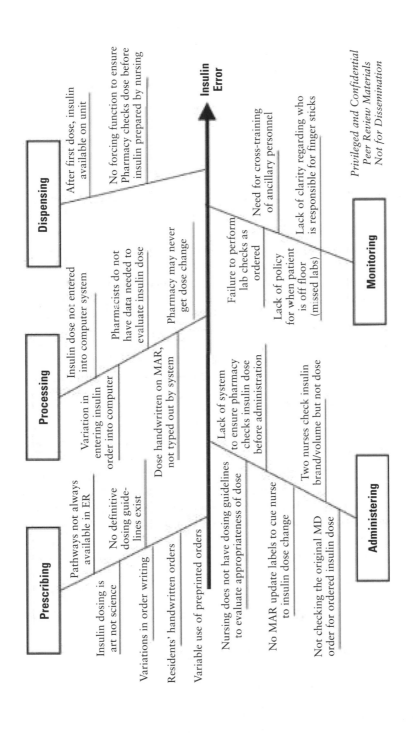

Figure 1. Sample fishbone diagram showing root cause forces contributing to an insulin error.

prehensive questionnaire developed by the Institute for Safe Medication Practices (ISMP). The ISMP *Medication Safety Self-Assessment* evaluates the current status of a health system at a particular point in time. It forces an institution to evaluate how well safety is incorporated into its medication processes (ie, how technology is used, how medications are securely stored, how well-lit drug-preparation areas are). It is recommended that the survey be completed by a multidisciplinary team as honestly as possible. Individual questions are weighted and scored directly by ISMP. Once a baseline is established, it can be used as an internal comparison from year to year. **Figure 2** demonstrates how an institution used the survey's recommendations to increase their score over a period of time. This tangible feedback should then be shared with the entire organization to reinforce efforts. Specific changes in the individual item scores of the ISMP assessment can also be used to focus quality improvement efforts.

Staff Surveys

One last key area of critical information regarding high-risk practices or areas of vulnerability is the front line staff. No one knows the practices better than those individuals who use them every day. It is essential to real-ize that medication-use flow diagrams and self-assessment safety surveys rely on stated practices. Often, the true practice is different than the stated practice. While this may sound minor, the resulting weaknesses that this can introduce into the medication-use system can produce major vulnerabilities. For example, while the staff are required to scan every source bottle going into a total parenteral nutrition compounder, for the sake of efficiency, the staff may only scan the original bottle and either adjust solution volumes or use bar codes taped to a "cheat sheet" to change out bottles faster. Obviously, this can result in the wrong solution being added to a high-risk medication. Regularly surveying staff regarding where they see the greatest risks can uncover practices that are either overlooked or incompliant with policy—resulting in risk.

EXAMPLE OF IMPLEMENTING A SUCCESSFUL PATIENT SAFETY PROGRAM

Analyzing medication errors highlights a variety of prevention steps that can be taken to improve patient safety. An important prevention step is effectively informing patients about their medication. Most experts agree that informing patients of the name, indication, dose, frequency, and side effects of their prescribed medication

Date	3-04 (Baseline)	10-04	3-05	10-05	3-06	10-06	1–07
ISMP Score	607	643	664	693	730	757	883

Figure 2. Sample of ongoing results of Institute for Safe Medication Practices (ISMP) *Self-Assessment* used by a hospital as a quality improvement measure.

helps to prevent patient confusion, error, and the potential for adverse drug events.

In September 2005, the UPMC implemented a house-wide medication education program with specific roles for nurses, pharmacists, and respiratory therapists. With an emphasis on patient education to reduce patient medication errors, the program is called EPITOME (Enhanced Patient Safety Intervention To Optimize Medication Education). The goal of EPITOME is to reduce patient medication-related problems, reduce the number of medications prescribed, and improve patient satisfaction with medication education.

The EPITOME program design provides medication education to patients by pharmacists, nurses, and respiratory therapists. **Figure 3** illustrates the steps of EPITOME. Patients are educated on all oral and selected injectable medications prescribed by physicians during their hospital stay (Step 1); medication information sheets are printed from the hospital's information system (Cerner HNA Millenium, Kansas City, MO) (Step 2); nurses and respiratory therapists provide education to patients at each administration of oral or inhaled medication (Steps 3 and 4); assessing patient's comprehension of medication information; pharmacists educate patients at risk for medication non-compliance as determined by nursing assessment and number of medications prescribed or changed during a hospital stay (Steps 5 and 6). Patients are educated on the proper drug name, dose, frequency,

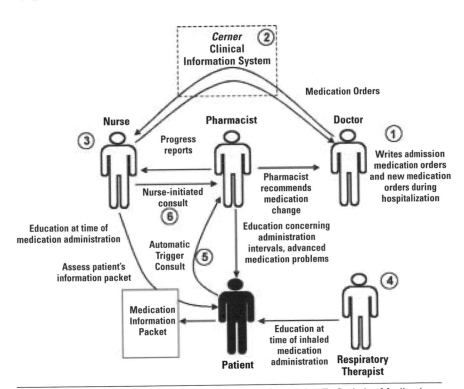

Figure 3. Overview of the Enhanced Patient Safety Intervention To Optimize Medication Education (EPITOME) project.

side effects, and significant drug interactions (both drug-drug and drug-food).

Education is provided by nurses, pharmacists, and respiratory therapists in the context of a health behavior change model, where patient autonomy in medication use is established along with assessing the patient's readiness to be compliant with their medication regimen. Caregivers providing education elicit information from patients regarding their medications, provide answers to their questions, while reinforcing and assessing readiness for change. This climate for patient learning and addresses patient ambivalence and resistance.

Health Care Provider Roles
Nurse and Respiratory Therapist

The unique aspect of the EPITOME program is that education is provided at each medication administration. This approach provides patients with many opportunities to ask questions and to clarify information regarding their medication. In addition, the nursing and respiratory staff can continually assess the patient's understanding of the medication regimen, referring the patient to a pharmacist if necessary.

Pharmacist

The pharmacist reinforces medication education by the nurses and respiratory therapists in patients at risk for medication noncompliance. Importantly, the pharmacist performs medication therapy management in these patients that involves simplifying dosage regimens to reduce patient confusion and error. Medication therapy management involves monitoring regimens for medication duplicates, optimizing drug selection and

dosages, reconciling the medication regimen, recommending a drug for an untreated condition, and discontinuing drugs that are not indicated. After educating the patient and reviewing the drug regimen, the pharmacist documents their activities in a progress note so that all caregivers are aware of their intervention.

Strategies for Implementation and Sustainability
Recruit Physician Champions

EPITOME was the championed effort of key physicians on the medical staff, making this program a high priority for clinical disciplines as well as hospital administration. The physicians recognized the importance of patients understanding their medication regimens and provided help with resistant physicians. Without their support and passion for this program, EPITOME would have failed.

Assure for Adequate Resources

The support of the hospital's Chief Operating Officer (COO) was vital to the implementation and sustainability of EPITOME. The COO provided resources for pharmacy support (1.5 full-time equivalent) and computer equipment for data collection.

An important focus was also to make the education a part of the daily work of the pharmacists, nurses, and respiratory therapists. Nurses and respiratory therapists provide education at the time of medication administration, and the pharmacists provide care directly to nursing units performing medication regimen review and education as a regular daily job function.

EPITOME Outcomes

EPITOME impacted the organization's safety culture by increasing staff and patient awareness of medication education and by simplifying medication regimens in patients at risk for noncompliance.

Increased Organizational Awareness of Patient Medication Education

EPITOME's comprehensive approach highlighted this program as an important patient safety initiative at UPMC Presbyterian. Progress was reported on and reviewed at the hospital medical executive and executive management committees. Ninety percent of the staff surveyed are aware of EPITOME and its role in patient safety.

Increased Patient Awareness of Medication Education

Patients are surveyed and asked, "How often have you been provided education on your medications?" Patient responses on a Likert Scale (1 to 5) have improved from "Not sure" (average 2.8) to "Very often" (average 4.7) over a 9-month period.

An Improved Medication Regimen in High-Risk Patients

Pharmacist medication therapy management has improved the quality of patient's medication regimens. Over a recent 4-month period, the medication regimens of approximately 500 EPITOME patients by pharmacists resulted in over 100 medication changes.

SUMMARY AND CONCLUSION

Medication-error prevention is an essential requirement for pharmaceutical care and must be a core mission of every pharmacy. The medication use process is extremely complex and as a result, error-prone. It is the responsibility of everyone in the process to work toward improving communication and clarity and take responsibility for their value in the system. Many health systems have worked to develop elaborate surveillance and data collection systems to track their medication errors. However, they fail to harness these data to drive change throughout their organization.

Successful implementation of a patient safety program requires an approach that recruits physician champions, designs an effective and efficient intervention, and can be readily evaluated to show their impact on the organization's health care quality.

REFERENCES

1. Bates DW, Cullen DJ, Laird N, et al. Incidence of adverse drug events and potential adverse drug events: implications for prevention, ADE Prevention Study Group. *JAMA.* 1995;274:29-34.

2. McDermott R, Mikulak R, Beauregard M. *The Basics of FMEA.* New York, New York: Productivity Press; 1996:3.

3. Cohen MR, Senders J, Davis NM. Failure mode and effects analysis: a novel approach to avoiding dangerous medication errors and accidents. *Hosp Pharm.* 1994;29:319-324,326-328,330.

4. Williams E, Talley R. The use of failure mode effect and criticality analysis in a medication error subcommittee. *Hosp Pharm.* 1994;29:331-332, 334-339.

5. Derosier J, Stalhandske E, Baglan JP, Nudell T. Using health care failure mode and effect analysis: the VA National Center for Patient Safety's Prospective Risk Analysis System. *JCAHO J Qual Improv.* 2002;28:254. ∎

Using Health Care Failure Mode and Effects Analysis for High-Risk Medications

Bruce Doepker, PharmD, BCPS*, and
Robert J. Weber, PharmD, MS, BCPS, FASHP†

The *Director's Forum* series is edited by Robert Weber and Scott Mark and is designed to guide pharmacy leaders in establishing patient-centered services in hospitals and health systems. This month's article focuses on a health care failure mode and effects analysis (HC-FMEA) to analyze the prescribing of high-risk medications. HC-FMEA can provide the pharmacy director with a powerful approach to directly changing processes to improve medication safety.

Continued major concerns of health care workers, payers, and patients are medication errors (MEs) and adverse drug events (ADEs). The most popular approach to eliminating MEs and ADEs involves using technology, such as computerized prescriber order entry (CPOE), bar code medication administration, robotic technology, and intravenous pump infusion system safeguards.[1] For example, a recent study showed that medication bar coding (bar code electronic medication administration record [eMAR]) significantly reduced medication administration errors and the potential for ADEs.[2] This study also showed that medication administration errors were not totally eliminated with the bar code eMAR, implying the need for continued refinement of the bar code eMAR process or a change in other processes associated with medication administration. Technology is not the only answer to the problem of MEs; others propose incorporating process and cultural changes as a multimodal approach in reducing MEs and ADEs.[3]

Process changes to minimize ADEs and MEs are accomplished by utilizing continuous quality improvement techniques that establish the "ideal" condition or system and point out areas of potential failure or error. This failure mode analysis (FMA) may also refer to the specific type of system failure and the degree of failure.[4] As a result, an FMA only addresses quality concerns in a system; for example, an FMA may be conducted on a brake system for an automobile to ensure all components work as specified. To assess the risk of these brake system failure modes on drivers, an FMEA (failure modes and *effects* analysis) must be conducted. FMEA discovers the potential risks in a system or process by determining the ways that the process or system might fail and the consequences of that failure.

A health care FMEA (HC-FMEA) analyzes the potential failure modes and associated risks in patient care, including medical devices, procedures, equipment, treatment protocols, and high-risk medications.[5] HC-FMEA has been used in health care since the early 1990s to prevent medication er-

*Specialty Practice Pharmacist, Critical Care; Associate Clinical Professor, The Ohio State University Medical Center, Columbus, Ohio. †Senior Director of Pharmacy, The Ohio State University Medical Center; Assistant Dean for Medical Center Affairs, The Ohio State University, College of Pharmacy, Columbus, Ohio.

rors from drug delivery systems. For example, Stanford Hospital & Clinics utilized HC-FMEA to improve patient safety in postoperative pain control. They analyzed 56 events occurring over a 12-month period and identified five major failure modes that were responsible for the majority of errors in patients receiving patient-controlled analgesia (PCA). Researchers determined the areas of failure were related to pump operation, pain medication orders, and side-effect monitoring. Changes in these areas improved the quality of PCA therapy; it is now considered the standard mode for parenteral opioid postoperative pain control.[6]

Most HC-FMEA involves devices or workflow processes. HC-FMEA may be used to improve the prescribing process of medications because these practices involve a systematic approach (eg, patient selection, drug dose, frequency, monitoring plan). However, there is very little published on using HC-FMEA to evaluate and analyze high-risk medications. As part of developing a patient-centered pharmacy service, the pharmacy director is concerned about the use of high-risk medications and should always be focused on reducing or eliminating the possibility for error with these medications, making errors visible and transparent, and minimizing the adverse effects of an error related to a high-risk medication.

The goal of this article is to provide a framework to the pharmacy director for the implementation of HC-FMEA in analyzing high-risk medication use. Specifically, this article will (a) describe the HC-FMEA process, (b) review past practices with HC-FMEA to evaluate medication use, and (c) apply HC-FMEA to a process of prescribing a high-risk medication at an academic medical center. It is hoped that the information in this article can be used to broaden the application of HC-FMEA throughout an organization's medication patient safety program. Active involvement in medication safety programs will continue to promote the pharmacy as a patient-centered clinical service.

HC-FMEA

HC-FMEA is a proactive, prospective quality improvement strategy that potentially identifies and assesses potential system errors, also called *gaps*.[7] Steps for a HC-FMEA include (a) selecting a focus area, (b) assembling a team, (c) mapping the process, (d) analyzing the harm associated with the process (eg, hazard analysis), and (e) developing action and outcome measures.

Selecting a Focus Area

The first step is to identify a focus area or process to review that is clinically significant, complex, or not commonly encountered. A review of essential department data such as reported MEs, as well as suggestions/concerns from staff around medication safety, may guide focus area selection. A comparison of an organization's reported MEs and ADEs versus national trends/information on high-risk areas can also help in selecting an HC-FMEA focus area. The case example in this article focuses on argatroban; it is deemed a high-alert medication because of the bleeding risk associated with it and the complex process in which it is utilized.

Assembling a Team

A multidisciplinary team is assembled to include clinicians from diverse backgrounds with experience and expertise in the HC-FMEA focus area. All information regarding the reasons for selecting the HC-FMEA focus area should be given to the team prior to the first meeting. Information includes, but is not limited to, ME and ADE details, expert opinions from consultants/peers, financial data, and other analyses related to the HC-FMEA focus area.

Mapping the Process

Mapping the process involves creating a detailed flow chart that identifies each step and failure mode in the process. This process is often facilitated by a person trained in quality improvement techniques of flow chart creation and observation. The facilitator leads the group with a series of questions such as: Tell me in detail each step of this process. What is your role in this process? Was this the process that was originally designed? If not, why?

Analyzing Potential Harm

Once the failure modes are identified, a hazard analysis can be completed in which the risk priority number (RPN) is calculated for each failure mode. The RPN is the ratio of the frequency of patient harm to the likelihood of detecting the failure mode. The RPN is calculated by multiplying the estimated frequency of occurrence by the detectability and the expected severity of the damage to the patient. A 10-point scale (1 being the lowest and 10 being the highest score) grades each failure mode on severity, detectability, and frequency. For example, the RPN for a failure mode may have a 10 (*high risk and severity*), 7 (*moderate to hard to detect*), and 2 (*low frequency*) for a calculated RPN of 140. The higher the RPN score, the

greater risk associated with the failure mode.

Developing an Action Plan and Outcome Measures

After the RPN score is calculated for specific failure modes, the action plan can be focused to address those issues with the highest RPN. For example, when an HC-FMEA is conducted on a PCA device, a high RPN score may be associated with device programming errors, specifically those addressing drug concentrations of pain medication in the PCA pump. Therefore, an action plan may be incorporated that provides a fail-safe in the programming process to prevent inadvertent entry of incorrect narcotic drug concentrations or to add a bar-coding capability to the device.

Another method commonly used by institutions to identify causes of serious adverse events is root cause analysis (RCA). RCA is performed retrospectively in response to errors that have already occurred. It reacts to recent failures within a system and is not an effective prospective error-prevention approach. It is used to identify major failure modes in the process as a result of an error and is often included as part of the HC-FMEA. Primarily, a detailed RCA is conducted when an event occurs that is serious or has a significant impact on the organization (eg, sentinel event).[8]

There are several ways that HC-FMEA can be successful. Clearly defining goals and focusing process review help to relieve the burden on busy staff in completing the HC-FMEA. Strong leadership and the involvement of individuals familiar with the current process are crucial to the success of the HC-FMEA. The appropriate people will provide a thorough review of all the intricate parts of the process, provide resources, and help eliminate barriers during implementation. HC-FMEA is a timely and sometimes costly process to which the team must be fully committed to thoroughly conduct the analysis. A financial focus on the HC-FMEA is helpful and provides a basis for justifying these resource expenditures. By preventing adverse effects, HC-FMEA can reduce harm to patients while decreasing health care costs.

In summary, HC-FMEA is an effective process for identifying faulty systems and processes. Changes made in the prescribing process as a result of HC-FMEA can reduce the potential for errors and minimize the effect of serious errors, but they do not guarantee that errors will be completely eliminated.

HC-FMEA AND MEDICATION USE

As stated previously, HC-FMEA typically analyzes a process or device, but specific uses of medications may not be generally applied to the HC-FMEA process. Very little published data describe the use of HC-FMEA to evaluate medication prescribing practices. In fact, a MEDLINE search from January 1990 to April 2010 revealed no published articles on HC-FMEA associated with prescribing a medication. A 2006 paper, however, described using HC-FMEA to prevent chemotherapy errors. The authors describe the entire HC-FMEA process as applied to prescribing, administering, and documenting chemotherapy. Recognized risk areas were the identification of patients for chemotherapy and verification of unclear or incorrect orders with respect to height, weight, body surface area, missing signatures, or administration dates. Uniquely, the

authors also added a post–HC-FMEA review (12 months) to determine the degree of sustainability of the action plan. The re-evaluation of this plan was an important step to ensure that process changes addressed all identified failure modes.[7]

Although there is a paucity of data about using HC-FMEA to review high-risk medications, The Ohio State University Medical Center (OSUMC) chose to apply HC-FMEA in reviewing anticoagulation practices related to The Joint Commission National Patient Safety Goal (NPSG) 3E, because of the high-risk processes associated with these medications. In general, anticoagulants account for 4% of preventable ADEs and 10% of potential ADEs.[9] Unexpected admission to the hospital from anticoagulant medication adverse effects (bleeding, blood dyscrasias) ranges between 10% to 15%.[10]

CASE STUDY: APPLICATION OF HC-FMEA TO IMPROVE ARGATROBAN USE
National Patient Safety Goal 3E

The Joint Commission under Patient Safety Standard LD.5.2 requires that institutions conduct a proactive review of at least one high-risk process annually to reduce sentinel events. In July 2007, The Joint Commission announced two new NPSGs to be implemented by January 1, 2009. One of these, NPSG 3E, required organizations to reduce patient harm associated with the use of anticoagulation therapy.[8,11] The primary process improvement initiative was to reduce morbidity and mortality associated with bleeding and thrombosis related to anticoagulation. The Joint Commission requested standardized practices to reduce the risk of these adverse events associated with the use of unfractionated heparin (UFH), low-molecular-weight heparin (LMWH), warfarin, and other anticoagulants. OSUMC's Quality Management and Operations Committee required that an HC-FMEA be performed on each of these medications, including argatroban, which was OSMUC's direct thrombin inhibitor of choice.

Application of HC-FMEA at an Academic Medical Center

OSUMC is a tertiary care academic medical center in Columbus, Ohio. The medical center is comprised of four hospitals—the Ross Heart Hospital, the James Cancer Hospital and Solove Research Institute, University Hospital, and University Hospital East (community-based hospital)—which contain over 1,100 beds. The six signature programs at OSUMC are oncology, critical care, cardiology, imaging, neuroscience, and transplantation. The pharmacy department employs approximately 130 pharmacists and more than 40 are considered clinical specialists. The clinical specialists practice in disciplines such as internal medicine, critical care, cardiology, oncology, and transplantation.

Problem description/selecting a focus area

FMEA was utilized to review each of the medications listed in the The Joint Commission's NPSG 3E. Argatroban was a major focus, because it was identified as a high-alert medication by OSUMC. It has an increased incidence of severe bleeding and a complex process for usage associated with the treatment of heparin-induced thrombocytopenia (HIT). A diagnosis of HIT carries with it catastrophic consequences such as limb amputation and life-threatening thrombosis.

OSUMC deemed it a priority to have a process in place for the recognition and treatment of HIT.

Assemble a team

A multidisciplinary committee was formed and charged with the responsibility of performing the FMEA. The committee was composed of experts in the field and medical professionals who worked in areas recognized as high-frequency users of argatroban. Included were physicians from hematology and cardiothoracic surgery, critical care nurses and pharmacists, laboratory personnel, hospital administration, information systems, and quality and operations improvement services. All adverse event reports that involved the use of argatroban or had any association with HIT were pulled for the previous year and were reviewed prior to the FMEA.

Draw the process

The first order for the committee was to create a detailed map of the current process at OSUMC for using argatroban (see **Figure 1**). Approximately 30 steps were identified. The process was broken down into seven stages: (1) diagnosing, (2) prescribing, (3) ordering, (4) dispensing, (5) administration, (6) documentation, (7) monitoring, and (8) discontinuation and follow-up. By breaking the process down into different stages, OSUMC was able to focus more on the individual stages and not be overwhelmed by the process as a whole.

The next task was to break down each step in the process and identify all of the potential failure modes associated with each step. It was important to consider every failure mode suggested by the multidisciplinary committee. The argatroban FMEA

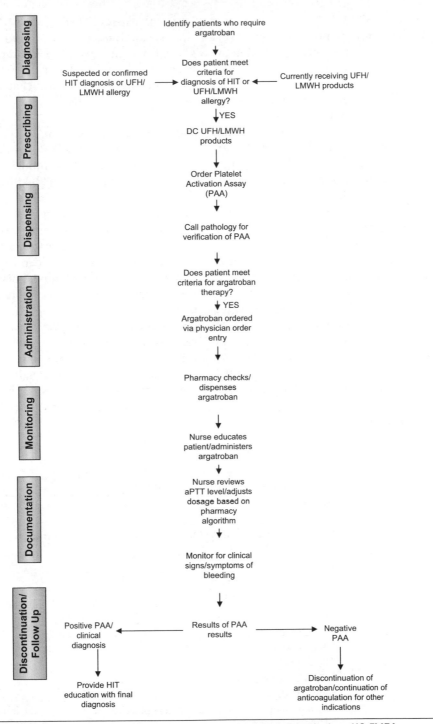

Figure 1. Argatrban flow chart. aPTT = activated partial thromboplastin time; HC-FMEA = health care failure modes and effects analysis; HIT = heparin-induced thrombocytopenia; LMWH = low-molecular-weight heparin; UFH = unfractionated heparin.

helped OSUMC identify weaknesses in their current process. The FMEA prompted several initiatives within the institution.

Conduct a hazard analysis

When the final analysis was completed, 38 potential failure modes were recognized in OSUMC's current process. After the failure modes were identified, RPN scoring was performed by each member of the group on each failure mode to determine the order of criticality. The RPN scores were then averaged and placed in order from highest to lowest. The top 10 failure modes are listed in **Table 1**. The failure mode with the highest RPN score (313.6), which correlated with the greatest risk, was the lack of pharmacy screening for concomitant UFH or LMWH products while a patient was suspected of HIT. In 2006, the US Food and Drug Administration designated UFH flushes as devices, not drugs; they are, therefore, not regulat-

ed by pharmacy. Through a medication use analysis, OSUMC found that several patients received UFH flushes even though they had a heparin allergy or during a time period that they were suspected of HIT.

Implement an action plan

Several initiatives were created in response to the failure modes that were discovered from the HC-FMEA. A timeline was created as a guide through the implementation process (see **Figure 2**). A HIT Practice Guideline was created as an educational tool for practitioners to use to identify patients suspected of HIT, guide them in the proper way to test for HIT, and treat patients with suspected or confirmed HIT. A retrospective analysis was done on all patients who received argatroban therapy within the past year. Initial dosages, steady-state dosage, time to therapeutic activated partial thromboplastin time (aPTT), percentage of aPTTs within the ther-

Table 1. Identified failure modes in argatroban prescribing

	Risk priority number score	Failure mode
1	313.6	Lack of pharmacy screening for UFH flushes/non–physician order entry areas (eg, operating room)
2	298.6	HIT test order falls off after 24 h
3	266.6	No standard HIT surveillance
4	261.7	Lack of screening for UFH products (eg, UFH coated catheters)
5	217	Lack of review of HIT test results by responsible physician
6	214.5	Lack on prebuilt monitoring parameters for procedure areas (eg, operating room) and emergency department
7	212.8	Allergies not consistently entered
8	210.8	Lack of or inconsistent documentation of initial dosage or dosage adjustments
9	203.8	HIT tests not performed by lab because of lack of physician coordination of lab draw
10	197.5	Lack of guidelines for holding argatroban prior to procedures or surgery

Note: HIT = heparin-induced thrombocytopenia; UFH = unfractionated heparin.

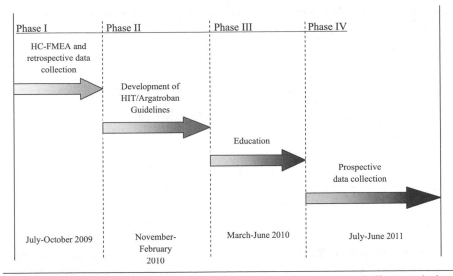

Figure 2. Implementation timeline. HC-FMEA = health care failure mode and effects analysis; HIT = heparin-induced thrombocytopenia.

apeutic range, treatment duration, bleeding rates, and risk factors associated with bleeding were collected. All of these outcomes were reviewed and adjustments were made to the argatroban dosing algorithm, initial dosages were reduced, holding parameters were specified for procedures, and aPTT goal ranges for treatment and prophylaxis were defined. An Argatroban Dosing and Monitoring Guideline was created as a reference for all of the changes to current practice. The CPOE was revised to include HIT as an allergy option and a "heparin pending allergy" was created to allow pharmacy to screen for UFH or LMWH products until the definitive diagnosis of HIT is confirmed or ruled out. OSUMC no longer routinely uses UFH flushes because of the increased rate of patients receiving them inadvertently and requires a physician order if UFH flushes are needed. Hospital-wide education will be completed on all of these changes and further

prospective review will be done after education and all changes to the process are in place. FMEA was used as a guide to improve the overall process of HIT management at OSUMC and to evaluate the process as a whole. The changes made to this process are intended to lower bleeding rates and prevent major adverse events related to HIT that have the potential to lead to catastrophic outcomes such as deep vein thrombosis, pulmonary embolism, and limb amputation.

Outcomes and measures

After implementation and education are complete, a follow-up analysis will be done as a quality initiative. Major outcome measures will include an evaluation of HIT test results, argatroban dosages, bleeding, and associated risk factors (see **Table 2**). These outcomes will be compared to the results from the retrospective analysis completed prior to the process changes from the HC-FMEA. The fo-

Table 2. A summary of selected outcomes measure to argatroban prescribing

Outcome	Measurement
Argatroban dosage	Initial dosage: dose started on day 1 of therapy Steady-state dosage: 3 consecutive aPTTs within the therapeutic range
Bleeding	Major bleed: any drop in hemoglobin $\geq$ 2g/dL $\geq$ $ 2 units of packed red blood cells transfused within a 24-h period, intracranial, retroperitoneal, or other life-threatening bleed Minor bleed: all other bleeds not described above

Note: aPTTs = activated partial thromboplastin times.

cus will be on reducing bleeding rates and streamlining argatroban dosing strategies.

USING HC-FMEA AS A MEDICATION SAFETY STRATEGY

The HC-FMEA process is a thorough review that will help reduce adverse events before they occur. It concentrates on the entire system and does not assign blame to individuals but on the process itself. Using HC-FMEA as a medication review process, institutions will be able to anticipate sentinel events and make changes to their current process to prevent these occurrences in the future. In medical laboratories, HC-FMEA is considered the method of choice in identifying potential failure modes and their effects within a system. HC-FMEA should be seriously considered by institutions for use in the medication review process prior to adding medications to formulary or to review high-alert medications already being utilized.

CONCLUSION

The HC-FMEA process may be time-consuming and tedious, however the overall benefit to patient safety outweighs the time and effort spent to perform the analysis. There are real advantages to using HC-FMEA for medication review. HC-FMEA allows the identification and prevention of potential adverse events related to the medication, but it also causes an examination of the entire system in which the medication is incorporated. Every hospital or medical institution has processes, resources, and methods that are different from other institutions. HC-FMEA helps identify those processes, obstacles, and gaps in the current system that may lead to catastrophic outcomes for patients. The HC-FMEA flow chart can be used as a template to identify and create solutions within the institution to ensure safe utilization, monitoring, and delivery of high-alert medications. HC-FMEA should not be used to review all medications, only those deemed to be high risk with complex processes associated with them. ME prevention is a continuous quality improvement process that requires commitment, dedication, and input from all disciplines in order to be successful. By using HC-FMEA, the pharmacy director can have a tremendous impact on medication safety and the development of patient-centered pharmacy services.

ACKNOWLEDGEMENTS

The authors acknowledge the following individuals who contributed to the HC-FMEA process at The Ohio State University Medical Center: Christine Chukajian, PharmD,

MS; Stacie Crosley, RN, BSN; Michele Dye, MS, RN, CCRN, CCNS, ANP-BC; Michael Firstenberg, MD, FACC; Anthony Gerlach, PharmD, BCPS; Trisha Jordan, PharmD, MS; Lisa Saslaw, MPH, RN, BSN; Ariane Schieber, PharmD, BCPS; Kevin Shively, MT(ASCP), MHA; and Anne VanBuren, MPH.

REFERENCES

1. Smetzer JL, Vaida AJ, Cohen MR, Tranum D, Pittman MA, Armstrong CW. Findings from the ISMP Medication Safety Self-Assessment for hospitals. *Jt Comm J Qual Saf.* 2003;29(11):586-597.

2. Poon EG, Keohane CA, Yoon CS, et al. Effect of bar-code technology on the safety of medication administration. *N Engl J Med.* 2010;362(18):1698-1707.

3. Smetzer JL. Managing medication risks through a culture of safety. In: Cohen MR, ed. *Medication Errors.* 2nd ed. Washington, DC: American Pharmaceutical Association; 2007.

4. Cohen MR, Senders J, Davis NM. Failure mode and effects analysis: a novel approach to avoiding dangerous medication errors and accidents. *Hosp Pharm.* 1994;29(4):319-330.

5. Senders JW, Senders SJ. Health care failure modes and analysis (Part I: Introduction to failure modes and effects analysis). In: Cohen MR, ed. *Medication Errors.* 2nd ed. Washington, DC: American Pharmaceutical Association; 2007.

6. Weir VL. Best-practice protocols: preventing adverse drug events. *Nurs Manage.* 2005;36(9):24-30.

7. Sheridan-Leos N, Schulmeister L, Hartranft S. Failure mode and effect analysis: a technique to prevent chemotherapy errors. *Clin J Oncol Nurs.* 2006;10(3):393-398.

8. Duwe B, Fuchs BD, Hansen-Flaschen J. Failure mode and effects analysis application to critical care medicine. *Crit Care Clin.* 2005;21(1):21-30.

9. Bates DW, Cullen DJ, Laird N, et al. Incidence of adverse drug events and potential adverse drug events. Implications for prevention. ADE Prevention Study Group. *JAMA.* 1995; 274(1):29-34.

10. Wu WK, Pantaleo N. Evaluation of outpatient adverse drug reactions leading to hospitalization. *Am J Health Syst Pharm.* 2003;60(3):253-259.

11. Chiozza ML, Ponzetti C. FMEA: a model for reducing medical errors. *Clin Chim Acta.* 2009;404(1):75-78. ∎

Understanding the Food and Drug Administration Risk Evaluation and Mitigation Strategies (REMS)

Matthew W. Eberts, PharmD, MBA*; Susan J. Skledar, MPH, FASHP†; and Scott M. Mark, PharmD, MS, MEd, FASHP, FACHE‡

The *Director's Forum* series is written and edited by Robert Weber and Scott Mark and is designed to guide pharmacy leaders in establishing patient-centered services in hospitals and health systems. As the Food and Drug Administration (FDA) approval process becomes more stringent with regard to postmarketing surveillance for medications, directors of pharmacy will need to understand expectations of inpatient pharmacy services to ensure patient safety and meet requirements. This article provides background information regarding the FDA Risk Evaluation and Mitigation Strategies (REMS) programs and potential implications for hospital pharmacy.

Today's pharmacy leaders are challenged with managing the financial, human resources, safety, technology, and regulatory responsibilities of their departments. Medication safety must take precedence, and following regulatory requirements and standards is a critical piece of this responsibility. In 2007, the US Food and Drug Administration Amendments Act (FDAAA) was signed into law, enabling postmarketing surveillance of safety risks of medications, whether they be newly marketed or already marketed.[1] The Risk Evaluation and Mitigation Strategy (REMS) programs for medications, which are a part of this Act, aim to ensure that patients and health care providers fully understand the risks associated with certain therapies before initiating treatment. The US Food and Drug Administration (FDA) has the authority to issue and enforce REMS by virtue of the FDAAA.[2] The challenges for pharmacy directors include understanding the requirements of the REMS programs, knowing which medications are part of newly designated REMS, finding the necessary resources to properly meet the REMS requirements, and building the process of implementing REMS requirements.

The goal of this article is to educate pharmacy directors regarding FDA-issued REMS and the necessary steps to maintain department compliance. Specifically, the article provides background information regarding the FDA and the REMS program, details regarding specific REMS implemented by the FDA including those most significant to hospital pharmacy, strategies for maintaining compliance with the REMS requirements, and information about the future of this program and how it will affect hospital pharmacy.

*Manager, Pharmacy Operations, University of Pittsburgh Medical Center, and Adjunct Instructor, Department of Pharmacy & Therapeutics, University of Pittsburgh School of Pharmacy, Pittsburgh, Pennsylvania; e-mail: ebertsmw@upmc.edu; †Director, Drug Use and Disease State Management Program, University of Pittsburgh Medical Center, and Associate Professor and Vice Chair, Department of Pharmacy & Therapeutics, University of Pittsburgh School of Pharmacy, Pittsburgh, Pennsylvania; ‡Director of Pharmacy, University of Pittsburgh Medical Center, and Associate Professor and Vice Chair, University of Pittsburgh School of Pharmacy, Pittsburgh, Pennsylvania.

OVERVIEW OF THE FDA AND REMS

The FDA is a regulatory agency of the US government. It is the oldest consumer protection agency in the country, started in 1848 to conduct analysis of agricultural products. The FDA began overseeing foods and medications after the passage of the 1906 Pure Food and Drugs Act.[3,4] Today the scope of FDA regulation includes roughly 25% of the gross national product of the United States.[5] Responsibilities of the FDA include protecting the public health by ensuring the safety, effectiveness, and security of human drugs, vaccines, and other biological products as well as disseminating accurate, science-based information to the public.[4]

The Federal Food, Drug and Cosmetic Act (FD&C Act) is the primary legal standard for medications used in the United States. Based upon the framework of the FD&C Act, the FDA develops regulations, which are considered law, that enforce and support the measures of the Act.[6] The authority by which the FDA creates the rules and regulations on behalf of the US government to enforce the FD&C Act is granted by the Administrative Procedure Act.[7]

In September 2007, the FDAAA was signed into law by President George W. Bush.[8] The FDAAA, an amendment to the FD&C Act, enhanced postmarket authorities of the FDA with respect to the safety of medications.[9] Specifically included in the Act was the authority of the FDA to implement REMS programs as a method to ensure that the benefits of a drug or biological outweigh its risks.[8,9] The REMS can be issued upon the release of a new medication or implemented for medications that are on the market.

REMS ELEMENTS

There are five standardized REMS elements. Table 1 lists those elements with definitions. A particular REMS program may use some or up to all five of the elements as determined necessary by the FDA.[4] Therefore, a particular REMS program may only require providing a medication guide or the REMS may include more complex components such as a patient registry, certification program for prescribers, and specialized training for prescribers.[9] One can think of a REMS program as a step between issuing a FDA safety warning letter for practitioner and, the most severe consequence, re-

Table 1. Risk Evaluation and Mitigation Strategy (REMS) program elements[9,10]

Element	Description
Medication Guide	Specific information that is to be provided to the patient that explains the risk associated with a particular treatment
Communication Plan	A plan the manufacturer will utilize to notify the health care community about changes the REMS put in place for the medication
Elements to Assure Safe Use	Specific steps put in place to ensure the safe use of a medication (eg, patient registries or health care provider education)
Implementation System	System to monitor and evaluate implementation for and work to improve implementation of Elements to Assure Safe Use
Assessment of REMS	Sets time table for assessment of the REMS. Normally three assessments are performed. 1st assessment: 18 months from approval 2nd assessment: 3 years from approval 3rd assessment: 7 years from approval

moval of a medication from the market.

Since becoming law in September 2007, 117 medication-specific REMS have been issued by the FDA. The most common REMS requirement is to issue a medication guide with each prescription of the designated medication. The medication guides are frequently included as part of the packaging from the manufacturer and are easily available on-line at the FDA's Web site.[10] Of the 117 REMS currently in place, 82 require only that a medication guide be included with the prescription, recommended at the time of first dispensing of the medication to the patient. Of the other 35, 23 require a communication plan from the manufacturer to health care professionals in addition to the medication guide. The remaining 12 require additional elements to ensure safe use (see **Table 1**).

From the perspective of the hospital pharmacy director, the most significant REMS program actions to be implemented are the recently issued directives for the erythropoiesis-stimulating agents (ESA), erythropoietin and darbepoetin, labeled as the ESA APPRISE (Assisting Providers and cancer Patients with Risk Information for the Safe use of ESA) Oncology Program.[11] The goal of this REMS is to support informed decisions between patients and health care providers considering treatment with ESAs for oncology-related conditions with regard to risks and benefits associated with the ESA treatment.[11] The specific requirements of ESA APPRISE are documented in **Table 2**. To date, the ESA REMS program is the most wide-reaching REMS program, as ESAs are very commonly prescribed. The pharmacy director or his/her designee will

need to determine a process that ensures all patients receive the medication guide, establishes a procedure to register the hospital and health care providers as appropriate, and develops a mechanism to obtain patient signed acknowledgment forms regarding ESA therapy.

The process of dispensing the medication guide can be carried out by the staff administering the medication or by pharmacists with the capacity to interact directly with the patient. The guide can be obtained from the online sources noted previously (FDA or manufacturer Web site) and be made available immediately from an electronic health record upon dispensing. Some sites are considering having the patients overview the material as part of their consent to the treatment process. In the community pharmacy, the medication guides are dispensed with the medication to the patients when they pick up their prescription. Documenting that the patients received the material is recommended, perhaps in the education section of the medical record or in the computer system. Sample data collection forms are available from the FDA and manufacturer to assist with this. A sample tracking form is provided in **Figure 1**. Efforts to meet the registration requirements should be interdisciplinary. Physician leadership should be involved in the process design to assist with holding the medical staff accountable for obtaining the proper registration for prescribing in cases where that is required, for example, oncology uses of ESA. The pharmacy should refuse orders from physicians who have not met the registration requirement where that step is mandated by the FDA REMS program. A process by which the patient signs the

Table 2. Requirements of the ESA APPRISE program[11]

Element	Requirement
Medication Guide	Outpatient hospital clinic or retail: include medication guide with each dispensing pack Hospital inpatient/physician office/clinic: dispense a medication guide each time the medication is dispensed to the patient
Communication Plan	Manufacturer will send communications regarding the REMS to the following: • Nephrology Professional Societies • Dear HealthCare Provider letter to medical staff that may prescribe the drug in patients with cancer • Dear Pharmacist/Administrator letter to hospitals • Oncology Professional Societies
Elements to Assure Safe Use	Health care providers who prescribe and dispense for patients with cancer in private health care settings will be specially certified. Health care providers who prescribe for patients with cancer in hospitals will be specially certified.[a] Hospitals that dispense ESA to patients with cancer will be specially certified.[a] ESA will only be dispensed by hospitals and providers once the patient with cancer has participated in a risk:benefit discussion about the treatment and have signed an acknowledgment statement.
Implementation System	Manufacturer will monitor compliance and intervene as necessary to improve compliance.
Assessment of REMS	8 months, 1 year, 18 months and every year thereafter

Note: ESA = erythropoiesis-stimulating agents; ESA APPRISE = Assisting Providers and cancer Patients with Risk Information for the Safe use of ESA; REMS = Risk Evaluation and Management Strategy.

[a]Certification specifics are found in the REMS located at reference 12.

acknowledgment form also needs to be implemented. Obtaining this information clearly is recommended, so the data can be compiled or demonstrated if an audit from the manufacturer occurs.

REMS AND HOSPITAL PHARMACY

The extent to which REMS are going to affect hospital pharmacy is still being determined. Some REMS specifically address hospital pharmacy actions and some do not. With REMS strategies becoming more prevalent, however, the hospital pharmacy director and pharmacy team must be proactive and determine their role to ensure patient safety, appropriate record-keeping, and patient monitoring. The pharmacy director needs to im-

Romiplostim (Nplate™ NEXUS Program Patient Tracking Log for Inpatients)

Institution = _____
Institution NEXUS ID = _____

Date admin	Patient name	DOB	Patient ID	Patient NEXUS ID	Health care provider name	Health care provider NEXUS ID	Dose	No. of vials used

Figure 1. Sample REMS Tracking Form.[13] DOB = date of birth

plement at least the minimum expectations for the appropriate REMS (eg, distribution of medication education guide, or registration of prescribers); to facilitate the process, he or she can leverage the FDA mandate to complete this task. Many individuals and organizations are trying to determine the role of the pharmacy department in the REMS programs, so it is important to conduct discussions on actions that are reasonable until the final recommendations are issued. At a minimum, distributing patient medication education guides at a patient's first exposure to the REMS medication is an important step to meet the spirit of the FDA REMS safety programs.

Many hospital pharmacy departments have elected to distribute the medication guides when specifically directed to do so, but further clarification is warranted and welcome. One of the top REMS priorities for the pharmacy director should be hardwiring in a process to distribute medication guides to patients. The number of REMS requiring this element are going to increase. If the organization has a plan that standardizes the distribution, it will be seamless to incorporate new REMS into practice as they are approved.

The enforcement of REMS is another critical aspect to understand. The FDAAA grants the FDA authority to fine manufacturers if they are out of compliance with REMS requirements; however it does not grant the same authority to the FDA regarding pharmacy compliance.[14] The manufacturers, however, may perform site audits to check documentation and monitoring compliance or ask that records be maintained, so the REMS programs must be handled seriously. If pharmacies are noncompliant with a REMS, they run the risk of misbranding violations and the associated punishments.[14] Because most hospitals do not participate in interstate commerce, there is debate as to whether the jurisdiction falls to the FDA or the hospital's state board of pharmacy. In light of this uncertainty, it is important that pharmacy directors stay current regarding how REMS are going to be enforced at the hospital level and by whom (manufacturers, FDA, or state boards of pharmacy).

REMS MOVING FORWARD

The utilization of REMS by the FDA is gaining momentum and attention. In the first 3 months of 2010, 14 REMS were approved by the FDA.[10]

Table 3. US Food and Drug Administration (FDA) Risk Evaluation and Management Strategy resources

Source	Web site address
ASHP Advantage	http://www.ashpadvantage.com/fdaaa/
ASHP Risk Evaluation and Mitigation Strategies Resource Center	http://www.ashp.org/Import/MEMBERCENTER/Sections/SectionofPharmacy PracticeManagers/Resources/REMSRDDS.aspx
FDA	http://www.fda.gov/Drugs/DrugSafety/PostmarketDrugSafetyInformationfor PatientsandProviders/ucm111350.htm

Note: ASHP = American Society of Health-System Pharmacists.

It is clear that more REMS are going to be approved, including many that impact hospital pharmacy practice. Pharmacy directors are going to need to stay current with new developments in order to maintain compliance. The resources listed in **Table 3** are useful for this purpose. It is recommended that pharmacy directors regularly utilize these resources so they can serve as knowledge leaders regarding REMS in their institution.

One of the upcoming REMS directives with the greatest potential to have a wide impact concerns opioids. The FDA is currently reviewing public and stakeholder input regarding the development of a REMS program for certain opioid products.[15] The FDA has also announced that the comment period has been reopened through October 19, 2010. Submit written comments regarding the opioid REMS to: The Division of Dockets Management (HFA–305), Food and Drug Administration, 5630 Fishers Lane, Room 1061, Rockville, MD 20852. Electronic comments can be sent to: http://www.regulations.gov. The FDA has indicated that the REMS may include long-acting and extended-release opioids containing fentanyl, hydromorphone, methadone, morphine, oxycodone, and oxymorphone. It is too early to predict what the REMS will be or when it will be implemented, but it is intuitive that the potential scope of these opioid-based REMS will be unprecedented compared with the current strategies in place.

Professional organizations such as the American Society of Health-System Pharmacists (ASHP) have been proactive in serving as knowledge experts on this issue and advocating for hospital pharmacists regarding the FDA's management of REMS. Keeping in touch with those professional organizations is a key method of staying informed. ASHP has a dedicated risk evaluation and mitigation strategies resource center available on-line. The specific address is included in **Table 3**.

CONCLUSION

It is clear that the utilization of REMS by the FDA is becoming an important tool for their ability to improve the safety of "high-risk" medications and those with new and emerging safety data. As the REMS program builds momentum, the impact on hospital pharmacy will continue to grow. The issuance of the ESA APPRISE REMS serves as an example of how REMS becomes the responsibility of the hospital pharmacy leader. It is important that the pharmacy director has up-to-date knowledge on the current state of REMS and utilizes resources available, including the FDA and ASHP, to stay current with this issue. The pharmacy director is expected to be the organization's medication management expert leading interdisciplinary team discussions of this subject, which is an FDA-driven initiative to improve the safety of medications.

AFTERWARDS

As a testament to how REMS are continuing to increase their impact on hospital pharmacy, since this manuscript was sent to the editor a new REMS regarding propylthiouracil was issued by the FDA.[16] Every patient who receives the medication must receive a medication guide. Pharmacy leaders need to develop procedures for executing the elements of REMS and make REMS compliance part of the medication dispensing and patient education process.

ACKNOWLEDGMENT

Jeffrey Little, PharmD, MPH, and Susan Guttendorf, PharmD, are acknowledged for their contribution to the background information of this article.

REFERENCES

1. US Food and Drug Administration. Regulatory information: legislation: Federal Food, Drug, and Cosmetic Act (FD&C Act): Food and Drug Administration Amendments Act (FDAAA) of 2007. http://www.fda.gov/RegulatoryInformation/Legislation/FederalFoodDrugandCosmeticActFDCAct/SignificantAmendmentstotheFDCAct/FoodandDrugAdministrationAmendmentsActof2007/default.htm. Accessed April 22, 2010.

2. US Food and Drug Administration. FDA Issues draft guidance on risk evaluation and mitigation strategies. September 30, 2009. http://www.fda.gov/NewsEvents/Newsroom/PressAnnouncements/ucm184399.htm. Accessed April 22, 2010.

3. US Food and Drug Administration. What we do: history. http://www.fda.gov/AboutFDA/WhatWeDo/History/default.htm. Accessed April 13, 2010.

4. US Food and Drug Administration. About FDA: FDA basics. http://www.fda.gov/AboutFDA/Basics/ucm194877.htm. Accessed April 13, 2010.

5. US Food and Drug Administration. News & events: newsroom: press announcements. http://www.fda.gov/NewsEvents/Newsroom/PressAnnouncements/ucm204236.htm. Accessed April 14, 2010.

6. US Food and Drug Administration: About FDA: FDA basics. http://www.fda.gov/AboutFDA/Basics/ucm194909.htm. Accessed April 13, 2010.

7. The Federal Register. Administrative Procedure Act: United States Code, Title 5, Part 1, Chapter 5 Subchapter II. http://www.archives.gov/federal-register/laws/administrative-procedure/552a.html. Accessed April 14, 2010.

8. Govtrack. Congress: legislation: HR 3580: Food and Drug Administration Amendments Act of 2007. http://www.govtrack.us/congress/bill.xpd?bill=h110-3580. Accessed April 13, 2010.

9. Traynor, K. Risk-Management plan for opioid drugs proves slow going. *Am J Health Syst Pharm.* 2009;66(14):1242-1243.

10. US Food and Drug Administration. Drugs: drug safety and availability: postmarket drug safety information for patients and providers. http://www.fda.gov/Drugs/DrugSafety/PostmarketDrugSafetyInformationforPatientsandProviders/ucm111350.htm. Accessed April 13, 2010.

11. Amgen. Aranesp REMS. http://wwwext.amgen.com/pdfs/products/ESA_REMS_Aranesp.pdf. Accessed April 15, 2010.

12. BL103951 *Aranesp* (darbepoetin alfa). http://www.fda.gov/downloads/Drugs/DrugSafety/PostmarketDrugSafetyInformationforPatientsandProviders/UCM200104.pdf. Accessed April 18, 2010.

13. About Nplatee NEXUS. http://www.nplatenexus.com/about.html. Accessed April 19, 2010.

14. ASHP Advantage. E-Newsletter. FDAAA. Winter 2010. http://www.ashpadvantage.com/fdaaa/fdaaa-winter-newsletter.pdf. Accessed April 19, 2010.

15. US Food and Drug Administration. Drugs: drug safety and availability: information by drug class. http://www.fda.gov/Drugs/DrugSafety/InformationbyDrugClass/ucm163647.htm. Accessed April 15, 2010.

16. US Food and Drug Administration. Drugs: drug safety and availability: postmarket drug safety information for patients and providers: FDA Drug Safety Communication: new boxed warning on sever liver injury with propylthiouracil. http://www.fda.gov/Drugs/DrugSafety/PostmarketDrugSafetyInformationforPatientsandProviders/ucm209023.htm. Accessed April 22, 2010. ∎

Patient Services and Related Issues

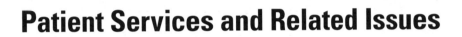

Establishing a Patient-Centered Philosophy of Pharmacy Practice

Robert J. Weber, MS, FASHP* and Michael Sanborn, MS, FASHP†

This article begins the *Director's Forum*, a series of articles designed to guide pharmacy leaders in establishing patient-centered services in hospitals. As stated in Dr. Cada's *Editorial* which introduces this series, we hope to answer key questions that pharmacy directors face and provide others with information to foster growth in pharmacy leadership. The articles in this column will build on one another and, when put together, will serve as a "tool kit" to develop patient-centered pharmacy services in hospitals of all sizes. Examples of topics in future *Director's Forums* will include establishing clinical service priorities, justifying clinical pharmacist positions, implementing a patient safety program, and budgeting for patient-centered services.

The first article of the *Director's Forum* describes a foundational element of pharmacy services in hospitals and establishes an approach to pharmacy practice that centers on improving the quality of patients' lives. This is accomplished by establishing a practice environment that operates the Pharmacy as a patient care department instead of a revenue center. We will briefly describe the importance of establishing a patient-centered service, and the steps that pharmacy directors can take to focus their departments on their most important assets—patients. By focusing on patients, we are not overlooking pharmacy's key internal customers—physicians, nurses, and other health care professionals. Nor are we ignoring our fiscal responsibility of operating our departments; in fact, we posit that a patient-centered pharmacy service almost always re-sults in a fiscally sound pharmacy department.

THE IMPORTANCE OF A PATIENT-CENTERED PHARMACY SERVICE

The role of pharmacists in improving the safety and efficiency of the medication-use system is well-documented; however, pharmacy departments that actually employ comprehensive patient-centered services are not widespread. An American Society of Health-System Pharmacists recent survey showed that over 75% of hospitals provided consultations on dosage adjustments, drug information, pharmacokinetics, and selection of antibiotics;[1] however another survey showed that the majority of hospitals monitored fewer than 50% of their patients.[2] In addition, approximately half of the hospital pharmacies provide nutrition support consultations and 40% or less provide fundamental services of patient teaching, anticoagulation dosing, and pain management.

From a systems perspective, only 58% of hospitals use automated dispensing devices, and less then 2% of hospitals employ bar code medication administration.[3] This statistic indicates that there is also an opportunity for developing a strategy for justifying expanded pharmacy technology in hospitals.

*Associate Professor and Department Chair, University of Pittsburgh School of Pharmacy, Executive Director of Pharmacy, University of Pittsburgh Medical Center, Pittsburgh, PA; †Health System Pharmacy Director, Baylor Healthcare System, Dallas, TX

Subscribers to the United States Pharmacopeia's (USP) MEDMARX program reported over 235,000 medication errors during calendar year 2003; recently the USP published its experiences of medication error reporting and analysis over a 5-year period. At least 2% of those reported errors resulted in significant patient harm.[4] There is also skepticism being raised by experts claiming few significant improvements in health care safety.

Pharmaceutical costs are an important area for hospital financial administrators. The national costs of pharmaceuticals, for example, have risen by 6% to 15% yearly, since 1997, with over 70% of those costs associated with new drug approvals.[5] Pharmaceuticals represent 4% to 7% of the yearly operating expense of most hospitals.[6] An additional consideration is that current medication systems cannot prevent all medication errors and adverse drug events (ADEs), which add to overall hospital and pharmaceutical costs.[7] This evidence and our own hospital experiences demonstrate the necessity for pharmacists to be directly connected to patients.

STEPS IN ESTABLISHING A PATIENT-CENTERED PHARMACY DEPARTMENT
Develop a Vision of Patient-Centered Services

Establishing patient-centered and innovative pharmacy services requires a clear vision of what patient-centered care means. It is important to understand that the vision does not provide a destination, but rather a direction in which the practice of pharmacy is guided. A practical approach is to talk with your staff about the daily impact of their job on patients. For example,

providing a double-check of a chemotherapy protocol directly protects patients from harm; performing nursing unit checks and removing dangerous floor stock medications can prevent a serious medication error. Additionally, teaching a patient about diabetes medications with an emphasis on recognizing the signs and symptoms of hypoglycemia can prevent an unnecessary hospitalization or emergency department visit.

Establish a Mission Statement for the Pharmacy

The importance of a clear and simple mission statement focuses the department's efforts on patient-centered activities. Examples of mission statements include: "The Memorial Hospital Department of Pharmacy is a patient-centered service that employs state of the art technology and expertise to promote the safe and effective use of medication;" "The Baptist Hospital Pharmacy Services strives to improve the quality of patient lives through interdisciplinary care around the medication-use process."

Appoint the Pharmacy Director as a Member of the Medical Executive Committee

The role of pharmacy director is critical in developing patient-centered pharmacy services, since they are responsible for representing Pharmacy across the organization. Important to patient-centered services are cooperation and collaboration with our medical staff colleagues and to actively participate in decision making at the medical staff level of the hospital. The active participation of the pharmacy director in the medical executive committee establishes a collaboration that extends itself to all aspects of the pharmacy service. For example, the pharmacy director may update the medical staff on pharmacy services on a regular basis, and point out the important role that the physicians play in medication use. From this relationship, physician "champions" for pharmacy can be recruited to provide additional support for important pharmacy programs and medication-use initiatives.

Establish a Plan

A plan and directions for a patient-centered pharmacy practice is essential to provide a focus to the department, which reduces staff and customer frustrations that result from an unclear strategy. Pharmacy is a clinical profession, and the overall practice philosophy must address the department's role within the organization. Some key questions to ask during the development of this philosophy are as follows:

- What should our practice model look like?
- What pharmacy services are considered to be essential and most valuable to the patients and to the organization?
- Are we serving the right patients?
- Where does technology fit in?

The plan for patient-centered pharmacy services should recognize and demonstrate that our primary responsibility is to our patients. The pharmacy should maintain focus on the patient and ensure the delivery of quality patient care. It should also promote collaboration with other health care professionals and pharmacy customers.

Consideration must be given to the department's ability to monitor medication use and outcomes to assure appropriate medication usage and measure the impact of the provision of patient care. It is also important to implement quality and process improvement tools to measure pharmacy service delivery and use of resources.

Technology must be planned and optimized to support and enhance the continual development of a progressive pharmacy practice model. Systems should be integrated to allow pharmacy personnel to promote seamless care.

The philosophy should also address the department's commitment to education and research. It is imperative to provide medication-use education to patients, caregivers, and other health care providers. The importance of staff retention and professional development should also be well-planned. Is there an expectation for the department to contribute to the body of medical and pharmacy literature through research, publications, and presentations? Should the staff be encouraged to participate in professional organizations to promote the practice of pharmacy? The balance between resources and staff development must be well-considered and integrated into the core philosophy.

Communicate the Plan and the Vision

An important part of establishing a patient-centered pharmacy service is to communicate the philosophy throughout the organization. For example, the pharmacy director, serving as the secretary of the Pharmacy & Therapeutics Committee and on the hospital's medical executive committee, can communicate this plan and its progress on a regular basis to the medical staff. The pharmacy director can use this opportunity to describe the pharmacy's services and how they improve the quality of patient care. Giving the medical staff confidence that your department is focused on patients' wellbeing is important in maintaining and developing patient-centered programs. Effective communication with department staff is critical to the success of the plan as well.

SUMMARY

Hospital pharmacists are uniquely suited to improve medication use in our patients. Establishing a patient-centered department is critical to a hospital pharmacy's mission, as traditional functions of a pharmacist in hospitals are being replaced by pharmacy automation or orders management technology (eg, computerized prescriber order entry). Developing and communicating a department vision, mission, and plan for delivery of care are critical steps to effectively delivering high quality, patient-centered care.

REFERENCES

1. Pedersen CA, Schneider PJ, Scheckelhoff DJ. ASHP national survey of pharmacy practice in hospital settings: prescribing and transcribing—2004. *Am J Health-Syst Pharm.* 2005;62:378–390.

2. Pedersen CA, Schneider PJ, Scheckelhoff DJ. *Am J Health Syst Pharm.* 2004;61:457-471.

3. Pedersen CA, Schneider PJ, Scheckelhoff DJ. ASHP national survey of pharmacy practice in hospital settings: dispensing and administration—2002. *Am J Health-Syst Pharm.* 2003;60:52-68.

4. Hicks RW, Santell JP, Cousins DD, Williams RL. *MEDMARX™ 5th Anniversary Data Report: A Chartbook of 2003 Findings and Trends, 1999-2003.* Rockville, MD: USP Center for the Advancement of Patient Safety; 2004.

5. Shah ND, Vermeulen LC, Santell JP, et al. Projecting future drug expenditures—2002. *Am J Health Syst Pharm.* 2002;59:131-142.

6. Pierpaoli PG. The rising cost of pharmaceuticals: a director of pharmacy's perspective. *Am J Hosp Pharm.* 1993;50:S6-S8.

7. Bates DW, Spell N, Cullen DJ, et al. The costs of adverse drug events in hospitalized patients. *JAMA.* 1997;277: 307-311. ∎

Promoting Patient-Centered Pharmacy Services Through Effective Facility Planning and Design

Scott M. Mark, PharmD, MS, MEd, FASHP, FACHE, FABC*;
Thomas Kirschling, PharmD, MS†; and Robert J. Weber, MS, FASHP‡

The *Director's Forum* series is written and edited by Michael Sanborn and Robert Weber and is designed for guiding pharmacy leaders in establishing patient-centered services in hospitals and health systems. Another specific goal of this column is addressing many of the key challenges that pharmacy directors currently face while providing information that will foster growth in pharmacy leadership and patient safety. A well-designed facility is an important component to providing patient-centered care. This *Director's Forum* article focuses on specific elements that should be considered when planning a new pharmacy facility.

INTRODUCTION

Hospital pharmacy departments require adequate space to dispense medications in a safe and effective manner. In fact, during their survey processes, many state health department regulators and The Joint Commission (TJC) evaluate the appropriateness of square footage devoted to pharmacy operations. Considerable fines may be imposed by state regulatory agencies and significant recommendations received from TJC if there is not adequate space in the pharmacy for meeting patient needs. As a result, facility planning and design should be a priority for all pharmacy directors. Furthermore, given the rapid changes that occur in the health care field, participation in facility planning and design will likely be required of pharmacy directors several times through-

out their careers. More importantly, the use of a "standard" facility plan for each hospital is not possible because of variations in physical layouts, differences in state regulations, and changing national standards. For example, in the Commonwealth of Pennsylvania, very specific information on required square footage is included in the Pharmacy Act, which specifies the following: minimum size of the prescription area must be at least 250 square feet; within the prescription area, there must be a prescription working counter of at least 10 linear feet in length and 2 linear feet in width. Moreover, if more than 2 pharmacists are on duty simultaneously, the minimum counter length should be increased by 5 linear feet for an additional pharmacist. Finally, proper facility design is important to patient safety, staff satisfaction, and positive quality outcomes.[1-3]

This article illustrates the steps in effective facility planning and design that promote patient-centered pharmacy services. Its aim is to describe the stages of facility planning, including (1) matching facility design to departmental services, (2) developing the architectural and business plan for the

*Director of Pharmacy, University of Pittsburgh Medical Center; Assistant Professor and Vice Chair, University of Pittsburgh School of Pharmacy; †Manager, Pharmacy, UPMC Presbyterian; ‡Executive Director of Pharmacy, University of Pittsburgh Medical Center; Associate Professor of Pharmacy, University of Pittsburgh School of Pharmacy, Pittsburgh, Pennsylvania.

facility design, and (3) implementing the facility plan. Finally, this article presents examples of facility plans at the University of Pittsburgh Medical Center (UPMC) as a guide for pharmacy directors in developing their facility plans. Hopefully, this text will provide pharmacy directors with a transferable framework for planning, designing, and developing a patient-centered pharmacy facility.

MATCHING FACILITY DESIGN TO DEPARTMENTAL SERVICES

Over time, pharmacy facilities become obsolete as a result of new and updated government regulations (eg, United States Pharmacopeia [USP] <797>), adoption of new technology, practice model changes, variations in workload, and/or aging structures and equipment. Thus, these facilities require modification and renovation. Improving pharmacy productivity through the implementation of new medication dispensing technology (such as robotics) or changing practice models (such as the recentralization of pharmacy services) allows some latitude in choosing the opportune time for, and scope of, renovation. Even the most well-designed space can become inefficient over time; as new technology is added, workflow can be adjusted to make room for larger equipment and additional workspace for staff may be added to address new services or to make room for a growing formulary. The unpredictable nature of regulations, technology, and pharmacy practice changes creates a tremendous need and opportunity for the pharmacy to redesign the current space and, importantly, negotiate for additional space.

The role of pharmacy in hospitals is ever changing, as evidenced by previous articles in the *Director's Forum* that focused on suggestions to pharmacy directors for implementing advanced pharmacy services and conducting strategic planning for critical functions (such as medication safety).[4–6] Strategic planning for departmental services employs feedback from department and organization stakeholders for developing services that meet the goals of the institution. When designing a new pharmacy space, a clear and specific departmental strategic plan is necessary for ensuring that facilities match departmental services.

For instance, a hospital's information technology strategy may detail plans for implementation of bar-code technology (such as for patient identification and medication administration). To successfully execute this organizational goal, the pharmacy needs to build space for extemporaneously packaging medications and assigning bar-codes to those products using manufacturer guidelines. Failure to plan for future services may necessitate the redesign of an already renovated facility to allow for bar-code packaging and processing; this renovation may generate unnecessary costs and further interrupt pharmacy workflow and patient care activities.

In the absence of a strategic plan, a pharmacy director should ask the following questions of the organization when designing a new facility:

1. Is the organization focused on innovation, service, or efficiency, and is this likely to change?
2. Is the space allocated, or is there potential for negotiation? Are there any options for a more centrally located space with access to multiple delivery paths or for sites that do not have as many ar-

chitectural limitations (eg, ceiling height)?

3. Who will carry what cost? Are there any funds allocated for regulatory mandates?

4. Are there services that are provided, or likely will be provided, to new customers that include other facilities? What are these services, and how might this affect automation planning or space allocation?

5. What hospital-specific policies (eg, a "green" hospital) might affect a pharmacy design?

6. Will other services in the hospital be moving? For example, are there plans to move any of the intensive care units (ICUs), which would make them geographically removed from the pharmacy?

7. Are there any plans for implementation of hospital technology that must be considered in the pharmacy plans? This may include the addition of a tube system, wireless networks or phones, or changes in security systems.

8. Are there any hospital strategic plans that may require additional services from the pharmacy? An example might be the opening of a sister hospital whose back-office infrastructure will be provided by the home hospital. This may require space for additional pharmacy billing, information technology personnel, and other staff who will support the new venture.

Answering these questions in lieu of a clear strategic plan will facilitate decision making that supports a sustainable pharmacy facility design.

DEVELOPING THE ARCHITECTURAL AND BUSINESS PLAN

Designing a facility begins with an understanding of the scope of services that are, or will be, provided. For instance, a facility that serves inpatients and outpatients requires different designs than one that only services inpatients. However, designs should give consideration to both whenever possible, such as a pick-up window that could also serve as an after-hours outpatient prescription service. Specific structural considerations are needed for open-architecture, sterile-product preparation; chemotherapy preparation; or high-risk-product preparation areas, such as ante areas, and for ample overhead space for heating ventilation and air conditioning (HVAC) requirements. Ventures that necessitate eyewash water and pneumatic tube stations require passageways for conduits. Subflooring consideration is needed when determining the location and feasibility of drain installation at eyewash stations, as well as installation of sinks, heavy equipment, and in-floor power or network outlets. Table 1 lists the scope of services that may be considered when designing a pharmacy facility. In addition, understanding the overall goal of the department is vital. The design for departments whose focus is maximization of operational efficiency will be different from those whose primary focus is clinical service or patient safety. As stated previously, it is essential that the department facility plan aligns with the overall hospital direction and, more specifically, the intended direction for the department of pharmacy.

The Architectural Plan

Once the scope of service has been identified, but before working with an architect, it is necessary to map the intended workflow to the allocated space. Workflow should be designed

Table 1. Scope of Services That May Be Considered When Designing a Pharmacy Facility

Advanced technician roles

Anticoagulation services

Automation (including oral and intravenous robotics)

Call centers

Chemotherapy preparation

Compounding

Consultation/drug and poison information services

Distribution model (including satellites and dispensing cabinets)

Drug-use and disease-state management programs

Educational programs, student precepting, inservices

Finance and inventory services

Indigent care medication programs

Information technology and informatics programs (with analysts)

Integration of distribution and clinical services

Investigational drug services

Machine-readable coding of medications

Management of automated dispensing cabinets

Management of investigational medications

Management of medication returns

Management of medication samples

Measurement of quality performance measures

Medication safety, surveillance, and adverse drug reactions

Order entry/review for ancillary areas (operating room, emergency department, etc)

Pharmacy technician training and certification

Practice model (including the inclusion of a unit-based pharmacy program)

Residency training program

Secretarial services

Student training program

Unit-dose distribution

for minimization of the number of steps in the flow and allowance of proper communication. In a central pharmacy operation, the workflow often follows the medication order and associated product. Therefore, the pharmacy should be designed for the efficient flow of orders in 1 direction, and the flow should follow a linear or curved path depending on the space layout. This means that as orders are processed, they should pass from one area to an immediately adjacent area; rework must be kept to a minimum. For instance, the most frequently used items (ie, drugs, solutions, paperwork) should be conveniently accessible from each work area. If given the option in new construction, a linear workflow is preferred for best facilitating the most efficient operations. A curved, near-circular workflow is often preferred for best facilitating face-to-face communication. In either choice of workflow design, an open architectural plan consisting of minimal barriers (ie, walls, corridors) that aids communication should be balanced with a plan that encourages sense of ownership in an employee's defined workspace.

The functionality required can affect structural requirements and design as well. For example, doors used to receive inventory may need to be larger, allowing for delivery of supplies on pallets. Consideration must also be given to the ergonomics of the area. Ergonomics require that the design of a space minimizes bending, lifting, stretching, or working in awkward positions for long periods of time. Lines of sight, or an individual's views of specific work areas, must be designed to ensure appropriate pharmacist oversight. This includes the abilities to observe work in the

IV room and to screen visitors at the pharmacy entrances. This is particularly important on evening and night shifts when fewer employees are at work.

Another key consideration in facility design involves the intended use of pharmacy automation. For instance, medication carousels are commonly employed for inventory control. It is important to know whether they will be used for filling first doses, automated dispensing cabinets, and crash carts. These functions can create bottlenecks in workflow if a workload analysis that determines the number of needed carousels is not properly done. At times, workflow is dictated by the placement of automation, and it will certainly change with the use of automation. Although understanding automation specifics is important for practical reasons—such as confirming the product size fits existing space, confirming power needs are met, and verifying weight capacity on floors does not exceed structural capacity—knowing the intended use of automation will also affect workflow.

Proactively planning for changes rather than retrofitting space in subsequent years is certainly easier and less expensive. For example, if the intention is installation of technology in subsequent years, it is wise to run additional network lines, increase capacity for power supply and emergency power, and reserve space. If future plans are unknown, construction using a modular concept is also prudent. In this manner, succeeding changes will only affect a minimal area. Examples may include mounting mobile, rather than permanent, shelving or installing temporary walls.

Extensive input should be sought from employees to ensure that any concerns are raised and that oversights are minimized. Development of a working drawing of the proposed project, which includes workflow, for internal use before meeting with the architects can be beneficial. This will increase efficacy of time spent with the architects.

Architects who use these working plans as a starting point for blueprints can draft scale drawings for discussion. They can ask specific questions related to design ideas, and the pharmacy team can raise questions that may have come up in the staff planning meetings. Furthermore, the architects can point out any design layouts that may not be possible because of structural constraints.

Often architects have experience in pharmacy design, but they will likely make errors of assumption. Because an architect's knowledge of the specific pharmacy may be unknown, inclusion of rationale behind each diagram placement and the strategic plan as it relates to necessary modular or scalable design is helpful. In planning an innovative pharmacy, there is a good chance the architect may not have experience with designs that best support emerging IV robotics or an open-architecture clean room, which does not require the traditional, laminar-flow workbench placement but substitutes an open, table-like workbench. Pharmacists may find themselves reworking drawings, which will potentially delay the ground-breaking. It is essential that the director ensures that the designs reflect the long-range vision of the department.

The architect and project manager must engage in a discussion of sufficient detail. Aesthetic considerations should be included in a written form so that details that may foster a sense of departmental pride are not placed at risk of omission. These may include items such as wood laminate flooring, local university colors, and murals. Likewise, details regarding equipment such as high-capacity shelving might specify electric power versus traditional hand cranks.

The Business Plan

Once the design plans are complete, it is essential to write a business plan that will codify the time-lines of the project and scope. Timelines are necessary for outlining the key particulars of the project and any critical details for interested parties and for allowing effective project management. Ultimately, a business plan scope is described by the current state and future state of the facility. Defining the scope provides necessary information, including project specifics that are crucial when the project is sent to contractors for bid. Contractors base cost estimates on the information contained in the request for proposal. Most importantly, business plans are needed as justification for the project itself. Executives who are considering funding for competing projects rely on the background and rationale portions of the business plan to gain a better understanding of the need for the initiative.

The background and rationale must also contain short- and long-term plans for the department with an emphasis as to how this planned facility renovation meets the needs of the organization and the pharmacy. Reviewers of the plan who may be less familiar with the overall scope benefit from understanding how this particular project fits into the general vision of the organization and the pharmacy.

The business plan outlines the goals, targets, and benchmarks of the effort, along with the time frame for completion. Larger projects must be phased, meaning that the work will occur in sections. Because most facility projects do not involve moving to a new space or acquiring new space, it is important to outline how services will be maintained during the project and how functional areas should be relocated during this time. In addition to the logistical implications, this is also valuable in terms of added cost to the project. Renovating an existing location is in many ways harder than building new space. Maintaining operations from a temporary work space or environment is stressful, unorganized, and inefficient (ie, the lack of space or storage may result in the need for further travel to retrieve stored items). During this time, safety can be compromised because normal systems are disrupted and regulatory controls may be inadvertently relaxed.

A key section of the business plan addresses cost. Along with the total expenditure for the project, this section outlines the specific costs related to the project. This includes details such as whether equipment is part of the project cost and whether the costs are budgeted to the pharmacy cost center or to another department (eg, facilities). Details such as the return on investment for the project, who is responsible for cost overruns, and the process for approving any changes that will result in additional cost or time delays are also contained within this plan.

IMPLEMENTING THE FACILITY'S PLAN

To effectively implement a pharmacy facility plan, the director of pharmacy must understand the facility planning process within the organization. This includes the processes for obtaining approval, budgeting, bidding, and hospital facility development. This also consists of any moves within the facility that may need to occur before the start of construction. For example, the project may necessitate moves by other departments to create available space or the completion of other projects to which teams are already assigned.

Other key stakeholders are regulatory agencies such as boards of pharmacy and departments of health; these groups are important for a variety of reasons. Most notably, they determine whether specific design elements are necessary in construction. For example, certain agencies may require a minimum amount of counter space or compounding area or a specific size sink. All applicable regulations should be reviewed. Moreover, construction documents must be filed, and inspectors may require a site visit or sign-off before the project begins. These lead times need to be incorporated into the overall project timeline. Internal approvals also will be necessary. This may be a simple process, or it could require several iterations and support from nursing, physician staff, and hospital administration.

Given the complexity of a renovation project, some departments choose to employ a consultant. Although this certainly brings additional expertise to the process, it is wise to clarify roles of authority and to consult references. The process is stressful and complex at best, and selecting the wrong consultant can exacerbate an already difficult time, as well as increase costs.

Regardless of whether a formal consultant is hired, site visits made to other pharmacies are recommended, especially those locally who may have undergone renovations. Inquiries should be made regarding problems encountered, lessons learned, and oversights. This will prove time well spent.

FACILITY PLAN FOR THE UNIVERSITY OF PITTSBURGH MEDICAL CENTER

The UPMC experienced obsolescence as a result of government regulations (USP <797>), workload changes (resulting from information system changes), aging facilities, and new medication dispensing technology (additional robotics), among others. These situations created strong business plan justification for renovations to the department of pharmacy. Furthermore, a corridor that divided pharmacy operations was deemed unnecessary, allowing for an unprecedented opportunity for alignment of facility design with departmental services. The pharmacy department already had acquired and operated space for good manufacturing-process packing operations and was in the process of relocating its existing robot to adjacent, noise-isolated space in preparation for complete renovation of the main pharmacies in its 2 campus buildings.

The scope of services at UPMC includes the elements listed in **Table 1**. As a result, many functional and structural considerations were required in the architectural plan. To manage the structural considerations, vendors were consulted on an as-needed basis as each working group completed their analysis of the impact of automation on workload and the subsequent placement of robotic equipment, medication carousels, and other devices. Engagement of staff occurred through direct feedback and assignment of point persons to collect and document input, ensuring all necessary parties were surveyed. A sight visit to a nearby facility was an important step in gaining different perspectives on workflow design, and the visit gave insight into structural considerations for open-architecture clean rooms.

Several workflow diagrams were completed and revised using information from various levels of management, staff, and vendors; and documents were then completed in conjunction with an architect as a concept materialized. Two curved paths best fit the confines of support columns and external walls; one counterclockwise curve for sterile products and another clockwise near-circle for nonsterile-product medications—both ending at delivery carts or a tube station. Similar to a checking station being the center of the action, other aspects of the central pharmacy operations surrounded the proposed "command center." This allowed convenient placement of frequently used items and action locations. See **Figure 1** for an example of the working plans used in the pharmacy department at UPMC Presbyterian.

To facilitate communication, many window requests were included in the design to ensure the preservation of overnight line of site into all areas of the pharmacy. The manager's office also had line of sight between offices and pharmacy operations for increased presence and visibility; blinds allowed optional privacy when needed. After relocation of robotic automation, placement of medication carousels

was one of the largest considerations; only the support pillars could not be moved once placed. Nearly all tables were modular to allow for unexpected changes or mandates.

In alignment with a strategic plan for excellence, education, and research, space was proactively allocated for 2 sterile-product preparation robots so that a comparison could be performed and studied in the near future. UPMC is currently in a stage of implementing the facility plan, and a phased renovation plan is being modeled and tested to predict challenges in renovating existing space. Despite the challenges encountered in temporary workflow during renovation, the finished product has been designed to compensate for these difficulties for many years to come.

CONCLUSION

With the combination of constantly changing regulatory requirements and the number of pharmacy facilities past their prime, it is likely that most pharmacy directors will be asked to redesign a pharmacy in the upcoming years. A working diagram developed internally by a pharmacy department can be an effective tool for conveying workflow concepts and details that match a strategic plan. Proper planning with many considerations— primarily, workflow, current and potential automation, and staff input detail—is essential for ensuring that the resulting space allows for growth and remains functional far into the future.

REFERENCES
1. Lin BY, Leu WJ, Breen GM, Lin WH. Servicescape: physical environment of hospital pharmacies and hospital pharmacists' work outcomes. *Health Care Manage Rev.* 2008;33(2):156-168.

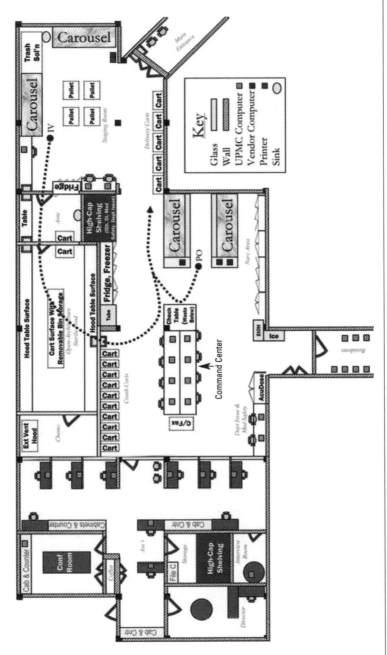

Figure 1. Revised floor plan for University of Pittsburgh Medical Center (UPMC) Main Pharmacy. Ass't = assistant; Cab = cabinet; Cap = capacity; C/Fax = copy and fax machines; Chemo = chemotherapy; Cntr = counter; Conf = conference; Dept = department; DI = drug information; IDS = alcohol; Ext = exterior; IDS = investigational drug service; IV = intravenous; Med = medication; Narc = narcotics; PO = oral; Prod = products; Sol'n = solution; Tube = pneumatic tube station.

2. Reiling J. Safe design of healthcare facilities. *Qual Saf Health Care.* 2006; 15(suppl 1):i34-i40.

3. PA Code Chapter 27: State Board of Pharmacy, §27.16 (b) (1) (i), Construction and equipment requirements. The Pennsylvania Code Web site. http://www.pacode.com/secure/data/049/chapter27/s27.16.html. Accessed July 18, 2008.

4. Mark SM, Weber RJ. Advanced practice programs in hospital pharmacy—investigational drug services. *Hosp Pharm.* 2008;43(2):143-148.

5. Mark SM, Weber RJ. Developing a medication patient safety program—infrastructure and strategy. *Hosp Pharm.* 2007;42(2):149-156.

6. Mark SM, Weber RJ. Developing a medication patient safety program—process and implementation. *Hosp Pharm.* 2007;42(3):249-254. ■

Strategies for Developing Clinical Services: Implementing a Decentralized Pharmacy Program

Michael Sanborn, MS, FASHP*

The focus of this *Director's Forum* is on the justification and implementation of a decentralized pharmacy practice model. This article is the first of three articles that will address the challenges that the pharmacy director must face when expanding pharmacist clinical practice opportunities. Two future articles will review advanced practice programs and the evaluation of clinical services. The goal of the *Director's Forum* throughout 2006 is to provide readers with information on all of the necessary core competencies of hospital pharmacy practice, comprising a "toolkit" in establishing a patient-centered pharmacy department.

There is plenty of evidence to support the impact that pharmacists can have when involved in collaborative care and patient interaction. A recent metaanalysis published in the *Archives of Internal Medicine* provides an excellent summary of the well-positioned pharmacist's potential impact.[1] Still, many hospital pharmacies do not provide services that place pharmacists in the position to make this type of positive contribution to patient care. Recent surveys continue to suggest that the majority of pharmacists are still "stuck in the basement," with significantly less than half of hospitals reporting that pharmacists have been redeployed to patient care areas.[2] Why does this paradox exist? There are many reasons given, including difficulties in recruiting pharmacists, lack of automation, inordinate dispensing-time constraints related to operations, and a misperception that decentralized services always require additional personnel.

Decentralized pharmacy practice is not a new concept, and was first described in the literature in 1965, partially as a means to promulgate the unit dose concept.[3,4] For the purposes of this article, decentralized pharmacy services are defined as traditional pharmacy services, such as order review and processing, formulary management, therapeutic drug monitoring, education, and other clinical services, provided by pharmacists outside of the department in patient care areas. It may or may not include some aspects of drug dispensing, and the goal of this article is not to delineate the detailed responsibilities of a decentralized pharmacist, but rather to review effective means to move pharmacists closer to the patient. It is important to note that fixed satellites are not required for a decentralized practice model, and can at times be a hindrance, since they can often create a situation where pharmacists are closer to a particular patient care area but are tied to a specific dispensing location that prevents them from fully-collaborating with other members of the health care team.

It is typically easier to recruit and retain pharmacists when the department structure is more progressive and allows them to be more proximal to the health care team. As long as salaries are competitive (but not

*Corporate Director of Pharmacy, Baylor Health Care System, Dallas, TX

necessarily at the high end) pharmacists tend to focus on their practice environment as well as their opportunity to have an impact on patient care. Decentralized models have been shown to improve pharmacist job satisfaction and increase opportunities to use clinical skills.[5-8] Another benefit, while not required by Joint Commission standards, is that the survey process is often easier in a decentralized environment, because pharmacists are more familiar with patients involved in the tracer methodology. They can also directly assist the unit in compliance issues over time, and positive pharmacist interaction with surveyors in patient care areas can often reduce the need for more focused pharmacy scrutiny later in the survey.

STARTING A DECENTRALIZED PROGRAM

Many pharmacy managers buy into the concept of decentralized services, but feel that they do not have the necessary full-time equivalents to make it happen. In my experience of implementing such programs at many large and small facilities, a decentralized service model can be initiated without any addition of pharmacy staff. Also, implementing this type of practice model cannot happen overnight and requires careful analysis and planning. In some cases, it can be accomplished in a matter of weeks, while in others it may take several months to fully-implement the service.

There are some key elements needed to move the department towards this type of practice environment, and they include: streamlining existing operations, planning for the process change, implementing a stepwise progression, and ongoing evaluation of progress. If the goal is to decentralize at least some

services without increasing staff, then each of these steps are critical, and thus, will be reviewed further.

STREAMLINING EXISTING OPERATIONS

One of the first steps towards an effective decentralization effort needs to involve a thorough and objective review of existing services. To free up time for decentralized services, the pharmacy must be operating at (or near) peak performance. A means to implementing a decentralized program starts with the effective division of labor with a focus on minimizing the time spent by pharmacists on drug distribution. The focus needs to be on the specific tasks that pharmacists and technicians spend their time on each day. What functions require the most pharmacist or technician time? Is there a way to streamline these processes? As an example, one hospital spent a significant amount of time throughout the day filling unit-based automated dispensing cabinets. Through a streamlining effort, the labor associated with this process was cut in half by optimizing cabinet inventories, par levels, and reducing the number of cabinet fills to no more than once per day or less. The time saved included both technician time associated with medication retrieval and delivery, as well as pharmacist time related to the checking process.

Another critical area to maximize is the use and deployment of existing technician resources. Are there functions that can be performed by technicians rather than pharmacists? For instance, some pharmacies require all chemotherapy be mixed by a pharmacist. There is no evidence to suggest that pharmacists can perform this time-consuming task better than a technician, and it is not an effective use of pharmacist resources. As long as state laws allow, technicians should be trained and their roles expanded to include all areas that do not require the professional judgment of a pharmacist. This can free up a significant amount of pharmacist time, which may be reallocated to the decentralization effort. Pharmacist workload must be refocused to increase the time allotted each day for the new decentralized practice model by leveraging technician time spent coordinating drug dispensing (with appropriate pharmacist checks).

It is also important to note that when it comes to pharmacy service decentralization, the automation surrounding the drug dispensing model (centralized, decentralized, or hybrid medication distribution) that exists within the institution is relatively unimportant. There are very effective decentralized pharmacy programs that have been developed with little, if any, automation. The overall efficiency of the distribution model in place, however, is critical to allowing the maximum amount of time for decentralized practice. All available automation must be effectively and fully-optimized to boost the probability of success.

PLANNING FOR THE PROCESS CHANGE

Large projects of this nature require effective planning to succeed. Creation of an internal decentralized team or task force can be very helpful in the project's planning process. The team can serve as an effective conduit to garner support and excitement for decentralized services and will also expand the ownership of the new program. Moreover, the team can assist in identifying operational improvements that can generate additional time to devote to the project. Team members will be different for each facility, but should include members of the pharmacy staff (pharmacists and technicians) that are knowledgeable regarding pharmacy operations, the pharmacy information system, clinical programs, and hospital logistics. As the department leader, it is important to communicate the vision of the service to the team in advance, so there is a clear understanding of the program goals, as well as the potential changes in day-to-day workload, expectations, and responsibilities.

After the team has a clear understanding of their goals, a useful technique is to conduct a SWOT (Strengths, Weaknesses, Opportunities, and Threats) analysis in a brainstorming type of format. Have the team identify all of the areas that could be potential problems, as well as environmental situations that could be leveraged for program success. For example, limited unit-based computer terminal availability is often an area that must be addressed, but there may be some units that have an unused terminal that can be used. Some pharmacists may be concerned about their abilities in a more clinical practice environment, but perhaps there are other staff members who can assist them in their own self-development.

Part of the planning process also needs to include detail surrounding specific pharmacist activities and program services. What will be the decentralized pharmacist's primary and secondary responsibilities? What are the feasible hours of operation for the decentralized service? Will the pharmacist carry a pager or cell phone for communication needs? What references are available or will be needed? How will new prescriber orders be communicated to the pharmacist? How many patient care areas or patients should a pharmacist be responsible for? Are there areas that will not be serviced by a decentralized pharmacist? What competing hospital projects should be considered when timing the roll out of the new service? These questions, and a myriad of others, should be resolved well before the decentralized program is initiated.

It is also important to involve nursing in the planning process. Often, a significant challenge is identifying an area on the floor that can serve as a "home base" for the decentralized pharmacist. Often, nursing will give up space on the patient care unit if it means that they will gain increased access to a pharmacist. Nursing can also serve as a tremendous advocate for the program and can be instrumental in garnering additional administrative support and resources.

IMPLEMENTING A STEPWISE PROGRESSION

As with any large project, a well-designed stepwise approach can set a strong foundation for success. This can mean different things, depending upon the size of the facility. In smaller hospitals, allowing a pharmacist to provide decentralized services for an hour or two a day may be a good lead-in step to full-decentralization. This strategy is especially effective in facilities with 100 or fewer beds, where pharmacist staff may only consist of one to three pharmacists per day. During this time, the pharmacist can identify and address any challenges or opportunities that may not have been identified during the planning stage.

In larger facilities, a great deal of information can be gained by conducting a decentralized pilot on a predetermined set of nursing units. Again, the information gleaned from the pilot can be invaluable for planning further service expansion. In many cases this small amount of progress can provide the necessary momentum and enthusiasm amongst nursing, pharmacy, and the medical staff to rapidly move the project forward.

Another effective technique prior to implementation is to set up a mock decentralization in the Central Pharmacy. To do this, divide up the workload from each of the nursing units between the pharmacists in the main pharmacy area, just as you would if they were fully-decentralized. This will allow you to measure the real time effects of the decentralized plan and can be an excellent indicator of projected pharmacist workload. It will also assist in identifying and addressing any design or productivity issues prior to actual decentralization.

There is no generally acceptable area to begin implementation of decentralized services, and the decisions surrounding initial locations will be hospital specific. In some cases, starting with Medicine and Surgery Units can be worthwhile. These areas allow for broader coverage of a large number of patients and can also provide good baseline information on order volume and what services will be needed. Intensive Care Units have advantages and disadvantages, because they tend to require more intense pharmacy services, but are atypical from most of the rest of the hospital with respect to patient turnover, medication load, and the large percentage of IV medications.

Throughout the program rollout, setting reasonable deadlines for each phase of the project is important.

Deadlines provide the staff with a milestone to look forward to and work towards, and also channel energy towards the effort. Once the implementation is underway, covered areas and hours of service can be gradually expanded. Initially, it may not be possible or logical to implement services either across the entire hospital or all at one time. Likewise, it is usually not possible to offer decentralized services throughout the entire 24-hour day. Gradual, organized implementation allows for a series of multiple wins for the pharmacy staff and can be a big motivator for new ideas, increased effort, and continued program expansion.

ONGOING EVALUATION OF PROGRESS

The importance of assessment and evaluation of progress cannot be understated. Despite a thorough planning and implementation process, there will always be opportunities for improvement and growth. As pharmacists become comfortable with their new assignments, their productivity will naturally increase. Because of their improved accessibility, there will be many new situations where pharmacists can become more involved in patient care (such as patient care rounds, medication reconciliation, advanced monitoring, etc) and these must be evaluated and encouraged. It may also be possible to further expand the technician's role to assist the decentralized pharmacist in their daily activities. Pharmacist performance expectations should likely be changed to reflect the new practice environment and encourage future professional growth.

There are also several tools available that can support decentralized pharmacists in their daily activities.

For example, there are software programs that can assist the pharmacist in reviewing and triaging patients by providing reports that are targeted at specific drugs or high-risk patient populations. This can increase both the efficiency and productivity of the pharmacist and allow him/her to manage several additional patients throughout the day. Other useful tools include: order scanning software that allows the pharmacist to receive and review written medication orders on a computer screen anywhere in the hospital, electronic intervention documentation systems, and numerous pharmacy applications for personal digital assistants.

At some point, it will probably be necessary to justify additional staff to further expand the program. Data collection regarding a variety of decentralized service outcome measures, including drug cost savings, medication safety improvements, and clinical interventions can be a significant asset to a formal business plan for additional full-time equivalents. Enlisting nursing and physician support can also provide a strong driver for program expansion.

SUMMARY

An effective decentralization effort can transform the pharmacy into a more dynamic practice environment that focuses on patient care. Implementing the process requires new operational efficiencies, careful planning, and a commitment to continuous improvement. The first stages of a decentralized program can often be implemented without any increases in staff, and the steps outlined in this article should assist pharmacy directors in moving forward with their own decentralization effort.

REFERENCES

1. Kaboli PJ, Hoth AB, McClimon BJ, Schnipper JL. Clinical pharmacists and inpatient medical care—a systematic review. *Arch Intern Med.* 2006:166;955-964.

2. Pedersen CA, Schneider PJ, Scheckelhoff DJ. ASHP national survey of pharmacy practice in hospital settings: monitoring and patient education—2003. *Am J Health Syst Pharm.* 2004;61:457-471.

3. Greth PA, Tester WW, Black HJ. Decentralized pharmacy operations utilizing the unit dose concept. II. Drug information services and utilization in a decentralized pharmacy substation. *Am J Hosp Pharm.* 1965;22:558-563.

4. Webb JW. MOSAICS. *Am J Nurs.* 1965;65:105–108.

5. Thompson DF, Kaczmarek ER, Hutchinson RA. Attitudes of pharmacists and nurses toward interprofessional relations and decentralized pharmaceutical services. *Am J Hosp Pharm.* 1988;45:345-351.

6. Cummins BA, Kvancz DA, Bennett DL. Evaluation of mobile decentralized pharmaceutical services in a community teaching hospital. *Am J Hosp Pharm.* 1987;44:324-332.

7. Weber RJ, Skledar SJ, Sirianni CR, Frank S, Yourich B, Martinelli B. The impact of hospital pharmacist and technician teams on medication-process quality and nurse satisfaction *Hosp Pharm.* 2004;39:1169–1176.

8. Janning SW, Stevenson JG, Smolarek RT. Implementing comprehensive pharmaceutical services at an academic tertiary care hospital. *Am J Health Syst Pharm.* 1996;53:542-547. ■

Advanced Practice Programs in Hospital Pharmacy: Anticoagulation Management

Joedell M. Gonzaga, PharmD* and *Robert J. Weber, MS, FASHP†*

The *Director's Forum* series is written and edited by Michael Sanborn and Robert Weber and is designed to guide pharmacy leaders in establishing patient-centered services in hospitals and health systems. Another specific goal of this column is to address many of the key challenges that pharmacy directors face today, while providing information to foster growth in pharmacy leadership and patient safety. This month's *Forum* focuses on specific ways to improve anticoagulation management in your hospital pharmacy department. This area presents an important opportunity for pharmacists to participate actively in improving patient safety.

The goal of *Director's Forum* is to provide guidance to pharmacy leaders on developing patient-centered services. As previously stated in this column, the role of pharmacists in this patient-centered approach (eg, pharmacist as part of a patient care team) improves the quality of care.[1] Medication patient-safety programs serve as valuable patient-centered services; recent information recommends the pharmacy director serve a leadership role in developing an institution's strategy and implementation plan for improving patient safety.[2] Steps in developing this plan include analyzing essential department and hospital data along with national information on medication errors. From these data, a patient safety strategic plan can be developed that focuses appropriate resources on high-risk patient care situations.

A significant area of patient risk and concern is anticoagulation (AC) therapy. Warfarin sodium, unfractionated heparin, and low-molecular weight heparin (LMWH) are commonly prescribed for a wide variety of thrombotic disorders.[3] The clinical challenge in using these medications is the close monitoring required to balance the risk of bleeding against the recurrence of thrombosis. Medication errors and resulting adverse drug events are reported; these are preventable and pose a major opportunity for pharmacists. According to the United States Pharmacopeia's National Reporting System (*MEDMARX*), unfractionated heparin and warfarin sodium are among the top 10 drugs associated with serious outcomes.[4] In most institutions, unfractionated heparin and warfarin sodium are often associated with severe bleeding events, some even fatal. Based on the types and causes of AC errors, pharmacists have the opportunity to be involved in systematically managing this therapy. Implementing an AC service has the potential to improve the understanding of AC management for staff and patients, maintaining updated procedures and protocol, and providing proper dosing and patient monitoring.

Improving the safety of AC dosing has also become a part of the na-

*Department of Pharmacy & Therapeutics, University of Pittsburgh Medical Center, University of Pittsburgh School of Pharmacy, Pittsburgh, PA; †Associate Professor of Pharmacy, Executive Director and Department Chair, Department of Pharmacy & Therapeutics, University of Pittsburgh Medical Center, Pittsburgh, PA.

tional patient safety agenda. The Joint Commission's (TJC) National Patient Safety Goals (NPSG) promote specific improvements in patient safety. The Sentinel Event Advisory Group, working with TJC, annually takes a systematic review of the literature and available databases to identify potential new goals and requirements. By making AC therapy a goal for 2008, TJC acknowledges the patient safety problem in hospitals and all health care facilities. The goals are published mid-year and approved by TJC Board of Commissioners in June. For accreditation purposes, these goals need to be met or a plan implemented. The expectation to meet the requirements for AC services is to be implemented by January 2009.[2]

The 2008 NPSG outline 11 steps to meet the goal of reducing patient harm associated with AC therapy.[2]

Meeting NPSG for AC will aid in the continuity of patient care. Pharmacists can provide an important service in educating and monitoring the patient during the hospital stay as well as after discharge. Studies have shown that pharmacist-monitored AC therapy improves international normalized ratio (INR) values and produces excellent outcomes.[4] The NPSG and welfare of our patients require pharmacy leaders to develop strategies to involve pharmacists in AC management. This poses the following leadership challenges: (1) How is a systematic and sustainable AC management program established within a hospital or health care organization? (2) What steps are necessary to justify funding for the service?

The goal of this article is to provide hospital pharmacy directors guidance in establishing warfarin and LMWH-AC services in both the in-and outpa-tient setting. The specific aims of the article are to: (1) Describe the role of pharmacy in AC management; (2) Review the recommendations for AC management as established by TJC; (3) List some strategies for implementing AC management services; and (4) Describe barriers and challenges in implementing these services.

ROLE OF PHARMACISTS IN AC MANAGEMENT

Pharmacists' roles in AC management have historically been focused on warfarin sodium dispensing. The complexity of warfarin dosing combined with its narrow therapeutic index requires close monitoring; pharmacists have provided expertise in appropriate management of warfarin demonstrating excellent outcomes. Witt and colleagues (2005) studied patients receiving AC care via centralized telephonic interactions with the Pharmacy-AC Service compared with the usual physician AC care. The results of the 6-month study showed patients were less likely (39%) to have an AC-therapy-related adverse event when seen by the pharmacy-AC service. In addition, patients had better control of their target range INR with 64% compared with 55%.[3]

Dager and Gulseth (2007) demonstrated successful collaboration with a hospital medical staff in implementing AC services. The University of California at Davis and St. Mary's Medical Center of Duluth, Minnesota both performed a review on prescribing misadventures related to AC therapy. The results, which demonstrated problems with prescribing ACs, prompted development of a protocol approved by the hospitals' Pharmacy & Therapeutics Committee. The success of this service justified other services such as monitoring programs for heparin-induced thrombocytopenia, LMWH management, factor concentrate dosing (eg, Recombinant factor VIIa), and phytonadione (vitamin K) antidote protocols.[5]

Additionally, the Health Alliance of Greater Cincinnati pharmacy program's goal was to provide a seamless transition of care for a variety of diseases and treatments, including AC. Using a medication-therapy management approach for their beneficiaries, Health Alliance was able to fund and provide continuity of care services in AC. An AC program coordinated by the Alliance maintained continuity of care for 300 patients receiving AC services.[6]

TJC'S NATIONAL PATIENT SAFETY GOALS AND AC

In June 2007, Board of Commissioners of TJC on Accreditation of Health Care Organizations approved the 2008 NPSG. In those goals, TJC addressed the safety needs associated with AC therapy. NPSG #3E states that for anyone given AC therapy, health care providers are to reduce the likelihood of patient harm associated with the use of AC therapy. The purpose of the NPSG is to promote standard prescribing practices to reduce the risk of adverse drug events from AC drugs such as heparin, LMWH, and warfarin.[2] The NPSG does not suggest specific guidelines for AC management except a conceptual framework for developing a systematic and sustainable approach to AC management. These strategy steps and TJC's framework are included in **Table 1.** Currently the Center of Medicare and Medicaid Services does not have a structured focused approach to AC therapy; however, the

Table 1. The Joint Commission's Framework for Meeting the Anticoagulation NPSG[2]

1.	The health care organization implements a defined AC-management program to individualize the care provided to each patient.
2.	When available, only oral unit-dose products and premixed infusions should be used in order to reduce compounding and labeling errors.
3.	Warfarin should be dispensed in accordance with established monitoring procedures for each patient.
4.	The health care organization should use approved protocols for the initiation and maintenance of AC therapy that is appropriate to medication, medical condition, and drug interactions.
5.	Establish baseline INR for all patients started on warfarin and for all patients currently receiving warfarin therapy; current INR should be available and used to monitor and adjust therapy.
6.	Dietary services should be modified, if provided, for all patients receiving warfarin and adjusted if necessary according to an established food/drug interaction program.
7.	The organization should use programmable infusion pumps when heparin is administered intravenously and continuously.
8.	The organization should establish a policy to address the baseline and ongoing laboratory tests that are required for heparin and low-molecular-weight heparin therapies.
9.	The organization should provide education regarding AC therapy to prescribers, staff, patients, and families.
10.	Patient/family education should include the importance of follow-up monitoring, compliance issues, dietary restrictions, and potential for adverse drug reactions and interactions.
11.	The organization should evaluate AC-safety practices.

AC = anticoagulation; INR = international normalized ratio; NPSG: National Patient Safety Goals.

Medicare Prescription Improvement and Modernization Act of 2003 suggests that beneficiaries who are at high risk for adverse events be provided medication therapy management.[7] In addition, the NPSG reinforce ASHP's 2015 Health System Initiatives, suggesting increased pharmacist involvement in high-risk medications.[7,8]

IMPLEMENTING PHARMACY-AC SERVICES

This section describes the steps in justifying and implementing pharmacy-AC services. In some hospitals, pharmacists are currently providing AC monitoring through routine medication order review and follow-up. However, implementing AC services requires 4 steps: (1) understanding hospital data on AC use; (2) designing an effective workflow for patient monitoring; (3) appropriate training for pharmacists providing AC services; and (4) tracking quality indicators for AC.

Review Hospital-Specific Information on AC

A justification of AC services requires that the hospital pharmacy director understand the patient outcomes related to AC as well as patient volumes. For example, the pharmacy director should know the number of medication errors and adverse events along with their type, cause, and severity. This provides a justification of the service as well as a baseline for measuring improvement in clinical indicators of AC once the program is initiated. Finally, it is strongly suggested that this information be reported through the medical staff executive committee to gain physician support for developing AC services.

Developing the Pharmacy AC-Monitoring Process

After essential hospital data on AC are reviewed, the pharmacy director should focus on developing a process for monitoring AC that does not interrupt the current pharmacy workflow. The University of Pittsburgh Medical Center (UPMC) operates an AC monitoring service for warfarin sodium and LMWH patients. The service, which is based on approved physician and pharmacist protocols, is a combination of patient visits (hospital discharge) and remote telephone management of INR values and warfarin dosing. The workflow employs both pharmacist and technician activities; an example of AC workflow is provided in **Figure 1**.

The pharmacists and technicians recruited to provide AC services must be specifically trained to deal with a variety of clinical situations, as they are often the first called for a patient experiencing an adverse event to AC.[9] A listing of the possible job functions of both the pharmacist and technician performing AC services is provided in **Tables 2** and **3**. Certification for pharmacists in AC is available through various online courses. The University of Southern Indiana College of Nursing and Health Professionals provides a 6-week interactive online certification course on AC therapy (http://health.usi.edu/certificate/anticoag/index.asp). The National Certification Board for Anticoagulation Providers (http://www.ncbap.org/index.aspx) provides certification for pharmacists.

The amount of pharmacist and technician full-time equivalents necessary to provide AC services varies; generally, a pharmacist can manage between 200 and 325 patients at any given time.[10,11]

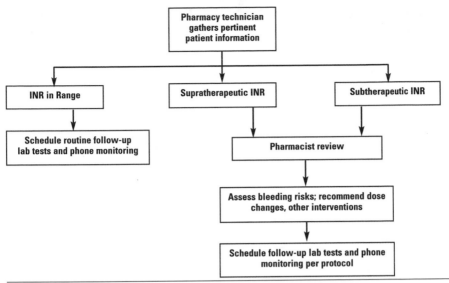

Figure 1. Example of a process workflow for anticoagulation monitoring.

INR = international normalized ratio.

It is critical that quality outcome indicators be tracked for the AC services. These indicators can be a focus on the operational, clinical, and financial aspects of the service. **Table 4** includes examples of quality indicators that would be tracked for an AC service. It is important to note

Table 2. Sample of a Job Description for an Anticoagulation (AC) Pharmacist

1. Provide pharmaceutical care activities to AC patients that are consistent with regulatory, accreditation, and professional standards. Activities include medication order review for safe and effective indication, dose, route, and scheduled administration.

2. Perform therapeutic interventions consistent with the evidence-based guidelines of the department's Drug Use and Disease State Management program.

3. Where possible, manage drug therapy through a collaborative-care agreement with physicians that is approved by the Pharmacy & Therapeutics Committee.

4. Electronically document and track interventions and provide a summary report of activities with calculated impact on patient care.

5. Actively participate in medication safety programs. Active participation means identifying opportunities to improve safety (reporting errors and adverse drug events, and implementing system-based changes as a result of those opportunities).

6. Educate health care professionals on the most current evidence-guiding drug use in AC therapy.

7. Participate in preparing drug-use evaluations, therapeutic-drug reviews, and designing evidence-based clinical practice guidelines.

8. Mentor pharmacy students and residents to support ongoing teaching programs and the missions of the Department of Pharmacy & Therapeutics and the University of Pittsburgh School's of Pharmacy.

9. Contribute to the general knowledge of AC-therapy pharmacy practice by publishing the results of practice innovations or research in the peer-reviewed literature.

Table 3. Sample of a Job Description for an Anticoagulation (AC) Technician

1. Assist the pharmacists by providing timely, regular reviews of patient medical information and pertinent laboratory results.

2. Assist the pharmacists in organizing patient medical information and proper storage.

3. Assist the pharmacists in scheduling patient appointments and phone interviews.

4. Assist the pharmacists in conducting patient bleeding risk assessment.

5. Update patient information in AC tracking database.

6. Assist in the preparation of drug-use evaluations and therapeutic-drug reviews.

7. Assist in the AC therapy education of health care personnel.

that the definition of quality parameters may differ among institutions; it is recommended that a consensus on what defines success in AC be agreed upon prior to implementing a program.

AC services can have very positive outcomes. At the UPMC, a significant cost savings has been demonstrated through AC services provided therein. In 2006, the AC service was able to show a cost savings of nearly $480,000 in LMWH based on inpatient days (590 days) saved in early discharge. From a clinical perspective, INR results (N = approximately 23,500) showed 64% of patients managed by the UPMC service were within the goal range for their indication on warfarin.

IMPLEMENTATION CHALLENGES

There are 4 challenges in implementation of AC services. The first is evaluating the organization's need to establish such a service. This would include the number of errors attributed to AC therapy or providing better patient-centered services for this high-risk population. Second is identifying the stakeholders; stakeholders need to see the justification for funding such a service. Moreover, funding can be limited based on whether or not the stakeholders agree on the purpose of the program. The third challenge is to recruit the right personnel to run the service. Last, leaders are faced with the challenge of continuously seeking new talent and service opportunities throughout the health care organization.

SUMMARY AND CONCLUSION

AC services can effectively support and establish a patient-centered focus for a hospital pharmacy department. The director of pharmacy must use a dynamic approach when developing AC services. The development and

Table 4. Example of Operation, Financial, and Clinical Quality Indicators for AC Services

Indicators	Type	Frequency	Data Source
Number of patients/FTE	Operations	Semi-annually	Pharmacy workload report
LOS cost savings	Financial	Monthly	Hospital finance system
Major bleeding rate	Clinical	Monthly	Medical error reporting system
Minor bleeding rate	Clinical	Monthly	Medical error reporting system
INR within goal range	Clinical	Quarterly	AC data system

AC = anticoagulation; FTE = full-time equivalent; INR = international normalized ratio; LOS = length of stay.

implementation involves using essential department data, collaborating with other health care professionals, and structuring a program evaluation based on the hospital's financial, operational, and quality missions.

ACKNOWLEDGEMENTS

The authors would like to acknowledge the contribution of the AC services staff of the UPMC for the content of this article. They include: Scott M. Mark, PharmD, MS; Bryan Yourich, PharmD; Deanne Hall, PharmD; and Bethany Helms, PharmD. They would also like to acknowledge Ted Rice, MS, BCPS, FASHP for his critical review of the manuscript.

REFERENCES

1. Kaboli PJ, Hoth AB, McClimmon BJ, Schnipper JL. Clinical pharmacists and inpatient medical care: a systemic review. *Arch Intern Medical.* 2006;166(9):955-964.

2. The Joint Commission: 2008 National Patient Safety Goals. http://www.jointcommission.org/PatientSafety/NationalPatientSafetyGoals/. Accessed November 20, 2007.

3. Witt DM, Sadler MA, Shanahan RL, Mazzoli G, Tilman DJ. Effect of a centralized clinical pharmacy anticoagulation service on the outcomes of anticoagulation therapy. *Chest.* 2005;127(5):1515-1522.

4. Santell JP, Cousins D, Hicks R. USP Drug Safety Review: Top 50 products involved in medication errors. *Drug Topics Health-System Edition.* December 2003.

5. Dager WE, Gulseth MP. Implementing anticoagulation management by pharmacists in the inpatient setting. *Am J Health Syst Pharm.* 2007;64(21):2279-2280.

6. Epplen K, Dusing-Wiest M, Freedlund J, Harger N, Kathman S, Ivey MF. Stepwise approach to implementing ambulatory clinical pharmacy services. *Am J Health Syst Pharm.* 2007;64(9):945-951.

7. Kuo GM, Buckley TE, Fitzsimmons DS, Steinbauer JR. Collaborative drug therapy management services and reimbursement in a family medicine clinic. *Am J Health Syst Pharm.* 2004;61(4):343-354.

8. American Society of Health-System Pharmacy—ASHP 2015 Initiative. http://www.ashp.org/s_ashp/cat1c.asp?CID=218&DID=255. Accessed November 20, 2007.

9. Weber RJ. Core competencies in hospital pharmacy: essential department data. *Hosp Pharm.* 2006;41(6):582-587.

10. Nutescu E. The future of anticoagulation clinics. *J Thrombosis and Thrombolysis.* 2003;16(1/2):61-63

11. Foss M, Schoch P, Sintek C. Efficient operation of a high-volume anticoagulation clinic. *Am J Health Sys Pharm.* 1999;56(5):443-449. ∎

Advanced Practice Programs in Hospital Pharmacy: Investigational Drug Services

Scott M. Mark, PharmD, MS, MEd, FASHP, FACHE* and
Robert J. Weber, MS, FASHP†

The *Director's Forum* series is written and edited by Michael Sanborn and Robert Weber and is designed to guide pharmacy leaders in establishing patient-centered services in hospitals and health systems. Another specific goal of this column is to address many of the key challenges that pharmacy directors face today, while providing information to foster growth in pharmacy leadership and patient safety. This month's *Forum* focuses on developing a pharmacy-based investigational drug service in a hospital pharmacy department. As part of a patient-centered pharmacy department, a investigational drug service can significantly contribute to the research mission of a hospital.

INTRODUCTION

Hospitals can be primary centers for clinical research investigations on new or investigational drugs; it is likely that hospital pharmacists will at some time be involved in the handling of these special drugs. The extent of the involvement will depend on the type of hospital facility, the willingness of the pharmacist to accept responsibility for investigational drugs, and the amount of service required. In order to carry out this role effectively, it is important for the pharmacist to know the laws governing the use of investigational drugs and the general methodology for handling and evaluating new drugs.

The development in recent years of new classes of drugs and new methods of creating drugs, as well as new regulations and guidelines related to research has produced an evolution in the way in which research is performed in the United States and in the role pharmacists play in carrying out research. The pharmacy director developing a patient-centered pharmacy service within a hospital can explore this role for pharmacists in developing and coordinating a pharmacy-based investigational drug service (IDS). In fact, the role of the pharmacist in providing IDS has been well-known and documented since the early 1970s.[1,2]

While the Food and Drug Administration (FDA) does not require that investigational drugs be stored and dispensed through a hospital pharmacy,[3] most hospitals require that all clinical investigational drugs be registered and stored by the hospital pharmacy for dispensing on orders from specifically authorized investigators. This policy provides control and monitoring of the security and storage of these medications. Finally, most hospitals have established a policy that no investigational drug be administered to a patient by a nurse or physician unless it bears a pharmacy department control or registration number. As a result of these policies, pharmacy departments

*Assistant Professor and Vice Chair of Pharmacy & Therapeutics, University of Pittsburgh School of Pharmacy, Director of Pharmacy, University of Pittsburgh Medical Center, Pittsburgh, PA; †Associate Professor and Chair, University of Pittsburgh School of Pharmacy, Department of Pharmacy & Therapeutics, Executive Director of Pharmacy, University of Pittsburgh Medical Center, Pittsburgh, PA.

should be actively involved in the dispensing of investigational drugs.

The objective of this article is to provide the pharmacy director with an introduction to developing pharmacy-based IDS. The specific aims of this article is to (1) describe key fundamental terms related to investigational drugs; (2) list the steps in developing pharmacy-based IDS; (3) describe the structure and operations of pharmacy-based IDS; and (4) list the metrics to measure the effectiveness of the service.

FUNDAMENTAL TERMS RELATED TO INVESTIGATIONAL DRUGS

At the present time the clinical investigation and marketing of new drugs is governed by the 1938 Federal Food, Drug and Cosmetic Act and the Kefauver-Harris Amendments of 1962. These statutes have been implemented by a series of FDA regulations that were published in the Federal Register and the Code of Federal Regulations. In essence, these laws and regulations define the conditions under which clinical investigational drugs may be shipped in interstate commerce and delineate the evidence for the claimed safety and efficacy of the drug, which needs to be provided prior to its marketing.[4] Federal regulations allow investigators to delegate these responsibilities to pharmacists and practice guidelines recommend pharmacist involvement with investigational studies.

Investigational New Drug Applications (INDs)

Any organization seeking to sponsor clinical trials with experimental agents must first submit an IND to the FDA. The IND is the legal mechanism under which experimental agent research is performed in the United States. No experimental agents may be administered to patients for research in the United States without an IND. All IND sponsors have obligations, which are specified in the regulations of the FDA. The initial IND submission by the sponsor to FDA is a lengthy document that sets forth the experimental rationale for human testing, including results of animal toxicology studies, manufacturing data, purity and stability information, and an initial plan of clinical investigation. The IND is the official record at the FDA of the sponsor's clinical research with the agent.

Phases of Clinical Drug Investigation

The clinical investigation of a new drug is divided into 3 phases and is directed toward producing substantial proof for the safety and efficacy of the drug.[5] Phase 1 trials determine a safe dose for subsequent trials and define acute effects on normal tissues. In addition, these trials examine the agent's pharmacology and may reveal evidence of biologic activity. The purposes of these studies include the determination of human toxicity, absorption, metabolism, elimination, pharmacodynamics, preferred route of administration, and safe dosage range. Phase 1 studies involve a small number of persons (20 to 80) and should be conducted under carefully controlled circumstances by qualified clinical investigators. Phase 2 studies are conducted by clinicians familiar with the methods of drug evaluation, as well as the disease being treated, and drugs currently in use for this condition. These carefully supervised studies are designed to demonstrate the new drug's efficacy and relative safety. Phase 3 studies are intended to assess the drug's safety, effectiveness, and most desirable dosage in treating a specific disease in a large group of subjects. The studies should also be carefully monitored, even though they are extensive. In each phase of a clinical drug trial the FDA receives continuous reports on the progress of each phase. If the continuation of the studies appears to present an unwarranted hazard to the patients, the sponsor may be requested to modify or discontinue clinical testing until further preclinical work has been done.

Qualifications of Investigators

The sponsor (usually a pharmaceutical manufacturer) of an investigational new drug will ask the clinical investigator to supply the following information before shipping the investigational drug to the investigator: a statement of his education, training, and experience as well as any information regarding the hospital or other medical institution where the investigation will be conducted; special equipment and other facilities. The training and experience required will vary, depending upon the kind of drug and the nature of the investigation. In Phase 1, the investigator must be able to evaluate human toxicology and pharmacology. In Phase 2, the investigator should be familiar with the conditions and the methods of human toxicology and pharmacology evaluation. In Phase 3, in addition to the experienced clinical investigators, other physicians not regarded as specialists in any particular field of medicine may serve as investigators. At this stage, a large number of patients may be treated by different physicians to obtain a broad background of experience with the drug.

Obligations of Investigators

The primary responsibility for disposition of investigational drugs in a clinical study is the responsibility of the principal investigator, usually a licensed physician. As a result, the investigator is obligated to obtain patient informed consent, maintain adequate records of drug preparation and dispensing, maintain study case and progress reports, and report adverse reactions.

FDA Authority in the Investigational Use of Commercially Available Drugs

The FDA has no authority over the practice of medicine and cannot require a physician to prescribe a specific drug for a particular illness. Many drugs are prescribed for conditions not approved by the FDA, or in an "Off Label" manner. Physicians are encouraged to submit an IND when they use a drug regularly for purposes other than those approved by the FDA. The FDA can then accumulate data on the safety and efficacy of the drug for such treatment and can share the information with other physicians. The University of Pittsburgh Medical Center has implemented a process for intensive review of Off-Label medication use through its Pharmacy & Therapeutics (P&T) Committee and as a mechanism for providing a cost and safety check for this type of medication use.[6]

Patient Informed Consent

Each patient should complete a document referred to as informed consent. The purpose of this document is to educate patients on the known risks of each therapy or procedure. Each informed-consent document must be protocol-specific and contain the elements required by Federal regulation. These regulations do not specify the language of the document but provide a list of elements that must be addressed in the text of the consent form. The description of expected adverse events in the informed-consent document must be complete and balanced and reflective of the treatment plan to be used. Adverse events of other modalities used in the study (eg, radiotherapy, surgery) must also be described.

Institutional Review Board (IRB) Approval

The IRB is a standing committee of a hospital that usually reports to the hospital's board of trustees. The purpose of the IRB is to review and approve research studies based on guidelines of the Department of Health and Human Services Office of Human Research Protections (OHRP). IRB approval is required in all situations where investigational drugs are used; a hospital or commercial IRB consists of both health care professionals and lay persons whose main mission is patient protection.

STEPS IN IMPLEMENTING A PHARMACY-BASED IDS

A pharmacy department's role in the handling of investigational drugs depends on the type of hospital, current facilities for handling investigational drugs, and the expertise of

Table 1. Basic and Specialized Pharmaceutical Services for Investigational Drugs

Basic Services
Maintain drug accountability logs
Medication computer order entry
Prepare dispensing procedures
Maintain specific logs wherever the drug is stored
Prepare drug monographs
Verify that the patient has signed the informed-consent document
Provide inservice education to pharmacy staff
Provide patient counseling predischarge
Provide inservice education to nursing staff
Obtain written prescriptions
Maintain patient profiles
Prepare patient reminder cards
Specialized Services
Compound special dosage forms
Generate randomization schemes
Assist in protocol development
Use special drug-delivery systems
Assist in subject recruitment
Review charts and collect data
Perform clinic audits and inspections
Administer doses to patients

pharmacy staff. The major steps in implementing pharmacy-based IDS include (1) determining the scope of service; (2) designing an adequate drug dispensing area; (3) developing an operational plan for the service.

Determining the Scope of Service

The basic role of the pharmacy in handling investigational drugs includes the registration, control, storage, dispensing, maintenance of disposition records, and drug information for these medications. **Table 1** lists both basic and specialized investigational drug services that can be provided by a pharmacy department. A basis for these activities is a P&T Committee-approved investigational drug service that should also be reviewed by the pharmacy director with the hospital's medical executive committee. In order for the hospital pharmacists to carry out even this basic role, it is imperative that the hospital adopt certain policies for the use and storage of investigational drugs.

The scope of the pharmacy-based IDS is determined by understanding the hospital's strategic plan for research and or innovative medical care. For example, an organization that has a medical staff with an affiliation to a large research university will require sophisticated pharmacy services; likewise, hospitals that have established research institutes not affiliated with an academic institution will also need a higher level of pharmaceutical service.

Some hospitals have developed innovative clinical practice committees that monitor the use of care processes that may not be totally supported by medical evidence. These processes may include medical procedures (use of devices, surgical procedures) or drug treatment (innovative off-label medication use). In this case, an intermediate form of pharmaceutical service may be required to include review and monitoring of off-label medication use or devoting part of a pharmacist full-time equivalents (FTEs) to handling investigational drugs. Finally, hospitals that do not deal with patients on investigational drugs may only need to have a policy and procedure for how to handle situations where patients are admitted to a hospital and receiving an investigational drug.

The following demonstrates a focused example of processes for investigational drug accountability and storage, and stresses that pharmacy directors must understand the full scope and detail involved in investigational drug dispensing as they plan for this service in the pharmacy department.

Specific accountability procedures for control of investigational drugs assist the responsible principal investigator in making certain that agents received are used only for patients entered onto an approved protocol. Importantly, these processes can be delegated to the pharmacy but still remain the responsibility of the principal investigator. **Table 2** lists specific accountability for investigational drug storage and control.

Designing an Adequate Drug Dispensing Area

For hospitals offering specialized services in dispensing investigational drugs, an adequate amount of space should be designated for drug storage and preparation. **Figure 1** shows an example floor plan for an investigational drug area of the pharmacy. The floor plan notes that the area is secured (using an electronic security sys-

Table 2. Examples of Investigational Drug Storage and Control Accountabilities

Store the agent in a secure location, accessible to only authorized personnel, preferably in the pharmacy

Maintain a careful record of the receipt, use, and final disposition of all investigational agents received

Maintain appropriate storage of the investigational agent to ensure the stability and integrity of the agent

Return any unused investigational agents to the pharmacy at the completion of the study or upon notification that an agent is being withdrawn

Each investigational agent should be stored separately by protocol. If an agent is used for more than 1 protocol, there should be separate physical storage for each protocol

Each agent should be accounted for separately by protocol. If an agent is used for more than 1 protocol, there should be a separate Drug Accountability Record Form (DARF) for each protocol

There should be a separate DARF for each agent in a multiagent protocol

Separate accountability forms should be maintained for each different strength or dosage form of a particular agent (eg, an agent with a 1- and a 5-mg vial would require different DARFs for the 1- and 5-mg vials)

The DARF has been designed for use at each location where agents are stored, eg, main pharmacy, satellite pharmacy, physician's office, or other dispensing areas

The DARF is also designed to accommodate both dispensing records and other agent transaction documentation (eg, receipt of agent, returns, broken vials)

tem through a card reader) and segregates the drug stock from other stock in the pharmacy (pharmacy supply storage). The floor plan also provides for an area for sterile compounding and other extemporaneous preparation (pharmacy workroom). In the design of the floor plan, adequate re-

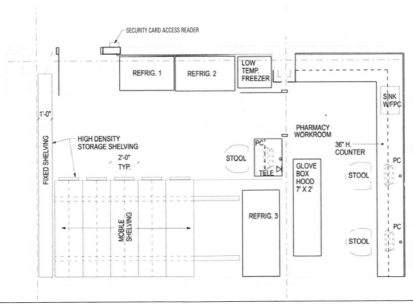

Figure 1. Example of floor plan for an investigational drug service.

frigeration must be considered along with data information capabilities (eg, computer, fax machines).

Developing an Operational Plan for the Service

A significant challenge to implementing a pharmacy-based IDS is to develop an operating budget and metrics for the service. This may be difficult initially; the budgeting and staffing of the service will most likely be the result of educated assessments of new and ongoing research study volumes. These data are most easily obtained by planning a strategy with all of the stakeholders in clinical research to include research investigators, industry sponsors, and program administrators. In planning the pharmacist and technician time to operate the service, the following functions must be considered: protocol receipt and review; protocol set-up and paperwork; developing the drug information monograph, establishing requirements for preparation, labeling and storage of medication, monitoring administration and documentation, and auditing for compliance. As a result, the department should establish a time standard for various types of investigational drug preparations, and calculate required FTEs based on volume of these investigational medication types. Table 3 lists common metrics a pharmacy director could use in monitoring the financial, operational, and quality aspects of pharmacy-based IDS.

MISCELLANEOUS CONSIDERATIONS FOR A PHARMACY-BASED IDS

Retention of Records

FDA regulations require that all research records (including patient charts, case report forms, x-rays, scans that document response, IRB approvals, signed informed-consent documents, and all agent accountability records) must be kept by the investigator for at least 2 years after an New Drug Application has been approved for that indication or the study has been closed.

Data Management and Statistics

Since most clinical trials involve professional staff other than the protocol chair, adequate collection of clinical data is a complex task that must be integrated into the medical practices of the institution. Furthermore, data collection is best done

Table 3. Workload Metrics for a Pharmacy-Based Investigational Drug Service

Indicators	Type	Frequency	Data Source
Number of active clinical research studies	Operations	Monthly	Daily workload statistics
Number of studies/FTE	Operations	Monthly	Daily workload statistics
Study openings and closings	Operations	Yearly	Daily workload statistics
Doses dispensed	Operations	Monthly	Daily workload statistics
Required pharmacist and technician man-hours	Operations	Monthly	Daily workload statistics
Total IDS revenue	Financial	Monthly	Hospital finance system
Number of medication errors	Quality	Monthly	Medication Error Reporting System

FTE = full-time equivalent; IDS = Investigational Drug Service.

as data are generated; this practice promotes protocol compliance and permits the protocol chair to monitor the study's progress. For these reasons, data management organized and supported at the department or institution level is usually more efficient and reliable than that which is left to the individual investigator. The patient recruitment goals of a study should be specified in advance, with a maximum number of patients explicitly stated. Justification for the target sample size, in terms of precision of estimation or levels of type 1 and type 2 error, should be provided. The accrual rate of eligible patients that can be realistically anticipated should be given as well. Finally, mechanisms should be in place for early stopping of negative trials.

Verification of Compliance to Study Procedures

Compliance to procedures ensures proper agent usage and is reviewed during site visits, which are conducted under a research sponsor monitoring program. Specifically, site visitors will check that the agent accountability system is being maintained and will spot-check the agent accountability records by comparing them with the patients' medical records to verify that the agents were administered to a patient entered in the recorded protocol.

Cost Justification

Most IDSs charge fees in an attempt to recoup the costs of the IDS as well as the dispensing pharmacists' time and supplies. These fees vary from study to study and among institutions but frequently institutions charge a study initiation fee, a quarterly maintenance fee, and a per-dose dispensing fee. Often, payment received from these charges is not sufficient to cover the cost of running the IDS. However, there may be other economic benefits. One benefit to an institution is cost avoidance, which has been defined as dollars that would have been spent to purchase medications but that were not spent because of a specific study-related intervention.

Another key benefit is regulatory and sponsor compliance. Failure to properly maintain records can place entire research programs at risk. For this reason, it is critical to outline key benefits to hospital administrators who may be hesitant to implement an IDS because the benefits are not readily apparent. Potential funding sources for the IDS include: (1) Fees charged to investigators; (2) Hospital support provided or costs absorbed; (3) Salary support provided through a research grant; (4) Fees charged to departments; (5) Designated funding provided through a research grant; and (6) Salary support obtained from a school or university.

SUMMARY AND CONCLUSION

A pharmacy-based IDS can effectively support and establish a patient-centered focus for a hospital pharmacy department in supporting innovation and new knowledge in medication use. The director of pharmacy must use a dynamic approach in developing pharmacy-based IDS. The development and implementation involves determining the scope of service, designing an adequate drug dispensing area, and developing an effective operational plan for the service.

REFERENCES

1. Kleinman LM, Tangrea JA, Gallelli JF. Control of investigational drugs in a research hospital. *Am J Hosp Pharm.* 1974;31(4):368-371.

2. Kleinman LM, Tangrea JA. Involvement of the hospital pharmacist in single- and double-blind studies. *Am J Hosp Pharm.* 1974;31(10):979-981.

3. Peltzman S. An evaluation of consumer protection legislation: the 1962 drug amendments. *J Polit Econ.* 1973;81(5):1049-1091.

4. LaFleur J, Tyler LS, Sharma RR. Economic benefits of investigational drug services at an academic institution. *Am J Health Syst Pharm.* 2004;61(1):27-32.

5. The Food and Drug Administration. Clinical testing for safe and effective drugs, DHEW Publication No. (FDA) 74-3015. US Government Printing Office, Washington, DC.

6. Ansani N, Sirio C, Henderson B, Smitherman T, Weber RJ, Skledar SJ, ZgheibN, Branch RA. Designing a strategy to promote safe innovative off-label use of medications. *Am J of Med Qual.* 2006;21():246-254. ∎

Advanced Practice Programs in Hospital Pharmacy: Pharmacy-Based Immunization

Deanne L. Hall, PharmD, CDE* and Robert J. Weber, MS, FASHP†

The *Director's Forum* series is written and edited by Michael Sanborn and Robert Weber and is designed to guide pharmacy leaders in establishing patient-centered services in hospitals and health systems. Another specific goal of this column is to address many of the key challenges that pharmacy directors currently face, while providing information to foster growth in pharmacy leadership and patient safety. This month's article describes providing immunizations in a hospital-based retail pharmacy. As the pharmacists' role in immunization evolves to one of procurement, advocacy, and immunizer, hospitals can provide a valuable public health service to patients using hospital-based retail pharmacies. Developing this program may also further develop more advanced-practice programs in patient medication education and medication therapy management.

INTRODUCTION

Pharmacy involvement in vaccinations began over 150 years ago with the advent of the smallpox vaccine.[1] Early pharmacists' roles initially consisted of procurement, storage, and distribution of the vaccines, as well as serving as a vaccine advocate to both patients and physicians.[2] The pharmacist's role as an immunizer began in 1994; Washington became the first state to grant pharmacists the authorization to administer vaccinations.[2] To date, 44 states have amended their pharmacy practice acts to allow pharmacists to administer immunizations.[3] This movement is helped by the American College of Physicians and American Society of Internal Medicine position paper on pharmacist scope of practice stating support of pharmacists as an "immunization information source, host for immunization sites, and immunizer."[4] Additionally, an increase in public health awareness of immunizations is promoted by the publication of *Healthy People 2010* that established goals to increase childhood vaccination rates to 80% and adult influenza and pneumococcal vaccination rates to 90%.[5] The potential for pharmacist involvement was quickly realized in many preventive care areas including immunizations.[6,7]

Pharmacists have been involved in hospital settings to promote vaccination compliance and education. The University of Pittsburgh Medical Center's (UPMC) pharmacy, as part of the Pharmacy & Therapeutics (P&T) Committee, coordinated a multidisciplinary effort in developing a procedure to improve pneumococcal vaccination rates among hospitalized patients.[8] Standing orders were developed to incorporate both risk assessment for vaccination and pharmacy order processing. Education was provided to staff that described the importance of providing pneumococcal vaccinations and reinforced a new vaccination procedure. This program improved the hospital's pneumococ-

*Assistant Professor, Department of Pharmacy and Therapeutics, University of Pittsburgh School of Pharmacy, Ambulatory Care Clinical Pharmacy Specialist, University of Pittsburgh Medical Center, Pittsburgh, Pennsylvania; †Associate Professor and Chair Department of Pharmacy and Therapeutics, University of Pittsburgh School of Pharmacy Executive Director of Pharmacy, University of Pittsburgh Medical Center, Pittsburgh, Pennsylvania.

cal vaccination rate to over 90% for qualifying patients.

Hospital pharmacy departments that also operate retail-based pharmacies (eg, clinic building, hospital lobby) can enhance the role of the pharmacist in public health by providing immunizations in this venue. Immunization delivery offers unique advantages to patients in this environment and furthers development of medication therapy management services.

The goal of this article is to provide guidance to directors of pharmacy with development of immunization services in a hospital-based retail pharmacy. The specific aims of this article are to: (1) describe the advantages of providing immunization services in a hospital-based retail pharmacy; (2) list the steps in developing an immunization service in a hospital-based retail pharmacy; and (3) describe the hospital-based retail pharmacy immunization program at the UPMC.

ADVANTAGES IN DEVELOPING IMMUNIZATION SERVICES IN A HOSPITAL-BASED RETAIL PHARMACY

Hospital-based retail pharmacies offer a unique opportunity to develop patient-centered pharmaceutical care programs. An immunization program can be effectively implemented in this setting based on the following: (1) hospital-based retail pharmacies are often located on hospital or clinic grounds and can be easily accessed by patients; (2) the pharmacy has a close proximity to the medical staff, which aids in the recruitment of a medical staff sponsorship for an immunization program; and (3) professional liability insurance for a pharmacist providing immunization may fall under the hospital's umbrella policy complementing the pharmacist's personal liability insurance.

STEPS IN DEVELOPING A PHARMACY-BASED IMMUNIZATION SERVICE

The steps involved in developing a pharmacy-based immunization service include: (1) obtaining proper certification and licensing to provide immunization; (2) evaluating pharmacy department resources; (3) understanding billing and reimbursement; (4) redesigning pharmacy workflow; and (5) safely administering vaccines. See Table 1 for a more thorough list of steps.

Certification and Licensing

The pharmacy director must be familiar with state pharmacy regulations related to vaccine administration

Table 1. Steps in Developing an Immunization Service in a Hospital-Based Retail Pharmacy

Analyze pharmacy resources (time, space, location)
Develop partnering relationships (physicians, employee health, employer groups)
Fulfill state licensure requirements
Train pharmacists (immunization delivery, cardiopulmonary resuscitation)
Obtain National Provider Identification (NPI) numbers (pharmacist and pharmacy)
Contact local Medicare office to become a mass immunizer for billing
Develop a collaborative protocol, if needed
Determine target population
Establish reimbursement mechanisms
Develop marketing plan and materials
Determine method of documentations (purchase software if needed)
Obtain needed supplies (eg, vaccine, syringes, needles, gloves, cotton balls)
Train staff on immunization workflow
Administer vaccines

since states have differing regulations and requirements. For example, some states have specific regulations regarding what types of patients a pharmacist may immunize (eg, patients older than 18 years of age); others allow certified pharmacy students to administer vaccines. These distinctions are important and impact the immunization-target population and the types of vaccines administered. Also, pharmacy work flow and resources may be impacted if nonpharmacist personnel (pharmacy interns) are permitted to administer vaccines. Additionally, some states require a state license while others may only require a certificate from an appropriate training course; as an immunization service is developed, licensing and the time involved in obtaining appropriate licenses affect implementation. Finally, state boards of pharmacy will outline the requirements regarding written protocols, prescriptions for vaccination, documentation of vaccine administration, and patient monitoring (including emergency procedures).

Evaluate Pharmacy Resources

Assessing and planning for immunization resources should occur early in the process as these changes, such as changes in workflow and/or physical space, often take the most time to implement. A survey of pharmacists providing immunizations revealed the need for availability of time, staff support, and dedicated space within the pharmacy as the top 3 initiation barriers.[9] As a director of pharmacy, there may be resources that can be used outside the department or even in the hospital. Developing immunization protocol, facilitating space, purchasing supplies, and marketing the service may take a tremendous amount of time and resources; these should be considered far in advance during the project planning.

Importantly, the hospital may not be able to justify the pharmacist's time away from dispensing responsibilities to provide immunization services. Using pharmacy interns or residents may also be a lower-cost alternative for completing the ground work as well as providing a learning experience. And finally, if the hospital is associated with a school of pharmacy, partnering with interested faculty may get the service started without taking pharmacist time away from dispensing activities until sufficient staff support can be attained.

Assess Space Needs to Provide Immunizations

Providing immunizations requires a private, patient-accessible area. Oftentimes, the floor plan of a hospital-based retail pharmacy may not account for this or may be an extension of the inpatient pharmacy with only a patient-accessible window. Incorporating dedicated patient-care space for immunizations should occur during the initial planning. Lack of adequate space in a hospital-based retail pharmacy should not be a deterrent to providing immunization services. Immunizations can be provided outside of the pharmacy for those with limited space flexibility. For example, remote locations throughout the hospital, such as the cafeteria, hospital lobby, physician clinics, and the employee-health clinic, can be used for vaccination. An additional innovative strategy is to design an immunization cart that can be transported from the hospital-based retail pharmacy throughout the hospital to nursing units and other care areas to improve the accessibility of immunizations. Finally, hospitals that are associated with universities or specific employer groups may also be able to provide remote clinics to improve immunization rates.

Solicit Physician Support for the Immunization Program

Gaining physician support for the immunization program is very important as most states require a written prescription or signed protocol by a physician in order for a pharmacist to administer an immunization. Physicians can also support the pharmacy-based immunization program with their colleagues and hospital administrators. Finally, physicians serve as an important referral source for patients to receive immunizations through a hospital-based retail pharmacy.

Train Pharmacists and Others to Provide Immunizations

Training programs for immunization administration includes vaccine administration and service implementation. Training programs are usually 1 to 2 days in length and may require offsite participation. Programs are offered by national and state pharmacy organizations as well as schools of pharmacy; most programs use the American Pharmacists' Association Pharmacy Based Immunization Certificate Training Program. In addition to the training program, pharmacists are also required to be certified in cardiopulmonary resuscitation (CPR), which can often be attained through a hospital's CPR certification program for employees. Lastly, prior to beginning the service, all pharmacy staff should be educated on the processes for administering the immunizations and answering patient's questions. **Table 2** lists available resources for

Table 2. Helpful Resources for Pharmacy-Based Immunization Programs

ASHP Guidelines on the Pharmacist's Role in Immunization. *Am J Health Syst Pharm.* 2003;60(1):1371-1377.

Center for Disease Control and Prevention. Prevention and control of influenza: recommendations of the Advisory Committee on Immunization Practice (ACIP). *MMWR*, 56(RR-6). July, 2007

American Pharmacists Association Immunization Resource Center. http://www.pharmacist.com/

Center for Disease Control and Prevention Vaccine and Immunizations. http://www.cdc.gov/vaccines/default.htm

Advisory Committee on Immunization Practice (AICP) Recommendations. http://www.cdc.gov/mmwr/

Immunization Action Coalition. www.immunize.org

Vaccine Adverse Event Reporting System. http://vaers.hhs.gov/

State and Local Health Departments

immunization programs, including pharmacist training.

Identifying a Targeted Population to Immunize

Determining a target-patient population for immunization allows the pharmacy to identify possible program partners, including physicians. Target population can be determined by reviewing the demographics of patients using the hospital-based retail pharmacy. For example, if the patients of the hospital-based retail pharmacy are primarily employees, then working with employee health or the hospital's employer benefits group may provide an avenue to secure resources such as space or reimbursement for services. Vaccinating hospital employees has proven very successful.[10] Determining a target population may also dictate the types of vaccines administered. For example, if an immunization service focuses on adults, a reasonable approach may be to begin with offering the influenza and/or pneumococcal immunizations.

Develop a Documentation System for Administering Vaccines

Documentation requirements must be addressed, as most available community pharmacy dispensing systems do not provide fields to document vaccine administration. The required documentation varies depending on individual state regulations. Documentation can be performed via a manual paper system, the hospital's electronic medical record application, commercial software,[11] or by Microsoft *Excel* or *Access*.

Develop a Marketing Plan for the Service

Marketing efforts for the immunization service depends on the target population; for example, promotional materials developed for employees may vary from those developed for non-employees. Using the hospital's e-mail or newsletters may be a route to target employees and partnering with an employee benefits group may be another. If targeting patients in the community, contacting a local newspaper or community-based physician offices may be of benefit. Because the department of pharmacy is part of a larger hospital organization, working with hospital's media relations department can assure effective and professional communication.

Understand Reimbursement Mechanisms for Immunizations

Pharmacy-based immunization services are reimbursed (vaccine and administration fee) by submitting individual or mass immunizing claim (Health Insurance Claim Form 1500) to insurers. Many insurers are also beginning to provide vaccine reimbursement through Medicare Part D, in which a claim may be adjudicated through the pharmacy's medication dispensing system. Some insurers may also provide a mechanism for direct invoicing. As reimbursement strategies may differ depending on the vaccine and are in a state of change, a specific process will not be outlined in this article. It is important to contact local insurers to determine the mechanism in which to submit claims as well as working with the hospital's billing department.

HOSPITAL-BASED RETAIL PHARMACY IMMUNIZATION PROGRAM AT UPMC

In July 2006, The Commonwealth of Pennsylvania approved pharmacy regulations allowing pharmacist-administered immunizations. A first step in developing the pharmacy-based immunization service was to review and understand the pharmacy regulations. According to Pennsylvania state law, pharmacists are only permitted to administer immunizations to patients older than 18 years of age; it does not authorize pharmacy interns to administer vaccines. Lastly, the state requires either a signed immunization order from a physician or a standing-immunization protocol approved by a licensed physician. Based on these regulations, the pharmacy developed a vaccine protocol (see **Appendix 1**) that was reviewed and approved by the hospital's legal department as well as the P&T Committee. The department also recruited a physician to serve as the sponsor to provide clinical oversight for the immunization program. The protocol provides for a broad range of vaccine administration.

The pharmacy department's hospital-based retail pharmacy is a 2,500-square-foot facility housed in the campus's main clinic building. The pharmacy was recently renovated and fills approximately 750 prescriptions daily for employees throughout the hospital as well as discharge and clinic patients. A space for clinical care was designed in the pharmacy plan to provide for medication therapy management and immunization services. The immunization service is provided by registered pharmacists licensed to administer injectables; initial training occurred in 2006 with a more detailed plan for training to prepare for the 2007-2008 influenza vaccination season.

Although the pharmacy has a dedicated patient care room for immunizations, it was realized that only a small number of patients would be reached by only providing vaccinations in the pharmacy. An evaluation of the resources within the hospital and university revealed partners to work with that could provide additional space. As a result, remote flu shot clinics were held at both the hospital and the university. For example, vaccinating pharmacists attended health fairs and arranged dedicated dates and times at varying locations throughout the hospital and university to provide the influenza vaccine. These sessions were in addition to regularly scheduled clinics through the hospital's employee health and allowed employees greater access to the influenza vaccine. In addition, using employee health e-mail reminders provided a way to disseminate information about when and where the sessions would occur as well as times

available at the pharmacy for the vaccinations. Partnering with the university's benefits office and the health insurance group assisted in increasing patients' likelihood of receiving an influenza vaccine by developing a process in which the pharmacy could directly bill the payer, rather than the current practice of the patient paying out of pocket and later submitting a claim. Lastly, the pharmacy worked with the medical school to provide vaccinations for medical students in the same manner, thus providing another mechanism for pharmacists to provide immunizations.

The immunization service through UPMC's hospital-based retail pharmacy provided over 600 influenza immunizations from November 2007 through January 2008. In addition, 15 of these patients were found to be eligible to receive the pneumoccocal vaccine on-site as well. During the 2008 year, the service is expanding to include the addition of pneumococcal, zoster, hepatitis A and B, and tetanus vaccines, as well as expanding the influenza and pneumococcal programs.

There were very few barriers to implementing the service at UPMC. The pharmacy department's long-standing history of patient-centered programs along with the established role of pharmacists as immunizers was instrumental in gaining appropriate leadership support. However, some barriers relating to pharmacist time to immunize, physical space for immunizing, and patient access were encountered. These barriers were addressed by collaborating with University of Pittsburgh School of Pharmacy licensed and certified faculty to serve as immunizers, developing a remote immunization service, and by marketing services with employees.

SUMMARY AND CONCLUSION

Pharmacists have long served a role as public health advocates. Hospital-based retail pharmacies offer a unique opportunity to expand this role by administering immunizations. The pharmacy director must develop a plan that meets the needs of the organization related to immunizations, solicit physician support, and document the impact of a pharmacy-based immunization program. If the program is successful, the department takes one more step in developing a patient-centered pharmacy service.

REFERENCES

1. Grabenstein JD. Pharmacists and immunizations: increasing involvement over a century. *Pharm Hist*. 1999;41(4):137-152.

2. Hogue MD, Grabenstein JD, Foster SL, Rothholz MC. Pharmacist involvement with immunizations: a decade of professional advancement. *J Am Pharm Assoc*. 2006;46(2):168-182.

3. American Pharmaceutical Association. Fact sheet. http://www.pharmacist.com/AM/Template.cfm?Section=Public_Health2&TEMPLATE=/CM/ContentDisplay.cfm&CONTENTID=6256. Accessed January 21, 2008.

4. Keely JL. Pharmacist Scope of Practice. *Ann Intern Med*. 2002;136(1):79-85.

5. US Department of Health and Human Services. *Healthy People 2010*. 2nd ed. With Understanding and Improving Health and Objectives for Improving Health. Vol 1. Washington, DC: U.S. Government Printing Office, November 2000.

6. Healthy people 2010: challenges, opportunities and call to action for America's pharmacists. *Pharmacotherapy*. 2004;24(9):2141-2194.

7. Babb VJ, Babb J. Pharmacist involvement in healthy people 2010. *J Am Pharm Assoc*. 2003;43(1):56-60.

8. Sokos DR, Skledar SJ, Ervin KA, et al. Designing and implementing a hospital-based vaccine standing orders program. *Am J Health Syst Pharm*. 2007;64(10):1096-1102.

9. Kamal KM, Madhavan SS, Maine LL. Pharmacy and immunizations services: pharmacists' participation and impact. *J Am Pharm Assoc*. 2003; 43(4):470-482.

10. Sanchez D, Breland BD, Pinkos L, Eagle A, Nowlin D, Duty L. Pharmacist-run influenza immunization clinic for health care workers. *Am J Health Syst Pharm*. 2003;60(3):241-243.

11. Center for Disease Control and Prevention. Comprehensive Clinic Assessment Software Application (CoCASA). http://www.cdc.gov/vaccines/programs/cocasa/default.htm. Accessed January 23, 2008. ∎

Appendix 1. Immunization Protocol Adapted From the University of Pittsburgh Medical Center.

Purpose: To protect people from preventable infectious diseases that cause needless death and disease, the pharmacist may administer the following immunizations to adult patients over the age of 18 years, according to indications and contraindications recommended in current guidelines from the Advisory Committee on Immunization Practices of the US Centers for Disease Control and Prevention and other competent authorities.

Policy: The following named individuals acting as an agent ("Pharmacist") for the undersigned physician, according to and in compliance with Article 27.401 of the State of Pennsylvania Pharmacy Practice Act, may independently determine if a patient should receive one or more of the vaccines listed below. This standing order shall serve as the prescription order for these vaccines as well as the standing order for epinephrine and other emergency measures as described below.

Pharmacist Name, with Pharmacy License # XXXX (Expires XX-XX-XX) and Authorization to Administer Injectables # XXXXX

Name of Immunization	Dose	Route Administration	Site of Administration	Comments
Pneumococcal vaccine (PPV23)	0.5 mL	IM (preferred) or subcutaneous	Deltoid	
Influenza vaccine	0.5 mL	IM	Deltoid	
Zostavax (zoster vaccine live)	0.65 mL	subcutaneous	Deltoid	
Hepatitis B (*Recombivax*)	0.1 mL	IM	Deltoid	3 injection series: Month 0, 3, 6
Hepatitis A (*Havrix*)	0.1 mL	IM	Deltoid	2 injection series: Month 0, 6-12
Tdap (*ADACEL*)	0.5 mL	IM	Deltoid	Adults 18 to 64 years of age if Tdap not received or no record of primary series
Td	0.5 mL	IM	Deltoid	

IM = intramuscular

In the course of immunizing, the pharmacist will adhere to Universal Precautions and Occupational Safety and Health Administration's blood borne pathogen procedures. The pharmacist will have completed a training course authorized by the Pennsylvania Pharmacy Board and maintain current certification in cardiopulmonary resuscitation (CPR) or basic cardiac life support issued by the American Heart Association or American Red Cross. Immunizations will be provided at the Falk Pharmacy Patient Care Center (Medication Therapy Management Services) or at other locations within the University of Pittsburgh and University of Pittsburgh Medical Center (UPMC) Oakland Campus.

Perpetual records of all immunizations administered will be maintained for a period of 2 years from the date of administration of the immunization. Before immunization, vaccine candidates will be screened regarding previous adverse events caused by vaccines, the receipt of blood or antibody products, pregnancy, and underlying diseases. All vaccine candidates will be informed of the specific benefits and risks of the vaccine offered and will be provided with a Vaccine Information Statement (VIS) as required by law.

The patient will be monitored following the immunization(s) for a suitable period of time, a minimum of 15 minutes. In the course of treating adverse events and/or anaphylaxis following immunization, the pharmacist is authorized to initiate emergency response, administer epinephrine, and/or CPR pending arrival of emergency medical services (EMS) as outlined in **Appendix A** (not provided). If such an event occurs, the patient's primary care physician will be notified within 24 hours of the reaction as well as the undersigned authorizing physician. In addition, a Vaccine Adverse Event Reporting System (VAERS) form will be completed and submitted to the Center for

Disease Control and Pennsylvania, to the undersigned licensed practitioner, and to the patient's primary care physician.

Upon accidental needlestick, the pharmacist will comply with UPMC's Post Exposure Control Plan Policy. The pharmacist will file an Injury Log report with the UPMC Employee Health Services, which includes the name of the injured person, date, type, and brand of device involved, where the injury occurred, explanation of the incident, and signature of the Executive Director of Pharmacy of the UPMC.

When the pharmacist administers an immunization to a patient pursuant to a prescription other than the authorizing physician in this agreement, the pharmacist shall notify the ordering prescriber electronically, or via fax, within 72 hours of administration. If administration occurs under this protocol, the pharmacist will transmit the administration records electronically, or via fax, to the participating authorizing physician of this protocol within 72 hours of administration.

Management of Severe Allergic/Anaphylactic Reactions

The administering pharmacist will take every precaution to minimize the risk of adverse events by taking a thorough history for allergies and prior adverse events before any immunization is administered. Patients who receive vaccines will be observed for a period of at least 15 minutes after vaccination and the patient will be reminded to report any side effects to the pharmacist.

Recognition of Severe Allergic/Anaphylactic Reactions

Symptoms include sudden onset of itching and redness, with or without hives, within several minutes of vaccine administration. The symptoms may be localized (area of the injection) or generalized (angioedema, bronchospasm).

Emergency Supplies

- Epinephrine USP, 1 mg/mL (1:1,000) supplied as adult *EpiPen* (4), ampules, or vials. Syringe and needle (or filter needle if ampule) for administration of epinephrine.
- Blood pressure cuff and stethoscope.
- Supplies will be verified before each session for presence and expiration date.

Procedures for Treatment of Allergic/Anaphylactic Reactions

Prepare for possible syncopal episodes or collapsing with adequate physical space to decrease potential for injury as well as to place the patient flat on a hard surface if CPR is needed.

Emergency Treatment:

1. If itching and swelling are confined to the extremity in which the immunization was administered, observe patient closely for a suitable period, watching for generalized symptoms. If none occur, go to step 6.
2. If symptoms are generalized, activate EMS; if within UPMC Presbyterian, UPMC Montefiore, Eye and Ear Institute, or Falk Clinic building call (7-2345) for a "Condition;" if outside of a UPMC building within the University, call Allegheny County 911.
3. Administer epinephrine at 0.01 mg/kg (max 0.5 mg per dose) intramuscular or subcutaneous to the anterior thigh or deltoid.
4. Monitor patient closely until EMS arrives. Perform CPR and maintain airway, if necessary. Keep patient in supine position unless he or she is having difficulty breathing. If breathing is difficult, patient's head may be elevated—provided blood pressure is adequate to prevent loss of consciousness. Frequently monitor vitals signs.
5. If EMS has not arrived and symptoms are still present, repeat dose of epinephrine every 5 to 20 minutes, depending on patient response.
6. Refer patient for medical evaluation, even if symptoms are completely resolved. Symptoms may reoccur after epinephrine wears off, as much as 24 hours later. After the event is concluded, complete a Vaccine Adverse Event Reporting System Form at http:www.vaers.org and notify the referring or participating physician.

Pharmacy Medication Therapy Management Services and Reimbursement Options

Lindsey R. Kelley, PharmD, MS*; Jessica Vink, PharmD†; and Scott M. Mark, PharmD, MS, MEd‡

The *Director's Forum* series is written and edited by Robert Weber and Scott Mark and is designed to guide pharmacy leaders in establishing patient-centered services in hospitals and health systems. As more pharmacy boards are approving and endorsing medication therapy, management directors of pharmacy will need to understand mechanisms for payment for these services. This article provides some initial information for pharmacy directors in developing a strategy for financial support of pharmacy cognitive services.

The US population is advancing in age, and health care expenditures continue to rise.[1] The Agency for Healthcare Research and Quality recently released a publication on chronic disease that claimed rates of hospital readmissions and annual costs per person are dependent on the number of chronic conditions a patient has. They also stated increased focus on these patients could significantly reduce readmissions and total hospital costs.[2] Medication therapy management (MTM) represents a new pharmaceutical care program and is a primary tool for targeting patients with chronic conditions. Payers are aware of the increasing cost of chronic disease and the result is an emphasis on continuity of care before and after hospitalization.

Providing excellent patient care in a revenue-generating environment represents a great opportunity for health-system pharmacy services. For example, many hospitals and health care organizations support retail pharmacy services for both patients and employees where MTM can be provided by pharmacists in addition to dispensing prescriptions. In addition, some pharmacy departments deploy pharmacists in hospital-based clinics to provide added support to physicians and nurses to identify and manage drug-related problems. Finally, many pharmacy boards are revising their practice regulations allowing pharmacists to collaboratively manage medications with other health care professionals. For example, at the University of Pittsburgh Medical Center, a specialist transplant pharmacotherapy manages a patient clinic of new and existing heart transplant patients. As part of their duties, the clinical pharmacy specialist actively adjusts dosage of immunosuppressant medications, monitors and manages metabolic effects of transplantation (eg, hyperglycemia, hypertension) and educates patients, families, and other caregivers.

To sustain these services as described above, however, a revenue

*Pharmacy Manager, UPMC Shadyside, University of Pittsburgh Medical Center, Pittsburgh, Pennsylvania; †Clinical Pharmacist, UPMC Shadyside, University of Pittsburgh Medical Center, Pittsburgh, Pennsylvania; ‡Director of Pharmacy, University of Pittsburgh Medical Center, Associate Professor and Vice Chair, University of Pittsburgh School of Pharmacy, Pittsburgh, Pennsylvania.

cycle around MTM should be managed and developed. As a result, this article of the *Director's Forum* provides directors of pharmacy an overview of billing and reimbursement for medication management services. The specific aims of this paper are to (1) define activities and outcomes associated with MTM, (2) provide a primer on billing in health care, and (3) list the current and future ways pharmacists can bill for clinical services with the intent of providing the director with tools to develop a strategy for approaching pharmacy clinical services billing.

The pharmacy profession has succeeded in advancing patient care from 3-minute window counseling sessions to half-hour appointments scheduled with a pharmacist. Accomplishments of such endeavors such as the Asheville Project, the Diabetes Ten City Challenge, and the Minnesota Experience Project on improving outcomes for patients with chronic disease not only stress the need for pharmaceutical services but also show the monetary value of the services.[3,4] Advancements in innovative services such as chronic disease state management provide exceptional patient care and serve as an avenue for compensation. These services include medication management of chronic disease states, laboratory monitoring, and immunizations.

Providing advanced services is professionally fulfilling, but barriers exist; obtaining compensation for cognitive services is difficult and time and resource needs are great.[5] Though pharmacist-provided MTM services (MTMS) have shifted over the past several years from acute medication provision toward consultation-type services for chronic medications and disease states, it remains difficult to

Table 1. Traditional methods of billing for pharmacist-provided medication therapy management services

Billing method	Definition
Facility fee billing	Provider operating within a hospital-based clinic bills via an ambulatory payment classification group. Common codes: 600, 601, 602.
Evaluation and management billing	Provider practicing with physicians may bill using "incident to" rules. Provider is compensated utilizing coding for the lowest level of billing (99211, 99201).

obtain contracting for these services.[6,7] Payer organizations plan to expand face-to-face pharmacist-patient interaction, but MTMS are still provided by a great variety of practitioners through a great variety of methods.[8]

To advance pharmacy practice, hospitals and community pharmacy organizations must work together to utilize the billing tools available and create services that will benefit patient outcomes. Traditional methods of billing include unique or "back door" mechanisms such as facility fee billing or low level evaluation and management codes also known as "incident to" billing (see **Table 1**).[9] Other billing mechanisms may exist if a provider is able to contract with payers within or outside of their organization. Contract options include employer-paid MTMS, reimbursement using *Current Procedural Terminology* (CPT) codes, or reimbursement under contract for defined services but not utilizing *CPT* coding.

PHARMACY MEDICATION THERAPY MANAGEMENT

In 2008, the American Pharmacists Association (APhA) and the

National Association of Chain Drug Stores (NACDS) published a consensus program on MTMS developed by 11 national pharmacy organizations. MTMS as described in the consensus model follow a model of patient-centered care previously described and do not include medication dispensing. This model has five core elements: medication therapy review (MTR), personal medication record (PMR), medication-related plan (MRP), intervention and/or referral, and documentation and follow-up. All core elements are to be included in the provision of MTMS as all elements are critical, but elements may be shifted or modified based on patient need.[10,11]

The core elements of an MTMS model gives a specific definition to each criterion. MTR is a systematic process of collecting patient-specific information, assessing medication therapies to identify medication-related problems, developing a prioritized list of medication-related problems, and creating a plan to resolve them. The PMR is a comprehensive record of the patient's medications (prescription and nonprescription medications, herbal products, and other dietary supplements). The MRP is a patient-centric document containing a list of actions for the patient to use in tracking progress for self-management. In intervention and referral, the pharmacist provides consultative services and intervenes to address medication-related problems, and, when necessary, refers the patient to a physician or other health care professional. Documentation and follow-up accounts for documenting the MTMS in a consistent manner and scheduling follow-up MTM visits based on the patient's medication-related needs or a transition in care settings.[11,12]

MEDICAID AND MEDICARE MEDICATION THERAPY MANAGEMENT REQUIREMENTS

Since the inception of the Medicare Prescription Drug, Improvement, and Modernization Act of 2003 (MMA), pharmaceutical services have been included in legislation as an appropriate service, and pharmacists have come closer than ever to receiving provider status. This provision states that each insurer acting as a Medicare Part D sponsor must incorporate into their services an MTMS provision. Unfortunately, the MMA was not specific as to the definition of MTMS and did not provide guidance on a specific model. Previous communications from the US Department of Health and Human Services Centers for Medicare & Medicaid Services (CMS) identified these services as professional services designed to promote the safe and effective use of medications. These services may be provided by pharmacists or other qualified providers, may distinguish between settings, and are coordinated with any care management plan for a targeted individual under a chronic care improvement program. There are several requirements established under 42 CFR x423.153(d) that must be met to be compliant.[12]

The federal requirements were updated in April 2009 to include new requirements such as establishing an MTM program (MTMP) that targets beneficiaries who have multiple chronic diseases, are taking multiple Part D drugs, and are likely to incur annual costs greater than the $3,000 cap predetermined by the Secretary. Also new, the MTMP must enroll those targeted beneficiaries using an opt-out method only and evaluate them at least quarterly during the year. The list of chronic diseases specified by CMS includes hypertension, heart failure, diabetes, dyslipidemia, several respiratory diseases, multiple bone diseases, and mental health diseases. Though providers may continue to target self-selected specific disease states, they must target at least four of the seven on the list of core chronic diseases to meet the new requirements (see box titled "Centers for Medicare & Medicaid Services Core Chronic Conditions"). Insurers may also continue to require that targeted beneficiaries meet an established threshold for a minimum number of Part D–covered medications, but they cannot require more than eight Part D medications.[13]

Also included in these updates are requirements that parallel the established core elements model. MTMS offered by Part D sponsors must include a comprehensive MTR by a pharmacist or other qualified professional and must occur at least annually. The comprehensive MTR must include a review of medications, offer a real-time, person-to-person interaction performed either in person or via another interactive method such as a telephone, and implement a systematic process to summarize the consultation and provide the patient an individualized written "take-away" such as a PMR, action plan, or reconciled medication history list. MTMS must also include ongoing monitoring via targeted medication reviews that assess medication needs, unresolved issues, and medication therapy since the last MTR. These follow-up interventions should be interactive and occur at least quarterly, but it is at the discretion of the sponsor as to how to implement the process. The MTMS must then propose an intervention to prescribers either interactively or passively. The last piece of all MTMS provided by Medicare Part D sponsors is measurement and analysis of MTMS outcomes through reports to CMS.[13]

MEDICATION THERAPY MANAGEMENT REIMBURSEMENT OPTIONS
Gratis Services
Performing MTM establishes an on-site professional service to promote safe and effective use of medications. Although pharmacists providing MTMS acknowledge the value to both insurers and patients, many are unsure where to begin billing and seeking reimbursement for the services they provide. Due to the complexity of paperwork, time constraints, and inconsistent reimbursement from third-party payers, many pharmacists have resisted the process to file claims for services. This leads to situations in which pharmacists provide services and simply do not charge for their time or efforts, which allows pharmacists on the front line to be engaged in clinical care opportunities that may not be available if financial incentives had to be in place first. Their services become part of routine care and are never captured as a specific component of a patient bill. Performing MTMS in this manner promotes opportunities to engage senior administrators and insurers in further conversations about potential MTMS participants, benefits, and ultimately reimbursements. Although this method is only available for fiscally sound institutions, it promotes the integration of pharmacy services with established clinics and promotes value of the pharmacy services to patients and other health care providers.

Indirect Billing
Indirect methods have been successful in the past in the recovery of

reimbursement, but in addition to only permitting low-level billing they have other limitations. Both methods of indirect billing, facility fee and "incident to," are broad in scope and therefore do not capture specific pharmacist MTMS. This lack of specificity prevents both tracking and reporting. The inability to track and report pharmacists' impact on patient care results in undervaluation of pharmacist-provided clinical contributions.

Facility fees represent one method of indirect billing available only to hospital-based clinics. Under this method of billing, the provider would utilize the hospital outpatient prospective payment system, which is a prospective payment system developed by CMS that uses median costs based on claims to set a relative payment for hospital outpatient services. It has two components–a professional fee and a technical or facility fee. The submitting organization defines the code criteria and submits the bill under an ambulatory payment classification (APC). The APC is designed to capture all diagnostics, procedures, and drugs. Codes 600, 601, and 602 correspond to low-, middle-, and high-level visits. Code criteria are determined by each specific hospital or institution.[9,14] The reimbursement is paid to the submitting institution. It then becomes imperative to work closely with finance department representatives to ensure revenue is returned to the department of pharmacy or department responsible for the providing pharmacist's salary.

A second method of indirect billing utilizes a provision under Medicare in which a physician may bill for nonphysician services; this is referred to as "incident to" billing because the services are billed as part of the physician

visit. With the implementation of the Health Insurance Portability and Accountability Act (HIPAA), each health care provider was required to obtain a National Provider Identifier (NPI). Under HIPAA, a health care provider is anyone who submits health information in an electronic form. An NPI is used to uniquely identify a provider in health care transactions, such as submission of billing claims.[15] Currently, even though a pharmacist can obtain an NPI, CMS and many other payers do not recognize pharmacists as providers of medical care and therefore do not reimburse for pharmacist-provided consultation. Because of this, many pharmacists providing MTM in physician offices currently employ "incident to" billing, which allows the nonprovider status pharmacist to bill under the physician's provider or NPI. Although there are strict criteria that must be met, this method of billing is easier to implement and requires very little modification to current billing methods. To bill "incident to" a physician, the service provided must be an integral component of the physician visit, must be provided under the direct supervision

Centers for Medicare & Medicaid Services Core Chronic Conditions

Hypertension
Heart failure
Diabetes
Dyslipidemia
Respiratory diseases (such as asthma, chronic obstructive pulmonary disease, or chronic lung disorders)
Bone disease/arthritis (such as osteoporosis, osteoarthritis, or rheumatoid arthritis)
Mental health disorders (such as depression, schizophrenia, bipolar disorder, or chronic and disabling disorders)

of the physician, must be something that is routine practice in a physician's office, and must be documented and medically necessary. Under "incident to" billing, pharmacists bill as a level 1, or low-level [99201(new visit) , 99211 (brief visit)], clinic visit. Examples of services billed this way include anticoagulation monitoring, diabetes management, lipid management, and smoking cessation.[9,16]

Direct Billing

For providers well-positioned to contract with payers, contracts may be negotiated. These contracts are generally developed between specific cohorts of pharmacist-providers. These relationships may exist with local employers or local managed care organizations. The Asheville Project represents a collaboration between the city of Asheville and the North Carolina Center for Pharmaceutical Care. The contract is a fee-for-service intervention that varies based on the level of intervention. Similar programs have been seen in Iowa and Tennessee. A primary market for these types of relationships is self-insured employers.[5] These services, though pharmacist-provider specific in their language, are not required to use pharmacist-specific codes. The insurer simply develops an agreement with the pharmacist-provider cohort to provide outlined services for agreed-upon fees.

Contracts may also be developed that describe services with a common coding language already utilized by health information management services and physician offices. In January 2008, the Pharmacist Services Technical Advisory Coalition successfully obtained three codes within the *CPT* language that are specific to pharmacist-provided services (see Table 2).[17,18] The pharmacy profession and health information technology providers have begun to identify components needed to accommodate these new codes and the amount of data created.[19,20] As these codes are specific, they apply only when the MTMS is performed by a pharmacist. If a physician or other provider performs a medication history or assesses medication therapy, it cannot be billed under these codes and will be captured under existing physician-billing structure.

CPT codes are recommended by CMS as the preferred method of billing for pharmacist-provided MTMS.[13] They may be used as time-based codes or can be translated into crosswalks. Crosswalks may be built based on assessment, identification, complexity of care (number of medical conditions), and/or face-to-face time.

Table 2. *Current Procedural Terminology pharmacist-specific codes*

CPT code	Service definition
99605	MTMS provided by a pharmacist, individual, face-to-face with patient, with assessment and intervention if provided; first-encounter service, new patient (up to 15 min).
99606	MTMS provided by a pharmacist, individual, face-to-face with patient, with assessment and intervention if provided; follow-up encounter with an established patient (up to 15 min).
99607	MTMS provided by a pharmacist, individual, face-to-face with patient, with assessment and intervention if provided; combined with 99605 or 99606 to bill for additional time in 15 min increments.

Note: CPT = Current Procedural Terminology; MTMS = medication therapy management services.

Criteria would then correspond to a unit of service and a rate. Appropriate metrics for MTMS clinics include employee satisfaction (if contracted with a health-system based insurance provider), reductions in quantity and severity of medication therapy events, and improvements in other clinical markers (blood pressure, hemoglobin A1c, low-density lipoprotein/high-density lipoprotein cholesterol).[4,21] Financial metrics include direct health care costs to insurers, lost productivity for employers, and a consideration for increased productivity based on increased overall wellness of staff.[3,14]

Another method of reimbursement that may or may not use *CPT* codes is a "superbill" or paper summary of all services rendered for a patient while at the clinic. This method wraps all services into one form, which is then provided to the patient at the end of their visit. These types of superbills may use *ICD-9* diagnosis codes, *CPT* codes, and any service performed that may not currently have a corresponding code. Documentation of all services gives patients information to follow-up for fees with their insurance carrier or correlate the information to their health spending account. Resources for creating superbills are available from APhA and NACDS.[22]

CONCLUSION

Pharmacy departments in hospitals have a unique opportunity to collaborate with other health care professionals in performing MTM services. MTM can be provided by pharmacists as a part of a hospital-based retail pharmacy or in hospital-based clinics. To establish a financially viable MTM model, pharmacists will need to begin using appropriate CPT codes to (1) determine volume of services and (2)

determine potential reimbursed costs for these services. As the pharmacy directors establish MTM services in their departments, it will be vital for them to continually interface with the organization's billing/finance departments on the effects of using the pharmacy CPT codes. Demonstrating both the cost-effectiveness and clinical benefits of MTM can only strengthen an organization's investment in this valuable pharmacy service.

REFERENCES

1. Centers for Medicaid & Medicare Services. Overview of national health expenditure data. Available at: http://www.cms.hhs.gov/National HealthExpendData/. Accessed March 10, 2010.

2. Agency for Healthcare Research and Quality. Chronic Disease: A greater number of different chronic conditions increases hospital readmissions and costs. August 2009. Available at: http://www.ahrq.gov/research/aug09/0809RA16.htm. Accessed February 10, 2010.

3. Bunting BA, Cranor CW. The Asheville project: long-term clinical, humanistic, and economic outcomes of a community-based medication therapy management program for asthma. *J Am Pharm Assoc (2003)*. 2006;46(2):133-147.

4. Fera T, Bluml BM, Ellis WM. Diabetes Ten City Challenge: final economic and clinical results. *J Am Pharm Assoc (2003)*. 2009;49(3):383-391.

5. Snella KA, Trewyn RR, Hansen LB, Bradberry JC. Pharmacist compensation for cognitive services: focus on the physician office and community pharmacy. *Pharmacotherapy*. 2004;24(3):372-388.

6. Barnett MJ, Frank J, Wehring H, et al. Analysis of pharmacist-provided medication therapy management (MTM) services in community pharmacies over 7 years. *J Manag Care Pharm*. 2009;15(1):18-31.

7. Thomas J, Zingone MM, Smith J, George CM. Feasibility of contracting for medication therapy management services in a physician's office. *Am J Health Syst Pharm*. 2009;66(15):1390-1393.

8. Schommer JC, Planas LG, Johnson KA, Doucette WR. Pharmacist-provided medication therapy management (part 1): Provider per-

spectives in 2007. *J Am Pharm Assoc (2003)*. 2008;48(3):354-363.

9. Christensen D. Hospital-based ambulatory pharmacy services. In: Vogenberg FR, ed. *Understanding Pharmacy Reimbursement*. 1st ed. Bethesda, MD: American Society of Health-System Pharmacists; 2006:103.

10. Pellegrino AN, Martin MT, Tilton JJ, Touchette DR. Medication therapy management services: Definitions and outcomes. *Drugs*. 2009;69(4):393-406.

11. American Pharmacists Association, National Association of Chain Drug Stores Foundation. Medication therapy management in pharmacy practice: core elements of an MTM service model (version 2.0). *J Am Pharm Assoc (2003)*. 2008; 48(3):341-353.

12. Centers for Medicaid & Medicare Services. The Medicare Prescription Drug, Improvement, and Modernization Act. HR 1/Pub. L. No. 108-173. Published December 8, 2003. Accessed 2010.

13. US Department of Health & Human Services, Centers for Medicare & Medicaid Services. Memorandum to all Part D Sponsors: Contract year 2010 medication therapy management program (MTMP) submission. April 10, 2009.

14. Snella KA, Sachdev GP. A primer for developing pharmacist-managed clinics in the outpatient setting. *Pharmacotherapy*. 2003;23(9):1153-1166.

15. Overview on National Provider Identifier Standard (NPI). Centers for Medicare & Medicaid Services Web site. http://www.cms.hhs.gov/NationalProvIdentStand. Updated October 28, 2009. Accessed February 10, 2010.

16. Zingone MM, Malcolm KE, McCormick SW, Bledsoe KR. Analysis of pharmacist charges for medication therapy management services in an outpatient setting. *Am J Health Syst Pharm*. 2007;64(17):1827-1831.

17. Medication therapy management service codes. Pharmacist Services Technical Advisory Coalition Web site. http://www.pstac.org/services/mtms-codes.html#codemodel. Accessed February 10, 2010.

18. Coding communication: medication therapy management. *CPT Assistant*. 2008;18(8):3-15.

19. McMahan R. Operationalizing MTM through the use of health information technology. *J Manag Care Pharm*. 2008; 14(2 Suppl):S18-21.

20. Millonig MK. Mapping the route to medication therapy management documentation and billing standardization and interoperability within the health care system: meeting proceedings. *J Am Pharm Assoc (2003)*. 2009;49(3):372-382.

21. Isetts BJ, Schondelmeyer SW, Artz MB, et al. Clinical and economic outcomes of medication therapy management services: The Minnesota experience. *J Am Pharm Assoc (2003)*. 2008;48(2):203-211.

22. Hogue MD, McDonough R, Bennett M, Bryner C, Thomas RA. APhA Academy of Pharmacy Practice & Management Medication Therapy Management Task Force. Development of a medication therapy management superbill for ambulatory care/community pharmacy practice. *J Am Pharm Assoc (2003)*. 2009;49(2):232-236. ∎

Developing Patient-Centered Pharmacy Services Through Residency Training

Katie McMillen, PharmD* and Robert J. Weber, MS, FASHP†

Hospital pharmacy directors are faced with the challenge of implementing patient-centered services, which often requirers changing the pharmacists' role in patient care. An approach to develop pharmacists focused on patient care is to support post-graduate training programs that provide the pharmacists with specific patient-care skills. This month's *Director's Forum* presents a brief overview of pharmacy residency training as well as practical tips for directors interested in developing a residency program.

INTRODUCTION

The role of the pharmacist has changed dramatically over the years. Pharmacists' primary focus has shifted from filling and dispensing medications to assuming the responsibility of using medications in the prevention and treatment of diseases. Pharmacists have integrated a complexity of services into the health care profession. Developments in technology help create more efficient and effective operations, enabling pharmacists to focus on providing pharmaceutical care. Clinical pharmacists have emerged as providers in comprehensive drug management to patients and providers. Studies have shown that the development of clinical pharmacist services has made an improvement in patient outcomes.[1] The mission of a pharmacist is to improve patient outcomes through the optimal use of medications. The American College of Clinical Pharmacy (ACCP) and American Society of Health-System Pharmacists (ASHP) are two professional organizations that endorse the development of clinical management leaders through activities and residency training.[2,3]

Every hospital pharmacy director must decide how to optimally utilize the resources available to provide superior patient care. Resident programs provide an avenue to assist institutions in improving the efficiency and quality of services they provide. Regardless of the size of your institution, the development of residency programs can help promote patient-centered pharmacy services.

This article reviews the importance of pharmacy residency training as an integral part of establishing patient-centered pharmacy services; it also provides hospital pharmacy directors information on residency training along with steps and strategies to develop a residency training program. The specific aims of this article are to (1) provide background information on pharmacy residency training; (2) describe requirement considerations for a residency program; (3) provide strategies for justifying a pharmacy residency training program; and (4) describe the structure of the pharmacy practice management residency at the

---

*Pharmacy Resident—Practice Management, University of Pittsburgh School of Pharmacy, University of Pittsburgh Medical Center; †Associate Professor and Chair, University of Pittsburgh School of Pharmacy, Executive Director of Pharmacy, University of Pittsburgh Medical Center

University of Pittsburgh Medical Center (UPMC).

HISTORY AND BACKGROUND ON PHARMACY RESIDENCY TRAINING

The development of residency practice has evolved since the early 1930s. Early residency training focused on the development of managers for hospitals. Since then, residency training has encompassed a vast array of specialty training with a focus on clinical practice.[4] Currently, there are almost 900 American Society of Health-System Pharmacists (ASHP)-accredited residency programs.[5] Residency programs have been developed throughout the country as a means of educating the profession's future practitioners and leaders. New ASHP accreditation guidelines categorize residency programs as either a post graduate year 1 (PGY1) or post graduate year 2 (PGY2). PGY1 residencies in pharmacy practice are organized, directed, postgraduate training programs that center on the development of knowledge, attitudes, and skills needed to promote rational drug therapy. The purpose of a PGY1 residency is to accelerate and strengthen the individual's development of clinical skills and knowledge. Examples of PGY1 residencies include pharmacy practice with or without an area of interest, community, and managed care. PGY2 specialized residency programs include an emphasis on optimizing patient outcomes in a focused area of health care and a commitment to prepare a new generation for leadership within the specialty area of the profession. A few specialty areas of interest include: ambulatory care, drug information, critical care, cardiology, infectious disease, oncology, and practice management.

REQUIREMENTS AND CONSIDERATIONS FOR PHARMACY RESIDENCY PROGRAMS

ASHP accreditation standards and requirements are important factors to consider when developing a pharmacy residency program. ASHP has an established process in place to ensure standards and the quality of the program. Whether you are implementing a PGY1 or PGY2 program will dictate the specific requirements. An initial assessment should be performed to determine if the necessary elements are in place to train residents. The next step is to devise a group of potential preceptors to support the program and begin the development of a residency structure. The pharmacy director should prepare a cost-justification analysis in support of the development of the residency program.

JUSTIFYING A PHARMACY RESIDENCY PROGRAM

The pharmacy director must be able to provide justification to support the clinical and economical impact of a pharmacy resident. Health care resources are becoming increasingly scarce with increased competition to secure funds. Pharmacy residents can provide clinical, staffing, managerial, and academic resources for a fraction of the cost of nonresident personnel. Residents participate in activities and projects that can improve patient care and decrease costs for their institution. Resident staffing is one approach to cost justification of a residency program. For example, at UPMC, residents are required to staff every other weekend and holiday; this accounts for 56 shifts or 448 hours. Residents may also provide coverage for staff meetings, vacations, and holiday breaks according to resident availability and department need.

Clinical practice is an emphasis and priority for all PGY1 residents. Residents can help research and recommend the safest, most efficacious, most cost-effective therapy to other members of the health care team. They help provide support to areas and programs that might not otherwise be provided. At UPMC, residents help to expand pharmacy rounding coverage and participate in the development of programs such as core measure monitoring. Accredited programs require that each resident complete one major research project for each year of residency training. The projects are specifically designed to benefit the department and/or institution through increased knowledge and the potential enhancement of services. Residents also provide benefits through publications, teaching, mentoring, and working with physician subcommittees, the Pharmacy and Therapeutics Committee, and the Quality Improvement Committees.

Table 1 describes an example of a cost justification for a pharmacy residency program. Importantly, the Center for Medicare and Medicaid Services (CMS) reimburses hospitals partially for pharmacy practice residencies as part of the graduate medical education financial support

Table 1. Sample Cost-Justification for a Pharmacy Residency

PROGRAM COSTS		
Item	*Frequency/Amount*	*Cost*
Resident salary	Four/yr	$136,000
OTHER COSTS		
Preceptor teaching time	Main Rotations: 8 preceptors at approximately 1,040 h (0.5 FTEs)	$45,000
Space	Desk space, office rent (approximately 300 sq ft) at $20/sq ft	$6,000
Equipment	Computers	$4,000
Estimated Total		$191,000
BENEFIT/SAVINGS		
Service	*Frequency/Amount*	*Saving*
Staffing	Base: 416 h ($40/hour) x four (x 2 yr) $66,560 ($133,120)	$66,560 ($133,120)
Management services (eg, human resources issues, project implementation)	Approximately 10 h/wk/yr	$104,000 (for 520 h over 1 yr x 4 residents @ $50/h)
Subtotal		$170,560
Medicare reimbursement (per resident)	$10,200	$40,800
Grand Total		$211,360

FTE = full-time equivalency

system of CMS. Advanced practice residency programs are not reimbursed by CMS; in our institution, approximately 30% of a pharmacy practice resident salary is recovered from CMS.

PHARMACY PRACTICE MANAGEMENT RESIDENCY AT THE UNIVERSITY OF PITTSBURGH MEDICAL CENTER

Table 2 describes the rotation structure for UPMC's practice management specialty residency. The resident experience combines a pharmacy practice residency and a specialty residency in pharmacy administration. This schedule can be used as a template to design a pharmacy practice residency. UPMC offers a 24-month specialty pharmacy residency in pharmacy administration with the opportunity to complete a health-related Masters degree (MPH, MHA). The program is divided into 2 years, representing PGY1 and PGY2 with the primary goal of preparing pharmacists to assume leadership positions in health care systems. Residents will be concurrently enrolled in the University Of Pittsburgh Graduate School of Public Health. A minimum of 38 credit hours of graduate course work and the successful completion and submission of a manuscript for publication of a residency research project are required for completion of the graduate program.

The PGY1 year is designed to teach the residents how to practice as a pharmacist. An emphasis on clinical practice is a priority during the resident's major rotations.

Residents are required to complete four clinical rotations, two central pharmacy operations rotations, and a Drug Use and Disease State Management (DUDSM) rotation. Residents will also complete four focused 1-week rotations in select management areas. Residency rotations are designed to develop the resident's skills, attitudes, and abilities necessary to independently and competently optimize pharmacotherapy outcomes through direct patient care and pharmacy practice management. During the first year, residents are exposed to the basic concepts of pharmacy administration. Residents participate in an array of activities that focus on leadership and management, such as scheduling, interviewing, teaching, training, and human resource management, that will continue through PGY2. Integration with the University of Pittsburgh School of Pharmacy will allow for interaction with faculty and students as well as other experiences necessary for success in an academic health system. Residents participate in the University of Pittsburgh School of Pharmacy resident platform presentations, journal clubs, research methodology discussions and work groups, and UPMC Pharmacy Management Special Management Topics Discussion Series.

The PGY2 year of the pharmacy management residency at UPMC provides opportunities for the resident to further develop leadership and expert pharmacy management skills in an academic medical center. Residents develop a strong foundation in pharmacy services management through 12 flexible rotations in health system pharmacy. Residents are assigned rotations with pharmacy administrators in hospital pharmacy operations management, community hospital pharmacy, information technology and automation, finance, purchasing and distribution, drug use management,

Table 2. Sample Rotations and Structure for a Pharmacy Practice Management Residency

Year 1—Pharmacy Practice

Month	July	Aug	Sept	Oct	Nov	Dec	Jan	Feb	Mar	April	May	Jun
	Orientation		Clinical Rotation 1	Clinical Rotation 2	Clinical Rotation 3	Central Pharmacy Rotation	Clinical Rotation 4	Drug Utilization		Central Pharmacy	Clinical Management Rotation 2	

Year 2—Practice Management

Resident	July	August	September	October	November	December
	Medication Safety	Community Hospital	Operations Management	Corporate Pharmacy	Technology and Automation	Midyear/Central Operations

Option 2
Longitudinal Rotation

Drug Use and Disease State Management

	January	February	March	April	May	June
	Inventory Management-Purchasing and Distribution HC Central	Finance and Budgeting	Contracts and Asset Management	Advanced Technology and Automation (elective)	Education/Development	Advanced Operations Management

and medication safety and education. Practice Management residents also provide administrative services to the department. Residents participate in activities such as manager-on-call, recruitment, teaching, training, mentoring, and special project management.

SUMMARY AND CONCLUSION

The development of a residency programs can provide invaluable benefits to any pharmacy department and institution. The director of pharmacy must design the ideal residency program based on their institution assessment as well as adequately cost-justify the program through the development of patient-centered programs through residency training.

REFERENCES

1. American College of Clinical Pharmacy. Mission statement. http://www.accp.com/about.php#mission. Accessed June 26, 2007.

2. American Society of Health-System Pharmacists. ASHP mission and vision. http://www.ashp.org/s_ashp/docs/files/ashp_mission-vision.pdf. Accessed June 26, 2007.

3. Kaboli PJ, Hoth AB, McClimon BJ, Schnipper, JL. Clinical pharmacists and inpatient medical care. *Arch Intern Med.* 2006;166:955-964.

4. American Society of Health-System Pharmacists. History of residency training. http://www.ashp.org/s_ashp/cat1c.asp?CID=3499&DID=5437. Accessed June 26, 2007.

5. American Society of Health System Pharmacists. ASHP residency directory. http://www.ashp.org/s_ashp/residency_index.asp. Accessed June 26, 2007. ∎

Strategies for Evaluating Clinical Pharmacy Services

Michael Sanborn, MS, FASHP *

These series of articles of the *Director's Forum* switch their focus from the core competencies of hospital pharmacy practice to programs that enhance the ability of the pharmacy to provide patient-centered services. In the September 2006 issue, decentralized pharmacy services were reviewed and recommended as an effective patient-centered strategy for a hospital pharmacy. In the October 2006 issue, strategies for developing advanced practice clinical programs were discussed. These services place the pharmacist closer to patients, enhancing their ability to be involved directly in all aspects of effective medication therapy management.

In today's era of declining healthcare reimbursement and increased cost containment, pharmacy resources continue to be scrutinized. Pharmacy directors must be able to readily justify their staff and consistently demonstrate a meaningful pharmacy return on investment for the hospital. Further, the desire and demand for clinical programs is often a significant challenge in light of the resources available. An important question, however, is: As a pharmacy director, how do I know that the clinical pharmacy services that my department provides are effective? An even more fundamental question is: What clinical services should my department be providing?

The intent of this article is to address both of these questions and to highlight practical methods that can be employed to evaluate the collective impact of pharmacy services provided, rather than to discuss the performance evaluation of individual pharmacists. Much of the research associated with pharmacy service evaluation was conducted in the 1970s and 1980s in an effort to justify the impact that a pharmacist can have as an active participant on the health care team. Since that time, many studies have been published that continue to demonstrate the impact that a well-positioned pharmacist can have on patient care.[1,2]

Pharmacist involvement in clinical activities continues to grow. A relatively recent survey of hospital pharmacies indicates that virtually all hospitals (95.3%) have pharmacists regularly monitoring medication therapy for patients; however, only 42.8% of respondents monitor therapy for more than half of their patients.[3] The majority of hospitals also routinely monitor serum medication levels (for aminoglycosides, vancomycin, and narrow therapeutic index medications) or their surrogate markers, although there was a statistically significant difference favoring larger facilities providing this service. The survey also found that the amount of time pharmacists spent on monitoring drug therapy increased over the years.

PROVIDING APPROPRIATE CLINICAL SERVICES

One of the most challenging dilemmas for a pharmacy director is resource allocation. Ideally, every hospital pharmacy department would consist of enough pharmacists and

---

*Corporate Director of Pharmacy, Baylor Health Care System, Dallas, TX

technicians to carry out all drug distribution activities *and* provide extensive clinical pharmacy services for every patient. Because this situation is rarely the case, decisions must be made regarding which patients benefit most from pharmacist involvement. In 1996, the American Society of Health-System Pharmacists published guidelines on a standardized method for pharmaceutical care; however, the intent and foci of this document is on patient monitoring, plan development, and solving patient problems as opposed to a listing of clinical services that can be provided.[4]

There are a variety of indicators that can assist with the focus of pharmacy services. Congruence with major hospital service lines, for example, should always be considered when developing clinical pharmacy programs and services. Other important factors include patient acuity, length of stay, and even available pharmacist expertise. Medications that pose a greater risk of patient harm, are prone to improper utilization, or that significantly increase pharmacy expenditures should also have a bearing on services provided. Additionally, there are pharmacy services that have been shown to have a significant impact on patient outcomes (eg, pharmacist-managed aminoglycoside or vancomycin therapy was associated with significant improvement in health care and economic outcomes[5]) and these should always receive high priority.

It is also important to mention the need for triage as it relates to clinical service offerings. Many hospitals have developed a list of medications or identified specific hospital areas such as critical care or transplant services that always require an advanced level of patient monitoring.

The most comprehensive analysis of prognostic criteria for patients requiring clinical pharmacy services can be found in a series of articles published by Young and colleagues in 1974.[6,7] The authors found that variables such as patient temperature, number of diagnoses, number of abnormal lab values, and type of admission were strong predictors for advanced pharmacist monitoring. Additional research in this area would be quite valuable. Using computerized, rules-based algorithms for decision support can also assist with the integration of electronic laboratory and pertinent patient data with medication profiles to identify patients that require more intensive monitoring or intervention. Often such screening can occur automatically within the pharmacy's information system, or there are a variety of software products available that are designed to correlate key patient data elements and identify potential patient problems.[8]

Because pharmacy service offerings can vary significantly based on all of the factors discussed, there is not one definitive list or menu of clinical programs, and new services are constantly evolving. Core services such as pharmacokinetic monitoring, renal dosing, intravenous (IV) to oral conversions, nutrition support services, patient counseling, and participation on the cardiopulmonary resuscitation team should always be considered. A previous *Director's Forum* article discussed advance practice services and specialty practice, and an example of establishing an advanced practice program for the ICU was reviewed.[9] Pharmacist participation on patient-care rounds can also be an effective way for pharmacists to review and make interventions at the time of prescribing. When designing and implementing any new service, a thorough review of the literature can be helpful in identifying successful elements of the program.

It is also important to frequently reevaluate the clinical services that the department provides and to set short- and long-term goals for future program development. One effective and newly available pharmacy evaluation resource is the ASHP 2015 Self-Assessment Tool, which is available online at http://www.ashp.org/2015/2015SA_tool.pdf. The tool is designed to quickly and easily measure compliance with the 6 goals associated with the 2015 Initiative.

EVALUATING THE EFFECTIVENESS OF THE SERVICES PROVIDED

Once clinical services are established, what is the best way to ensure that they are effective? There are numerous methods, both direct and indirect, to appraise the value of clinical services provided. The options available depend on the service under review and several examples of evaluation techniques will be discussed.

One of the most common methods to evaluate services is through the review of documented pharmacist interventions. Most hospitals have developed electronic documentation systems that are either integrated with the pharmacy information system or function as a stand-alone software product. A weakness of this measurement system is underreporting, in that clinical activities can occur but the pharmacist fails to document them. As a result, documentation of interventions has become more convenient, with some hospitals showing improvement in intervention capture using technologies such as handheld

devices.[10] Also, there is evidence to suggest that the reliability and validity of computerized pharmacist interventions, especially as it relates to coding, is limited.[11] Nonetheless, intervention documentation remains a mainstay of the phamacist's contribution to patient care.

Most intervention systems can be customized so that activities associated with a specific clinical program can be documented easily. For example, most systems include categories for pharmacokinetic consults, renal dosing, and participation in rounds. Analysis of these categories can be very useful in the review and justification of a particular service. When possible, pharmacists should be encouraged to provide some level of detail when documenting the intervention so that the specifics are clear. To illustrate, rather than simply documenting "renal dosing," which gives little information about what actually transpired, the pharmacist should list "renal dosing: CrCl = 50 mL/min so dose decreased to 250 mg." Likewise, listing "patient-care rounds" is less helpful than individually listing the recommendations and consultations that occurred during the rounding process.

With respect to interventions, it is important to focus on the quality of interventions more than the quantity documented. The data should be reviewed regularly and analyzed for trends, cost effectiveness, acceptance rates, and new opportunities to improve a particular service. For instance, the number of physician-requested, aminoglycoside, pharmacokinetic consults can be compared with the total number of patients on aminoglycosides for the same period. Using this data and the documented patient outcomes, it may be possible to gain approval to expand the service to automatically cover all patients on aminoglycosides without a physician request.

Another method to measure the effectiveness of a particular service is to survey those directly affected by the service. This survey can involve patients, physicians, or other health care professionals, and can often provide important information regarding the success of the program as well as uncover potential opportunities for improvement. Koffler and colleagues, as an example, surveyed providers before and after participation in an ambulatory family medicine consult service and found that the service was beneficial to both providers and patients of the clinic.[12]

Benchmarking services against other programs can also provide worthwhile information regarding program effectiveness. For example, comparing the ratio of oral to IV doses of a particular drug with those of other facilities can suggest whether an IV to oral program is operating at peak performance. External benchmarking can be quite difficult because of variations between facilities and the integrity of the datasets; however, useful information can often be obtained despite these limitations.[13] Internal benchmarking comparisons can also be useful, and can be made within particular diagnoses related groups, medical services, by pharmacist, or using a variety of other variables.

Direct measurement of program effectiveness using a control group can also provide useful information and successfully demonstrate the impact of a pharmacist on patient care. This type of analysis can be more complicated and, in some cases, may require

approval by the hospital's institutional review board. As a case in point, Jill True Robke and colleagues evaluated the effectiveness of a pharmacist-led pneumococcal vaccination program and demonstrated a statistically significant improvement in the immunization of at-risk patients versus a control group.[14] The authors also identified several opportunities for improvement as part of the trial.

Another way to evaluate programs is to measure the impact of a particular program on drug expenditures or drug utilization. This can be accomplished through a formal drug utilization review or by measuring the amount spent on a specific agent before and after implementation of a program. When using this method, it is important to adjust for differences in patient population, volume, acuity, and other variables where appropriate.

Other methods of evaluation include direct observation, peer review, and audits. Each has its own advantages, disadvantages, and varying levels of utility depending on the service under review. With each method there exists an inherent amount of variability depending on the observer, reviewer(s), or audit tool. Like some of the other tools discussed, however, these methods can be used to assess both the quality and the effectiveness of the program under review. Depending on necessity, the methods can be conducted on a regular basis to measure the consistency of performance or used intermittently as a one-time evaluation tool.

Some examples of these types of evaluation could include shadowing pharmacists during patient-care rounds and observing the interactions and impact that they have. Querying residents regarding their rounding experience with a particular pharmacist would be another way to obtain this type of information. Peer review groups can be effective in analyzing specific pharmacist recommendations or interventions. Chart audits can be conducted by reviewing pre-selected charts based on drug use or patient population and evaluating departmental performance as it relates to programs such as therapeutic interchange, nutrition support consults, renal dosing, or IV to oral conversions.

SUMMARY

Choosing the right clinical programs to implement depends on a variety of hospital and patient-specific parameters. There are many ways to evaluate clinical program performance, and an organized review strategy is important to the assessment of overall department operations. Moving pharmacists closer to patients, developing clinical and advance practice programs, and regularly measuring the effectiveness of these programs are critical elements of a high-performance pharmacy department.

REFERENCES

1. Kaboli PJ, Hoth AB, McClimon BJ, Schnipper JL. Clinical pharmacists and inpatient medical care: a systematic review. *Arch Intern Med.* 2006;166:955-964.

2. Morrison A, Wertheimer AI. Evaluation of studies investigating the effectiveness of pharmacists' clinical services. *Am J Health Syst Pharm.* 2001;58:569-577.

3. Pedersen CA, Schneider PJ, Scheckelhoff DJ. ASHP national survey of pharmacy practice in hospital settings: monitoring and patient education—2003. *Am J Health Syst Pharm.* 2004;61:457-471.

4. American Society of Health-System Pharmacists. ASHP guidelines on a standardized method for pharmaceutical care. Am J Health-Syst Pharm. 1996;53:1713–1716.

5. Bond CA, Raehl CL. Clinical and economic outcomes of pharmacist-managed aminoglycoside or vancomycin therapy. *Am J Health Syst Pharm.* 2005;62:1596-1605.

6. Young WW, Bell JE, Bouchard VE, Duffy MG. Clinical pharmacy services: Prognostic criteria for selective patient monitoring, part i. *Am J Hosp Pharm.* 1974;31:562-568

7. Young WW, Bell JE, Bouchard VE, Duffy MG. Clinical pharmacy services: Prognostic criteria for selective patient monitoring, part ii. *Am J Hosp Pharm.* 1974;31:667-676

8. Cohen MR. Patient data monitoring: Watchdog technology that detects impending adverse events. *Hosp Pharm.* 2003;38:818-819.

9. Weber R. Strategies for Developing Clinical Services—Advanced Practice Programs. *Hosp Pharm.* 2006;41: 987–992.

10. Nystrom KK, Foral PA, Wilson AF, Christenson CM, Miller CK. Personal Digital Assistant (PDA) clinical intervention documentation system: Development, implementation, and comparison to a previous paper-based system. *Hosp Pharm.* 2006;41:143-150.

11. Cousins D, Gerrett D, Luscombe D. Reliability and validity of hospital pharmacists' clinical intervention data. *Am J Health-Syst Pharm.* 1997;54:1596-1603.

12. Koffler AB, See S, Mumford J, Johnston B. Implementing and evaluating a pharmacy consult service within a family medicine residency program. *Am J Health Syst Pharm.* 2002;59:1200-1204.

13. Knoer SJ, Couldry RJ, Folker T. Evaluating a benchmarking database and identifying cost reduction opportunities by diagnosis-related group. *Am J Health Syst Pharm.* 1999;56:1102-1107.

14. Robke JT, Woods M, Heitz S. Pharmacist impact on pneumococcal vaccination rates through incorporation of immunization assessment into critical pathways in an acute care setting. *Hosp Pharm.* 2002;37:1050-1054. ∎

Index

Page numbers followed by "f" denote figures; those followed by "t" denote tables.

tips on being responsible and
accountability, 151–152
tips on growing and developing people,
152–153
Leapfrog Group, 30
Low-performing employees, 137–138

M

Medical device manufacturers, 190–197
See also Industry relationships
Medicare and Medicaid, 64, 66
health information technology for,
185–186
medication therapy management
requirements of, 280–281
Medicare Prescription Drug, Improvement,
and Modernization Act, 280
Medication administration record (MAR)
bar-code systems and, 26, 27
electronic, 27, 39, 216
handwritten, 22, 26, 39
Medication carousels, 2, 3, 5–6
Medication costs, 1, 75–76, 76t, 82t, 83,
195, 234
Medication electronic order entry
medication order review and, 86, 91
by unit-based pharmacy technicians,
123–124
Medication errors (MEs), 68–69, 234
with anticoagulants, 253
assessing severity of, 202
bar-code medication administration
for reduction of, 3–4, 12–13, 15,
21–29
"blame-free" culture for reporting of,
201–202, 202t
central pharmacy automation for
reduction of, 1–11
determining causes of, 202
root cause analysis, 209–210, 211f
effectiveness of methods for prevention
of, 204t, 216
electronic prescribing for reduction of,
30–38
health care failure mode and effects
analysis for reduction of, 210,
216–224
medication order review for detection
of, 87
medication patient safety program for
reduction of, 199–215
infrastructure and strategy for
development of, 199–205

process and implementation of,
207–215
organizational safety culture for
prevention of, 199–200
pharmacists' interception of, 1
proposed national agenda for prevention
of, 199
rate of, 21, 199
smart pumps for reduction of, 54–61
traditional pharmacy dispensing and,
1, 3
unit dose dispensing automation for
reduction of, 12–19
Medication guides, 228
documenting patient receipt of, 228–
229, 229f
pharmacy distribution of, 226, 228
sources for, 228
Medication order processing time, 82t,
83–84
unit-based pharmacy technician model
and, 118–119, 119t
Medication order review, 86–92
compared with drug dispensing and
medication electronic order entry,
86
definition of, 86
medication errors detected by, 87
mental checklist for, 89, 90t
patient care and, 87
programs for enhancement of, 89–91
information systems, 91
University of Pittsburgh Medical
Center Drug-Use and Disease-
State Management Program,
89–91, 91t
as safety check, 87
standards for, 86
steps in, 87–89
dose, route, frequency, and duration,
88–89
drug selection, 88
monitoring and evaluating therapeutic
outcomes and side effects, 89
patient and physician identification,
88
Medication override, 87
Medication patient safety program,
199–215
"blame-free" culture for medication
error reporting, 201–202, 202t
effectiveness of medication error
prevention methods, 204t

steps in development of, 270–273, 270t
  assessing space needs, 271–272
  certification and licensing, 270–271
  developing documentation system, 273
  developing marketing plan, 273
  evaluating pharmacy resources, 271
  identifying targeted population, 272–273
  soliciting physician support, 272
  training immunizers, 272
  understanding reimbursement mechanisms, 273
  at University of Pittsburgh Medical Center, 273–274, 276–277
Physician identification, in medication order review, 88
Pneumococcal vaccination, 269–270
Preventing Medication Errors, 199
Privacy regulations, 64
Pro forma, 175, 176t
Probabilistic risk assessments of medication errors, 210
Professionalism and industry relationships, 193
Profit and loss statement, 175, 175t
Pure Food and Drugs Act, 227

Q

Quality indicators
  for bar-code medication administration, 26, 27t
  for electronic prescribing, 36
  for pharmacy anticoagulation services, 257–258, 258t
Quality issues
  essential quality data for pharmacy director, 82t, 84
  evaluating effectiveness of central pharmacy automation, 8
  role of Pharmacy and Therapeutics Committee in, 105

R

Recovery Accountability and Transparency Board, 182, 183t
Regulatory compliance, 1–2, 63–67
  accreditation agencies and, 66
  federal agencies and, 63–65
    FDA and REMS, 226–232
  state agencies and, 65–66

Reimbursement
  for medication therapy management services, 279, 281–284
  for pharmacy-based immunizations, 273
Resource allocation, 292–293
Resource Conservation and Recovery Act (RCRA), 64
Return on investment, 174, 175t
  for central pharmacy automation, 9–11
    definitions of elements in, 9t
    example of, 10f
  for unit dose dispensing automation, 18–19
Risk Evaluation and Mitigation Strategies (REMS), 226–232
  elements of, 227–229, 227t
  enforcement of, 226, 230
  for erythropoiesis-stimulating agents, 228, 229t
  hospital pharmacy and, 229–230
  medication guides, 228
    documenting patient receipt of, 228–229, 229f
  moving forward with utilization of, 230–231
  number issued by FDA, 228
  for opioids, 231
  overview of, 227
  resources for information about, 230t, 231
Robotic dispensing systems, 2, 3, 4–5, 15–16, 216
Root cause analysis
  of adverse drug reactions, 218
  of medication errors, 209–210, 211f
"Rounding" on employees, 128, 136–137
Rural health care, 184–185
RxHub *MEDS,* 33

S

Salaries, 141, 247–248
Scheduling options for staff, 139
SharePoint software, 47–53
  alternatives to, 52
  for ancillary department ordering, 49–51, 51f
  announcements on, 48
  capabilities of, 48
  charge pharmacist report on, 49, 50f
  for department calendar, 52
  for document storage, 48
  host department projects on, 49
  for inventory issues, 51